The Psychoanalytic Study of the Child

VOLUME FORTY-TWO

The Psychoanalytic Study of the Child

VOLUME FORTY-TWO

New Haven
Yale University Press
1987

Designed by Sally Harris
and set in Baskerville type.
Printed in the United States of America by
Vail-Ballou Press, Inc., Binghamton, N.Y.

Library of Congress catalogue card number: 45–11304
International standard book number: 0–300–04057–1
10   9   8   7   6   5   4   3   2   1

Contents

FREUD AND THEORY BUILDING

APPLIED PSYCHOANALYSIS

PSYCHOANALYTIC EDUCATION

PSYCHOANALYTIC VIEWS
OF PLAY

The Many Meanings of Play
Introduction

PETER B. NEUBAUER, M.D.

THE ATTEMPT TO DEFINE PLAY LEADS EITHER TO A CONCEPT SO broad that the borders between other mental and physical acts disappear, or to one so narrow that its usefulness is limited. Thus it may be of help to postpone the answer to the question, "What is play?" and to explore instead the role of play as we see it when we observe and analyze children.

There are, as has been pointed out, two interlocking components, a mental act and a conscious or unconscious fantasy and wishes, and a physical act which carries these into an observable enactment. These two components alone would not allow us to differentiate play from work. In games and in work, an idea or an attempt to fulfill a wish is also carried into physical achievements. Play therefore must have an additional quality which we might refer to as "trying on," an exploration, an attempt to resolve a problem in order to achieve a new level of competence or developmental organization. At closer inspection, even this characteristic insufficiently differentiates it from work. The carpenter, the artist, or the inventor may be hard at work to "try on" new solutions and to experiment in action and thought. Thus it is essential to stress what seems to be self-evident—that the necessary additional characteristic of play is the *awareness* that what is enacted is *not real*. The act is accomplished on a level of symbolic meaning; however close at times it may be to reality, it is after all "play." We assume that the child knows that the teddy

Clinical professor of psychiatry at the Psychoanalytic Institute, New York University; Chairman emeritus at the Columbia University Psychoanalytic Center for Training and Research.

3

bear is not real, that the tower he builds and then destroys is not a real tower, nor is the destruction a true destruction. The infant functioning on a presymbolic level does not play. One needs to explore here at what time in development the infant is able to enter the world of play. At what age can we expect the baby to be aware of the difference between wish and reality? It has been suggested by Eugene Mahon (verbal communication) that the child's early exercises, practicing the evolving ego apparatus, is closer to work than it is to play. The peek-a-boo "play" may thus be a forerunner of play which will later become hide-and-seek play, the experimentation with loss and reunion, loss and re-trieval, with the accompanying anxiety and the capacity to learn to anticipate events.

Freud (1930) clarifies our issues further: "Another technique for fending off suffering is the employment of the displace-ments of libido which our mental apparatus permits of and through which its function gains so much in *flexibility*. The task here is that of shifting the instinctual aims in such a way that they cannot come up against frustration from the external world" (p. 79). Here Freud speaks about those mechanisms which lead to sublimation as a protective device. Play stays too close to the drives to qualify as sublimation, but there are aspects of play which lead in this direction.

Freud then pursues the striving to achieve some indepen-dence of the external world: "the connection with reality is still further loosened; satisfaction is obtained from illusions, which are recognized as such without the discrepancy between them and reality being allowed to interfere with enjoyment. The re-gion from which these illusions arise is the life of the imagina-tion; at the time when the development of the sense of reality took place, this region was expressly exempted from the de-mands of reality testing and was set apart for the purpose of fulfilling wishes which were difficult to carry out" (p. 80). Freud uses this line of thought to explore art; much of it is applicable to the role of play. Imagination is trying on in the mind, to antici-pate new solutions, to elaborate possibilities in contact with fan-tasies. Play demands, in addition, enactment. It is this demand which gives play its special place in psychic life and its rich oppor-tunity for psychoanalytic interventions, especially in children. When the child invites the analyst to join *his* or *her* play, we participate only in the role assigned to us, precisely because it is understood to be a make-believe act. The analyst finds himself in a different position when the child asks him to play ball, or hide-and-seek, or a game, for the analyst then acts according to his intentions, unless the child assigns to him every step of interaction.

Freud (1930) adds another dimension: "The boundaries of this primitive pleasure-ego cannot escape rectification through experience. Some of the things that one is unwilling to give up, because they give pleasure, are nevertheless not ego but object. . . . One comes to learn a procedure by which, through a deliberate direction of one's sensory activities and through suitable muscular action, one can differentiate between what is internal—what belongs to the ego—and what is external—what emanates from the outer world. In this way one makes the first step towards the introduction of the reality principle which is to dominate future development" (p. 67).

This statement documents that play follows the pleasure principle, but nevertheless serves in an experimental way to pursue the road to reality. When the same play continues over a long period, because no appropriate solution is found, then we recognize that there is regression to or fixation on a point of pathological conflict or developmental deviations.

This process varies greatly in the economy of psychic life. At times, it is close to drive expressions. The ego, so to speak, has lost itself in the enacting of fantasy, while at other times the play attempts to reach more and more of reality and the concreteness of experience.

From a structural point of view, we also find great variations, dependent on, among other variables, the ego's capacity to regress, to tolerate drive expression and anxiety. From a topographic view, we see the capacity to tolerate preconscious states and to elaborate preconscious fantasies in conscious acts. Often, there is no sharp border between fantasy and thought as preparation for functioning in reality and those trial thoughts and actions which belong to the area of play.

From the viewpoint of drives, play can be studied as to the admixture of libidinal and aggressive strivings, with the discharge to be considered the aim but without a need to consider reality consequences, the reaction of the outside world, and

therefore without guilt from the side of the ego or superego.
Thus we can study the changing role of play from all the metapsychological consideration in the course of analysis.

A 6-year-old boy played over many months with blocks representing either swords or cars which fought and crashed against
each other. The fight was deadly. After this, the young patient
asked the analyst to be a zoo keeper who captured dangerous
wild animals. By treating them nicely, the analyst could tame
them to be gentle; he then was asked to demonstrate the animals
in their new behavior to the observing patient. I do not need to
discuss the meaning of the change of this patient's play, nor do I
need to outline the expected succeeding changes which will lead
to the child's taking over the taming of the animals and to the
child becoming the tamer of his own aggression. A point for
further consideration is the degree of displacement; whether it
shifts from the primary objects to other objects or to animals or
to inanimate objects. Are the differences in the shifts significant
on a symbolic level, and do they represent a noteworthy reflection of the defensive maneuvers which are seen in the need to
establish distance from the primary objects?

One aspect of this child's play is noteworthy. When he was not
playing during the sessions, he sought affectionate contacts with
the analyst. He often regressed to prephallic libidinal experiences. During the play, as we have seen, he asserted himself, took
control, and advanced in his psychosexual struggle. In the safe
make-believe world of his imagination he could pursue his developmental progression—that which he did not dare to express
in reality. This leads me to a question which I should try to
answer: To what degree can one resolve conflicts by play without
the correction of displacements and without bringing into
awareness the primary relationships? I have often been surprised at the progress children in analysis can make without
"primary interpretations." I mean by that term those interpretations that address themselves to the patient's relationship to primary objects.

Samuel Ritvo (1978) referred to this same technical consideration: "One of the major tenets of technique in child analysis is to
offer interpretations in the idiom of the play and to choose
carefully the time and setting when interpretations are offered
directly because the child is so intolerant of them. The child is

prone to become anxious, uncomfortable, and uncomprehending in response to a direct interpretation, and to break off the communication by fantasy play" (p. 301). Even in the psychoanalytic situation play cannot be viewed as an aberration which leads the child away from reality; it is a normal activity which may be endowed with pathological features. The child's playing during the analysis, that is, in the presence of the analyst, can be seen as a mode of communication. The degree to which the analyst is experienced as part of the play varies greatly. There are children who, at certain phases in the analysis, seem to exclude the analyst; for others, the analyst is a prime collaborator. This by itself is indicative of the child's object relationships, his transference, for even the exclusion of the analyst is a significant statement about the child's object relationships. Often, the psychoanalyst is made to be an ally of the child's wishes and fantasies—a part of the displacements or detours which are necessary so as not to face reality, and to find solution under the control of the child's ego; at the same time, the analyst is seen as an object who does not deny drive expressions.

When we follow the developmental line from play to game to work, we follow the ascendance of the reality principle. As Anna Freud (1965) pointed out, each developmental line intersects with others to bring about new developmental organization and reorganization. We can often observe the overlapping of phases or the coexistence of conflicts from one phase with those of another. Therefore, a child may "play a game," that is to say, the rules are changed according to the needs and wishes of the child. The analyst and the patient may share the recognition that they continue to "pretend," that they are engaged in a game while it has become a play. Similarly, a play can have significant features of a game. Rules are introduced—those that reflect ego controls and those which stem from the demands of the superego. There are toys, such as lego, which lead the child to consider reality and guide him toward work. As I mentioned before, this developmental line should lead from the preplay phase to play, to game, to work.

When I spoke about play being either close to drive expressions or to reality, I was simplifying the clinical function of play; I treated it as if it were a unit reflecting *one* dynamic, structural, and economic condition, when in fact play may combine many aspects side by side or move from one to another. In the continuous search for solutions, there may be more fantasy at one time and later more reality.

There are similarities and dissimilarities between dream and play analysis. We listen until the dream is completely told, for the outcome of the dreamwork reveals the capacity to resolve problems and the degree of anxiety connected with the inability to achieve it. Similarly, it may be advisable to wait until we know the outcome of the play, its gestalt, before we can usefully interpret the manifest and latent meaning. This does not exclude questions about the play's details. An early intervention during the play may not only evoke annoyance or disapproval of the psychoanalytic process, but may also deprive the analyst of the understanding of the complete function of play. Like the interruption of daydreams, it is experienced as an interference, an interruption which may lead to discontent.

Play has three characteristics: it is an expression of wishes and fantasies; it is an enactment of these wishes in search of fulfillment; and it is an awareness of its nonreality. These characteristics play a role on the road to reality, though it is difficult at times to maintain the distinction between reality and nonreality. There are also many variations in the degree of translating fantasies into enactments. Playing with words, the substitutions of acts by words—an aim of the psychoanalytic process—can often blur the distinction between words and acts. The verbal assignment of a fantasy role to the analyst may at times be enough, and therefore the boundaries between play and fantasy, play and words, play and drawings are not always distinct.

The intensity with which children and adults play, that is, the earnestness of intention of the psychic investment, reflects a sharp difference between play and playfulness. It seems that this characteristic of play—the nonreality of it, the symbolic displacement—allows it to occur. The lowering of the demands of the superego and the ego's acceptance of preconscious and unconscious drive derivatives, their libidinal and aggressive discharges in action, give play a dramatic fervor that could not be tolerated when it was directly expressed within the context of primary relationships or when reenacted as the *original* events.

In addition to the trying on of new solutions, and the change from a position of passivity to activity, those drive discharges have their therapeutic value. Since pathological conflicts may be interwoven with normal capacities or may coexist with them, it appears to be important, as in all conflict, to speak of both components. Which aspect of play should come under psychoanalytic scrutiny should guide the analytic work at any given time, though it also depends on the analyst's insight. We know that play cannot be viewed as totally pathological; rather, certain components may serve pathological or healthy strivings.

This short outline confirms the notion that play has a special, unique place in psychic life, particularly in the world of the child. I have referred to some of the technical implications and have raised many questions. In addition, one wishes to follow the various transformations of childhood play in adult life. One has to question the notion that the steps in the developmental line from play to work follow discontinuities as seen in the sequence of the libidinal phases. Rather we see the transformations into complex mental acts which either still reflect the earlier demands of plays or are offshoots from it with many branches which link wishes, imagination, and fantasies into sublimated functions. Calvino (1986) gives an example of it: "it has generally been said that the fable is a profane story, something that comes after myth. . . . My argument leads to the conclusion that the making of fables precedes making of myths. . . . Myths tend to crystallize instantly, to fall into set patterns, to pass from the phase of myth-making into that of ritual. . . . The game can work as a challenge to understand the world or as a dissuasion from understanding it . . . the boundary is not always clearly marked, and I would say on this score that the spirit in which one reads is decisive."

BIBLIOGRAPHY

CALVINO, I. (1986). *New York Times Book Review.* September 7, p. 31.
FREUD, A. (1965). Normality and pathology in childhood. *W.*, 6.
FREUD, S. (1930). Civilization and its discontents. *S.E.*, 21:59–145.
RITVO, S. (1978). The psychoanalytic process. *Psychoanal. Study Child*, 33:295–305.

Some Functions of Play and Playfulness
A Developmental Perspective

GEORGE S. MORAN, Ph.D.

FREUD (1908) STATED THAT THE OPPOSITE OF PLAY IS WHAT IS REAL (p. 144). Anna Freud (1965) viewed play as a precursor of daydreams, wherein the wishes which were formerly put into action with the help of objects are reshaped in the form of fantasy activity. She also drew attention to the advances in ego development and drive control which play helps to consolidate and which appear as forerunners of the individual's acquisition of the capacity to work. In this view play and reality are juxtaposed, and play can be seen as crucial for the child's acquisition of the capacity to differentiate "me" and "not-me" experiences, self and object representations, and fantasy and reality.

Play and the early infantile developmental processes which foster it are known to have a number of important psychological

Staff member at the Anna Freud Centre, London, which is at present supported by the G. G. Bunzl Charitable Foundation, London; the Freud Centenary Fund, London; the Anna Freud Foundation, New York; The New-Land Foundation, New York; the Leo Oppenheimer and Flora Oppenheimer Haas Trust, New York; and a number of private supporters.

I wish to acknowledge the many helpful contributions to this paper made by the members of the Study Group of Developmental Disturbances, including H. Kennedy (Chair), D. Bandler, P. Cohen, G. Fitzpatrick, A. Gavshon, B. Grant, J. Hodges, S. Marans, F. Marton, E. Phipps, D. Roditi, and J. Szydlo, and Nancy Brenner and Manna Friedmann, teachers in the Anna Freud Centre Nursery School.

The paper was presented at the International Conference on "A Psychoanalytic View of Play and Trauma," at Hebrew University, Jerusalem, March 1986.

functions. Early play makes an important contribution to the infant's libidinization of his own body (Hoffer, 1949) and his mother's body. At first, he is unable to draw a distinction between the two (Anna Freud, 1965; Mahler et al., 1975). Transitional objects (Winnicott, 1953) become important as he gradually develops the capacity for mutuality (Erikson, 1950) and creates, with the help of an inanimate object, a safe "no-man's land" in which to express affect-laden experiences. Thus, play with inanimate objects enlarges the scope of, and enriches the child's relations with, the animate world. Earlier, transitional objects aid the child in building up an inner world of increasingly stable self and object representations, with transitional phenomena deepening the child's investment in the world of inanimate objects.

Play objects become important from the time the infant begins to manipulate things. Play facilitates emerging ego functions, such as the establishment of body boundaries; or the acquisition of sphincter control (e.g., through toys which involve filling and emptying); or motility (movable toys). One can argue the point that these are only forerunners; there are activities which would only later lead to play as symbolic functions become available. The information-processing activities associated with play exercise and enhance the development of cognitive schemas from the sensorimotor phase through to the development of formal operations (Piaget, 1945). Play material helps the child to discharge instinctual trends in bringing things together (constructive activities) and dispersing them and breaking them apart (destructive activities). With the advent of the oedipal phase, dramatization and fantasy play, accompanied by various props, become increasingly complex. The universal appeal of games allows for a symbolic and highly formalized expression of a wide range of psychic conflicts in latency. Anna Freud (1965) and Peller (1954) have described these stages in the development of play, while Erikson (1950, 1977) and Plaut (1979) have extended the developmental sequence of play activity through to maturity.

Fraiberg (1974) convincingly described the way in which the play of mothers and fathers with their blind babies can express a wide range of unconscious motivation and conflict. She points out how the conventional disguises of play can provide harmless as well as detrimental influences on the child's development. In a more recent paper Fraiberg (1982) described pathological reactions of infants in the preverbal period and characterized them as defensive behaviors. These phenomena, though distinct from the later development of defense mechanisms proper, were understood as cut-off devices in perception whereby the child selectively edits the mother's face or voice in the service of warding off painful affects. She concluded by drawing attention to the important question of the relationship between defensive modes of behavior originating in infancy to cope with behavioral aspects of parental psychopathology and the development of defenses proper in later childhood.

Kennedy et al. (1985) drew attention to the many influences which the mother's attitude may exert on the young child's *capacity to play and use fantasy in the service of intrapsychic adaptation.* When these influences work against progressive development, they may contribute greatly to developmental psychopathology, that is, to unevenness and disharmony in the child's development, and result in what Anna Freud (1974) referred to as the fertile breeding ground for later structuralization of conflict and pathological defenses. Thus we became interested in studying whether there was a connection between playful interaction between the child and his parents and the child's later capacity to use fantasy for adaptive purposes. Furthermore, this led us to examine the role of playfulness in normal development.

In providing or failing to provide the appropriate opportunities and circumstances for age-adequate play, parents facilitate or impede the child's progress on various lines of development. Crucial in this respect is the parents' own capacity to suspend their consideration of reality and to pretend. Another important factor concerns the extent to which the parents initiate and actively participate in their child's play and thereby provide essential stimulation and pleasure. Limits and control, and the manner in which these are implemented by the parents, contribute greatly to the development of the child's capacity to play and the degree of safety or anxiety associated with play and the fantasy activity which underlies it. Excessive participation by the parents may take the form of overstimulation, intrusion, or rigidity. Much as children need others to participate in reciprocal play, they also need the opportunities and conditions, external and intrapsychic, which promote solitary play. How much direct involvement by the parents and how much scope for solitary play are required will be determined by the child's developmental phase, the constellation of his siblings, and his own individual inclinations.

As we thought about the child's developing capacity to play and the effects of parental influence, it became clear to us that the qualities which characterize family interactions and the atmosphere in the home are broad-ranging, often subtle, and change over time. There are enormous differences, for example, in the tone of the interaction between mother and infant, the value placed on mutuality, and preferences for visual, tactile, or auditory modes of interaction (Stern, 1974). Such parental inclinations are linked with empathy for the child's own needs as well as internal and unconscious determinants of their preferences. For example, the mother of an infant may choose to soothe or amuse her infant by using various devices to prevent crying. These form a sequence of repetitive and predictable stimulation which alternates with the introduction of novelty. Later on, the mother's wish to avoid battles and harsh confrontations of the toddler with the limits of his power to control motivates her to use a variety of playful distractions and diversions. Entering the animistic world of the toddler by personifying the inanimate is a common example. Instead of ordering the child to eat, the mother may say that the food wants to go in his tummy. She may use imaginative face-saving devices to help the child to avoid humiliation and ward off narcissistic hurts, and to cushion the child in the recurrent frustration of his wish to be big and grown up.

In examining the ways in which playful, empathic parents may foster ego development and tone down the harshness of superego precursors, we found that we relied increasingly on the notion of playfulness. In helping the child to progress developmentally, while at the same time intermittently and selectively diminishing the pressure on the child for more advanced forms of functioning, playful parents make the demands of reality more acceptable and indulge the child by sanctioning the pleasure principle.

As a working definition, we viewed playfulness as a quality

associated with lightheartedness and an empathic understanding of what the child feels which could be used by the parents to
attain various ends, not the least important of which may be to
"manage" the child successfully. Parents may generate mutual
pleasure by playfully gaining the child's cooperation and thereby reducing the unpleasure associated with frustration. We
knew of children who used playful techniques to cope with
frustration, disappointment, and anxiety, and we wondered to
what extent this was based on an identification with parental
style. We also knew of children who lacked the quality of playfulness, and we decided to examine whether or not this might
stem from an imbalance in the pleasure-unpleasure series at
critical periods during the child's development.

The Study Group on Developmental Disturbances at the
Anna Freud Centre has examined in depth a number of prelatency children whose early development was followed in one or
more departments of the educational unit of the Centre and who
were later in intensive treatment. Recorded observations of
babies in their homes, the well-baby clinic, the mother-toddler
group, and the nursery school were compared with subsequent
diagnostic formulations and detailed records of analytic treatment. We endeavored to examine where and why development
began to deviate from the expectable norm and to what extent
progress had been delayed or distorted. We were mindful of the
interaction of constitutional, maturational, and environmental
factors; the relative strengths of the psychic agencies and the
degree to which their development is in harmony. We were
concerned with the effects of parental psychopathology on the
developing child and the interplay between the impact of parental disturbance and the child's own responses at different phases
of development. In examining the importance of play and playfulness, we used observations of so-called normal children as
well as material from prelatency children in analysis.

Playfulness in Normal Development

We have found the notion of playfulness difficult to define. In
the broader sense we have in mind a pleasure-oriented flexibility. In this sense playfulness is a natural response of parents to

their young children's instinctive orientation to pleasure. Because of the biological bond of parents to their children and associated psychological processes, parents readily identify with the needs and frustrations of their children and will at times endeavor to lessen environmental interference and regulation to enhance the child's enjoyment. Playful parents find many inventive ways to lighten the demands which they make on the child. In the case of infants, playful parents will try to enhance the infant's feeling of competence and mastery. They may, for example, let their baby hold the bottle and attempt to put it into his own mouth, coming to the baby's aid at the appropriate moment. Such parents will protect their child's nascent frustration tolerance by endeavoring to minimize interference with the child's pursuit of pleasure. Playful mothers may contort themselves while changing a nappy or dressing their babies. Such parents will invent playful interactions to mediate a large variety of tasks. Manifestations of parental flexibility which enhance the child's pleasure or fun are so common that to comment upon them is to list the obvious: suggesting the child go to the window to wave bye-bye to mitigate anger and anxiety at separation; pretending to drive a bus upstairs on the way to putting the child to bed; arousing curiosity and anticipation about future pleasures to try and gain a child's cooperation in an activity which was previously rejected.

Parents also spend a great deal of time disidentifying with their children's unremitting orientation to pleasure. They themselves represent to the child the demand for adaptation to reality and do so more or less benignly, more or less consistently, and more or less angrily. Individual parents vary in the extent of their indulgence according to the stresses and strains of their own daily lives.

With the progressive stages of language acquisition and of emotional object constancy in the latter half of the second and during the third years of life opportunities begin to arise for parents and children to interact playfully in the more limited sense in which we use the term. Circumstances may be spontaneously exploited to blur the border between fantasy and reality in a preconscious effort to tone down the demands of the reality principle and the harshness of the child's introjects. Thus in a limited way, some degree of pleasure may be reestablished.

It is more difficult to gather observations of interactions between parent and child which not only enhance the child's pleasure in complying with parental wishes but which also playfully distort reality in terms of the child's immediate experience. We believe that loving parents who are in tune with their children playfully react to the child's anxieties with highly specific, well-timed interventions. Such responses are empathic, but the link between the parents' behavior and the child's anxiety remains preconscious for both parties. Such parental responses aim to ease the child's dilemma by introducing a modicum of enjoyment and thereby increasing the child's options for mediating or solving conflict.

Consider the following observations of Karen, a 4-year-old girl in the nursery school at the Anna Freud Centre. At the time of the observations Karen was, overall, functioning well in school, but she was also coping with considerable difficulties at home, including the impending break-up of her parents' marriage. She showed, at times, some difficulty in separating from her mother. During the day at the nursery school she occasionally became distant and found it difficult to involve herself in play. The following two observations were recorded independently by different teachers on two consecutive days:

> Karen spilled some milk on her clothes during lunch. No one is upset or cross, though Karen cries loudly for her mother. I say that the milk can easily be wiped up and I tell Karen that she can change her shirt if she wishes. I wipe her up, but she continues to cry and is miserable. She is unable to drink her milk or eat her yoghurt. Karen then goes out and gets her soft toy, a furry dog, which she cuddles. She then decides to take off her T-shirt and I provide her with another. Although she rallies later in the day, her upset and longing for her mother continue and are out of all proportion to the situation.

On the following day, another teacher recorded this observation:

> When Karen loses interest in a Lotto game, where she is one of three children, and nothing else seems to be of interest, I ask her to suggest what she would like to do. She has a long think during which time my attention is focused on her, and this she clearly enjoys. She still has no idea, is pale, and looks bored. Her mood changes when I say jokingly that the doll which was dripping wet

on the chair "has done a wee." Karen laughs and enlarges on the topic of weeing on the floor and speaks of pooing, etc. I say the doll must have had a bath and the water is still inside her. "No," says Karen, though I show her where the water comes out; "no, she did a wee," repeats Karen. This topic released Karen's boredom and she was quite lively afterwards. She knew, of course, that it was a joke.

The first observation reveals the teacher's concern about Karen's reaction to spilling her milk; it also suggests to the psychoanalyst-observer important determinants of Karen's conflicts and how these might contribute to her difficulties in separating from her mother. The second observation details an intervention in which the teacher playfully addresses what appears to have been at the heart of Karen's current conflict. The intervention was not therapeutic in its formulation or intent, but its therapeutic effect is obvious. The teacher's preconscious awareness of the nature of the little girl's conflict allowed her to focus on the child's problem. By playfully distorting the border between fantasy and reality, the teacher allowed the child to express in displacement and under the guise of a joke the persistence of her wish to wet and mess. The categorical imperative of sphincter morality is temporarily overcome by the blurring of reality by pretense. The appeal to the child's own sense of playfulness permits expression of her instinctual wishes while at the same time she does not feel belittled, as she might do, for example, if she were told in a therapeutic context that, like a baby, she wanted to do a wee-wee on the floor and that this made her think that her mommy would not like it.

Without being aware of it, playful parents address their child's conflicts in similar ways to those of the teachers in the above observations. Such playfulness creates an atmosphere of acceptance and increases the child's tolerance of id derivatives within himself and others. This relief is particularly important before the establishment within the child of a repression barrier. Before the setting up of defense mechanisms proper, at which time the child gains a new distance from awareness of instinctually derived wishes and a new capacity to modulate affect, he can do little more than try to turn attention away from his wishes. When the parents or others playfully invite the child to turn his attention toward prohibited or repudiated wishes under the guise of pretense or via displacement, the solutions for conflict open to the child are broadened.

Some children can mitigate their distress by finding inventive and imaginative solutions to painful situations. Karen's own sense of playfulness was repeatedly evident; for example, in her adaptations to the distress engendered by separating from her mother. Karen's teacher recorded the following observation in a period during which Karen was experiencing particular difficulties in separating from her mother.

> Karen makes me the "mummy" in her game all day long. This means that she goes and plays with friends but relates back to me periodically—to tell me something or to have a hug, kiss, or cuddle. When Karen's mother arrives, she says, "I have two mums here." Karen, her mother, and I all smile.

The observation is more than an illustration of displacement of dependence from her mother onto a substitute object. By pretending that her teacher is her mother and playfully relating to her as such, Karen creates a sense of enjoyment which is shared between herself, her mother, and her teacher.

PLAYFULNESS AND DEVELOPMENTAL PSYCHOPATHOLOGY

We have studied a number of prelatency children who have shown evidence of a serious interference with the capacity to enjoy fantasy play and to engage in playful interaction with others. In studying the early observational material in conjunction with the later analytic material, we have sought to understand the causes for inhibitions in the child's play and why, in some cases, fantasy play became associated with disapproval, anxiety, and shame. In the cases we have studied, disturbances of the child's capacity to use play in the service of intrapsychic adaptation could be seen to reflect, in some measure, parental attitudes toward play and the extent of parental flexibility.

In certain cases disturbances in the child's capacity to play appeared to be rooted in the interaction of mother and child from very early on. This certainly appeared to be the case with Scott who showed a long-standing reluctance to please his mother, and whose mother had shown little evidence that she had tried to induce him to please her by making it gratifying or enjoyable to do so.

The relative absence of shared pleasure which characterized Scott's early development was apparent from his infancy. By the age of 4 months he was described as a grizzling, uncuddly baby who was often unhappy unless feeding or sleeping and who appeared to prefer eye contact to being held by his mother. There were indications over his first 18 months that he had a narrow range of pleasures. As an infant Scott had been largely restricted to his cot because the family's new house had not yet been carpeted. The first time he pushed himself up on his arms it was at the home of a relative. Partly perhaps on account of such restrictions on his motility, he relished locomotion. However, his mother responded to his exuberance and wishes to explore as if they were aggressive intentions to misbehave. For example, at 13 months his mother wanted to teach Scott to use a pull toy, but he wanted to put the wobbly antennae of the toy caterpillar in his mouth. He made determined efforts, while his mother frustrated him by persistently keeping the toy out of his reach. He yelled in anger until his mother removed the toy from his sight. In another instance, although his mother did not close the toolbox, she forbade him to play with its contents. Scott put some screws in his mouth which his mother then had to remove. Later when he was a toddler, she felt that he should be able to take his toys into a room and stay there quietly occupied, thus revealing her inflexible expectations.

When Scott was 16 months his mother began to express her concern that his aggression toward other toddlers derived from her own rough handling of him in infancy, tossing him up in the air, for example. In the toddler group, over the course of the next year, she was seen to be excessively rough when, for example, she was dressing him. When she played football with him in the garden, she would become lost in her own performance, repeatedly kicking the ball too hard until he gave up. She did not believe in helping toddlers after a fall, and he was seen to suppress his tears after falling off a tricycle at the age of 17 months. While encouraging him to be tough, she locked away toy soldiers and would not let him have a toy gun. The feelings of dissatisfaction and aggression between Scott and his mother escalated to the point where he was uncontrollable at home; she retaliated by shouting, smacking, and locking him in his room. In the mother-toddler group he could not play. He was often observed to distance himself from his mother, baby sister, and others in the group and produce ear-shattering banging with a wooden hammer. It was striking that he could not express regressive wishes or jealousy in fantasy play.

In Scott's analysis opportunities for play and playful interaction with his analyst were adjuncts to verbalization and interpretation of conflict. By pretending he was the baby feeding from a bottle, a monster in the toilet, or a rival to his daddy for the love and affection of his mother, he was able to work through and master some of his conflicts and to structure new defensive adaptations. Interpretation of the underlying love and longing, expressed in the transference, freed Scott to act more positively toward his mother and eventually ushered in the development of positive oedipal wishes. Scott's fear of monsters was resolved and his tendency to be aggressive and unfriendly with other children changed dramatically. He did, however, remain a serious little boy whose pleasures were largely restricted to educative activities, such as reading and visits to museums.

Parents who are intolerant of id derivatives and who defend strongly against their own fantasies may influence their children to do the same. Instead of facilitating or sharing playfully in their children's play, they need to control and place an exaggerated emphasis on reality.

Mrs. A. sought help for her problems with her son William, aged 2½ years, "to prevent difficulties for him such as I experienced while growing up" (Gavshon et al., 1984). Over an initial period during which she received guidance for her son's difficulties, many frightening fantasies emerged about her son. At different times she had feared that he was mentally defective, brain-damaged, psychotic, hyperactive, and gifted. He had from infancy suffered from ear infections which were associated with intermittent hearing loss. Upon referral for analysis at 3¼ years, his mother was concerned about his poor articulation and was frightened by his aggression.

Our first observations of Mrs. A.'s interaction with William showed her to intrude upon his play and to put a premium on achievement. The parents, both competent professionals, repeatedly expressed their need for William to do things which would reflect his high ability. At home, he was even provided with real tools instead of toy ones, and this resulted on one occasion in an injury to his little sister whom he hit with a hammer. Consequently, William regarded play as a task he was obliged to complete. "I will play tomorrow," he would say to his analyst in the early days of treatment.

William's parents placed an exaggerated emphasis on cognitive achievement. They exerted constant pressure on him to acquire knowledge. William liked to be read to from certain books and in this way stayed close to his objects. He would sit beside them or dress up in outfits which matched in every detail the storybook characters. These outfits were often made by his mother. Her active support of William's efforts to imitate storybook characters by providing realistic props was a way in which she could feel involved in William's play and exercise some control over it. Through imitating the storybook characters and dramatizing elements of the story, he was able to gain his parents' approval by conforming to their expectations of him as clever.

Part of William's defensive maneuvers involved accumulating "reality" details and facts which were ineffective in the mastery of anxiety-arousing situations. In this accumulation of details and serious, sometimes frantic efforts to assemble props, William behaved very much as did his parents in their response to anxiety-arousing situations. Thus he repeatedly prepared games which he never came to play. Mrs. A.'s successful efforts in making his costumes and William's pleasure in the outcome derived from their shared defensive need for real achievement and their anxiety in the face of more loosely structured play or fantasy expression. In the areas of avoidance of anxiety through placing an exaggerated importance on reality and in the attitude of overcontrol with regard to imagination, William modeled his defensive style on his objects. In addition, he may have clung more to reality details because of his history of unreliable hearing, and his consequent difficulty in understanding and being able to experience the world as known and reasonably predictable.

The defensive characteristics which William developed were well illustrated during his treatment by his consuming interest in certain books. These featured aggressive, masculine heroes, who, one assumed, provided William with a measure of vicarious gratification of his aggressive wishes. Being read to kept him in control of events, and to this extent it was used as a resistance against anxiety-provoking material which might emerge if play were less structured. Initially, when his analyst read to him, William demanded that she read every word of certain sections of a story and skip other sections; if she left out a sentence which he wanted included, he would immediately recognize this. It was striking, however, that he had difficulty in using his identification with fictional heroes as a catalyst for the elaboration of his own fantasies as most young children do.

Consequently, his analyst had to devise ways to foster William's play so that she could gain access to his anxieties and conflicts. By providing him with admiration instead of explanations and allowing him to be passive instead of active and by recognizing his dependency needs, the therapist provided relief to William. She told him that although he felt he had to do something in treatment, there was nothing he really must do, and this permissive attitude gradually freed the boy, who began to work at his own slow pace.

Play became a pleasure instead of a burden as William began to delight in the escapades of naughty Anthony, the storybook character who splashed water about. The therapist's acceptance of the mischievous boy in the story enabled William to permit himself to identify with his pranks. For the first time in analysis he involved himself in fantasy play, which provided real excitement and pleasure. His parents observed that, at home, William's play had become "joyous." They described his slightly naughty, pleasure-filled ploys as "naughty but charming."

Subsequently, William began to paint more freely. He turned a feather from his Indian headdress into an Indian pen and "wrote" invisibly. He was playful and confident that the invisible writing could not fall short of anyone's expectations—and when his analyst eventually suggested that it was a pity the Indians only had invisible ink, William could dip his Indian pen into the paint and set about painting uninhibitedly. His therapist praised his work/play and helped him to consolidate his new-found freedom. By building up an atmosphere in which fantasies and their derivatives became acceptable to his therapist, then to himself, and finally to his parents, William became able to bring fears and fantasies to treatment where they could be analyzed.

As he progressed in the nursery school, William's previously very poor peer relations improved considerably, until he was at a stage in which he could easily move from constructing things with other boys to pretending to be the father in "playing mummies and daddies." However, in contrast to his ease with other children, William continued to show apprehension in the face of expectations, real or imagined, of the adults in the nursery school. He remained on guard when asked to perform in ways of which he felt himself to be incapable. The teacher reported, "When William plays with children and no adult is involved, he is boisterous and free. When an adult is involved, he becomes unsure of himself and feigns tiredness so that he won't have to perform and fail." The teacher felt that William's insecurity derived from his mother's persistent anxieties about his gaining admission to a prestigious school and, after his acceptance, about whether he would perform adequately in primary school.

Joseph's mother exerted a similarly inhibiting influence on his capacity to use fantasy play in the service of intrapsychic adaptation by entering into his play and turning it into a real experience (Roditi, 1985). When she noticed Joseph playing with a toy tea set in his analytic session, she began to organize a breakfast tea party in the waiting room, using a miniature service of plates, cups, and saucers. In fact, she served real food on toy dishes at a table which was only 2 feet off the ground, while sitting herself on a tiny chair, instead of merely playing and giving him tea in a less literal fashion. In this way she intrusively entered and controlled his fantasy play and unwittingly destroyed the quality of playfulness.

Fantasy play offers opportunities to gratify wishes and work through conflicts which are not permitted gratification in reality. For playful interaction between parent and child to be pleasurable, the child must experience, on one level at least, a distortion of reality which is fun and not frightening. Whereas it may be helpful when the parents selectively respond to the child's enjoyable blurring of the border between reality and fantasy, there are parents who confuse and distort the child's developing capacity to test reality. Some parents do this by sharing their own fantasies with the child, while others exploit the fantasies of the child in such a way as to undermine reality appraisal.

Elena was referred for treatment at the age of 4¼ years because of her poor language development in her mother tongue as well as English. Both parents came from rigid, superstitious, and materially and emotionally deprived backgrounds. However, they were devoted to their daughter and lavished gifts on her which they could ill afford, thus providing her with what they had felt deprived of in their childhoods. The mother found it difficult to say "no," and the child became increasingly successful in dominating and controlling her parents by refusing to eat or sleep or use the toilet. In response, her desperate parents would threaten or try to frighten her. When Elena had a tantrum in a shop, her mother told her the police would come and take her away. When she would not eat, she was told she would die. If she wanted to eat with dirty hands, her mother told her she would be poisoned. At nighttime, the parents would actually contrive to make noises of footsteps in the corridor which they said belonged to the bogeyman who was coming to take her away if she did not go to sleep. The manner in which the little girl presented her confusion, her preoccupation with aspects of reality which she could not understand, and her readiness to work toward untangling her confusion are vividly described in a paper by Szydlo (1985). In treatment, Elena learned that her parents' outlook on reality was different from that of others in her environment, and her parents responded in good faith to guidance they received from Elena's therapist.

While Elena's parents had increased her anxieties by trading on her fears and making it difficult for her to build up and maintain reality testing, Andrew's parents could barely contain their own anxieties (Phipps, 1985). They were unable to provide him with consistent handling and safety. They repeatedly heightened his anxiety by using elaborate explanations of reality which failed to reassure him. For example, when the boy confided his fear of fires raging out of control, his father introduced him to the idea of "spontaneous combustion." Similarly, when Andrew worried that the house would fall down, he was given complicated explanations concerning the unlikelihood of such an occurrence. Andrew was highly intelligent, serious, and pedantic. These qualities in his personality were understood to reflect in part his need to be vigilant rather than playful in observing the difference between reality and fantasy in the absence of adequate auxiliary ego help.

Teasing is often humiliating for a child and is not to be confused with genuine playfulness. A story which the mother of Jenny, aged 4, told at the time of referral illustrates this point (Bandler, 1980). At lunch Jenny was teased by a relative who offered her bread when she wanted cake, saying the bread was cake. Jenny ate the bread unsmilingly. Later, when the adult offered her the actual cake, Jenny declined, saying that she had already eaten the cake. Jenny's refusal was probably in part an expression of pride insofar as she fought back and hid her disappointment rather than submit to the humiliation. Regardless of how she perceived the teasing, e.g., whether as a condemnation of her greed, or an insult to her intelligence, her reaction indicated a habitual response to the delay in gratification.

Jenny's mother was inconsistent, rigid, and intolerant. From the time Jenny was a toddler, her mother had threatened and condemned her. Jenny herself was an overcontrolled, demanding child who complied with her mother's demands for obedience. Parallel to her "overcontrol" were her frequent battles and temper outbursts with her mother.

From her analysis, we understood the complexities behind these characteristics. What at first appeared as a persistence of greedy demandingness from the oral stage, and obstinacy from the anal phase, could later be seen as deriving in part from a precocious structuring of the personality. Her personality was characterized by a self representation in opposition and resistant to the unreasonable demands of her introject. Jenny's frequent outbursts and battles with her mother reflected her despair in the face of categorical internal prohibitions which were reexternalized.

DISCUSSION

In describing playfulness in parents and children, I have emphasized both a general disposition of pleasure-oriented flexibility and more specific ways in which parents and children exploit circumstances to blur the border between reality and fantasy. Both types of playfulness on the parents' part may help to tone down the demands of the reality principle and the harshness of the child's introjects. As the observations on Karen show, the associated pleasure gain helps the child to find adaptive solutions to conflicts and to cushion the move from conformity to the pleasure principle toward conformity to the reality principle. Playfulness does not derive solely from the need to adapt to instinctual demands. It also helps the child greatly to come to terms with feelings of humiliation associated with dependency and compliance. For example, a child may use playfulness as a face-saving device when unwilling to relinquish control to the adult or as a means of avoiding narcissistic hurts.

Our clinical research suggests that parents' disposition toward their child's fantasy play may be of crucial significance in facilitating or impeding harmony between psychic structures before the establishment of the repression barrier. The cases reported in this study were all first-born babies, and this may be one of the reasons why the impact of parental psychopathology was such a significant feature. In the prelatency children in analysis whom we have studied there was a diminished capacity for enjoyment as well as a poor capacity to use fantasy in the service of intrapsychic adaptation. Although treatment helped these children to work through their anxieties and find better conflict solutions, they did, with the exception of Elena, develop personalities characterized by a restricted range of enjoyment. They were limited in their tolerance of id derivatives in themselves and others and showed a narrowly circumscribed range of pleasures.

Parents are, in the child's early years, the mediators of their children's play. They give license to the child to express fantasy in play, and they are responsible for providing guidance and limits. The clinical case vignettes illustrate some of the ways in which parents may discourage their child from relying on fan-

tasy play and playful interaction to mitigate anxiety and mental
pain. Parents may be rigid and maintain developmentally inappropriate expectations, like Scott's mother. They can, because of
their intolerance of their own inner world, place an exaggerated
emphasis on reality, like the parents of William or the mother of
Joseph. They may exploit the child's fantasies, like Elena's parents, or share their own anxieties, as did the parents of Andrew.
Parents may also be disapproving of certain trends in fantasy
play, such as aggressive ones, and they may be intrusive, controlling, overstimulating, frustrating, or even denigrating like Jenny's mother.

Such attitudes may contribute to inhibition of the child's play
and lead to a situation in which fantasy play, and later fantasy
itself, becomes a source of anxiety and shame. However, we do
not have proof that such attitudes on the part of parents will
necessarily stifle the child's later capacity to use fantasy adap-
tively, though such attitudes may cause the child to indulge in
fantasy only secretly. Furthermore, we do not know to what
extent playful children develop this quality in imitation of or
identification with their parents, and what the critical period is
for its development. Nor can we be sure of the importance of
links between the earliest repetitive pleasurable interactions between mother and child and the later development of the capacity for playfulness.

The enjoyment that becomes attached to play and playfulness, though essential, may be conceived of as secondary to
its defensive aim of avoiding unpleasure. The pleasure gain associated with playfulness is necessarily linked to the experience
of mutuality, whether the interaction occurs with the external
object or between internal representations of self and object.
Where playfulness involves teasing, clowning, craftiness, or de-
ception, it may easily overstep its mark and become tiresome,
exploitive, or sadistic. Then it fails in its function as protector of
self and object. Thus many complex factors, such as the ability
to gauge the object's response in particular circumstances, decide whether a playful device is successful.

Finally, every so-called normal child will develop his own
unique style of tempering reality with pretense. The way in
which different children do so varies greatly. For example, some
children continue to prefer play enactments while others be-

come humorous or witty, and still others alter reality more privately by indulging in daydreams. Because of the immaturity of the mental apparatus of young children, they must rely to some extent on action and objects to express their fantasies. Consequently, they provide us with the opportunity to observe psychic processes before these are obscured by the mechanisms of repression.

BIBLIOGRAPHY

BANDLER, D. (1980). A year's analysis of a five-year-old girl. *Bull. Hampstead Clin.* 3:213–228.
ERIKSON, E. H. (1950). *Childhood and Society.* New York: Norton.
———— (1977). *Toys and Reasons.* New York: Norton.
FRAIBERG, S. (1974). The clinical dimension of baby games. *J. Amer. Acad. Child Psychiat.,* 13:202–220.
———— (1982). Pathological defenses in infancy. *Psychoanal. Q.,* 51:612–635.
FREUD, A. (1965). Normality and pathology in childhood. *W.,* 6.
———— (1974). A psychoanalytic view of developmental psychopathology. *W.,* 8:55–74.
FREUD, S. (1908). Creative writers and day-dreaming. *S.E.,* 9:141–153.
GAVSHON, A., HODGES, J., & MORAN, G. S. (1984). Interactive influences on the development of defence and language in a three-year-old boy. *Bull. Hampstead Clin.,* 7:271–286.
HOFFER, W. (1949). Mouth, hand and ego integration. *Psychoanal. Study Child,* 3/4:49–56.
KENNEDY, H., MORAN, G. S., WISEBERG, S., & YORKE, C. (1985). Both sides of the barrier. *Psychoanal. Study Child,* 40:275–283.
MAHLER, M. S., PINE, F., & BERGMAN, A. (1975). *The Psychological Birth of the Human Infant.* London: Hutchinson.
PELLER, L. E. (1954). Libidinal phases, ego development and play. *Psychoanal. Study Child,* 9:178–198.
PHIPPS, E. (1985). Report on the analysis of a 4-year-old boy. Read at the Anna Freud Centre.
PIAGET, J. (1945). *Play, Dreams and Imitation in Childhood.* New York: Norton, 1951.
PLAUT, E. A. (1979). Play and adaptation. *Psychoanal. Study Child,* 34:217–234.
RODITI, D. (1985). Report on the analysis of a 4-year-old boy. Read at the Anna Freud Centre.
STERN, D. (1974). The goal and structure of mother-infant play. *J. Amer. Acad. Child Psychiat.,* 13:402–421.
SZYDLO, J. S. (1985). Developmental help. *Bull. Anna Freud Centre,* 8:23–38.
WINNICOTT, D. W. (1953). Transitional objects and transitional phenomena. *Int. J. Psychoanal.,* 24:89–97.

Trauma, Play, and Perversion

JACOB A. ARLOW, M.D.

IN THIS PRESENTATION I PROPOSE TO DISCUSS SOME OF THE CON-
nections between trauma, play, and perversion. These connections became apparent to me while I was analyzing some unusual
character traits in several male patients. These character traits
had come to replace earlier perverse practices. By way of analogy to character neurosis, I refer to such traits as character perversion (Arlow, 1971). Among the several things which these
patients had in common was a history of playing certain games
that were manifestly unpleasant in content, in addition to a specific type of sexual play in front of the mirror.

The many functions that play may serve in the mental economy have been discussed by Waelder (1933), Alexander (1958),
and many others. The spirit of the psychoanalytic approach to
the understanding of play was clearly enunciated by Hartmann
(1948) when he wrote,

> There is a biological theory of play whose clearest formulation
> views it as a kind of exercise with the function of preparing the
> child for situations it will have to meet in its future life. The
> analytic theory considers play according to its content, the expe-
> rience the child may master in this way, the roles of the pleasure
> principle and repetition compulsion in it, and how, according to
> the developmental level, the contributions of these factors vary.
> Here again, the theories are not on the same plane. The rôle of
> analysis in explaining the play of children is analogous to the
> one it performs in explaining anxiety. In both, analysis tends to
> substitute a dynamic-genetic explanation for a teleological one.
> [p. 387].

Dr. Arlow is professor of clinical psychiatry, New York University College of
Medicine.

Summarizing the psychoanalytic contributions to the theory of play, Waelder (1933) pointed to the function of mastery, wish fulfillment, and assimilation of overpowering experiences, taking leave from reality and from the pressures of the superego. Each of these elements enters into any consideration of trauma, play, and perversion.

All play has at least one root in the function of fantasy. Concerning the latter, Freud (1911) said, "With the introduction of the reality principle one species of thought-activity was split off; it was kept free from reality-testing and remained subordinated to the pleasure principle alone. This activity is *phantasying*, which begins already in children's play, and later, continued as *day-dreaming*, abandons dependence on real objects" (p. 222). Freud went on to liken the world of daydreams to a national park preserve, the original state of nature kept in its pristine form. Daydreaming, as we know, is a universal activity, and fantasies are vehicles for derivatives of the instinctual drives. The pleasure premium in play is generally taken for granted.

Fantasies and play of an unpleasant nature seem to offer a challenge to this view. It must be borne in mind, however, that such fantasies and games are in themselves derivative representations of unconscious fantasies. They constitute acceptable conscious expressions of conflicts worked out at an unconscious level. Analysis of unconscious fantasies demonstrates the contributions of wish, defense, and guilt. Each of these components of the psychic structure plays some role in the organization of the unconscious fantasy; therefore, each of these tendencies of the mind finds expression in conscious fantasy and play (Arlow, 1969).

Depending upon the nature of the compromise formation effected, the manifest results of the influence of unconscious fantasies may take many forms, ranging from adaptive, sublimatory activity to character, neurosis, and perversion.

Most of the fantasy life is enjoyed in solitude. The individual plays by himself. And, in turn, the individual plays with himself, because some sort of fantasy becomes an indispensable component of masturbation. In fact, the major component of the guilt associated with masturbation stems from the contents of the fantasy, rather than from the conflict over the specific form of manipulation of parts of the body. Sometimes it is possible to observe how the fantasy component of this form of play is repressed and is replaced in consciousness by patterns of delinquency (Anna Freud, 1949) or by character traits and symptom formation (Arlow, 1953).

Fantasy play is a common activity of children everywhere. Sharing fantasies with others is a step away from solitude toward socialization. Daydreams shared in common mark the beginning of a process of artistic creation or artistic appreciation (Sachs, 1942) and constitute one of the foundations of myth, religion, and group formation in general (Arlow, 1961). In particular, Sachs emphasized how sharing fantasies in play helps alleviate the sense of guilt connected with the repressed conflictual wishes the fantasies convey. Fantasy play quickly becomes a primitive form of theater, complete with the rudiments of plot and a stage, very often enhanced by costumes and props. It seems most logical, therefore, that literature created to be staged should be called "plays." In this connection, Freud (1908) wrote,

> Might we not say that every child at play behaves like a creative writer, in that he creates a world of his own, or, rather, rearranges the things of his world in a new way which pleases him? It would be wrong to think he does not take that world seriously; on the contrary, he takes his play very seriously and he expends large amounts of emotion on it. The opposite of play is not what is serious but what is real. In spite of all the emotion with which he cathects his world of play, the child distinguishes it quite well from reality [p. 143f.].

A few observations should be made about play and reality. Since the child distinguishes play from reality quite well, he is in a position, should he be challenged, to disavow the implications of his play. He may repudiate the implications of his fantasy wishes by saying, "I was only playing. It was just a game. It really doesn't mean anything." Furthermore, it is comforting and reassuring to know that the game, like the play on the stage, ultimately comes to an end. In fact, the game may be broken off at will, just as the spectator may leave the theater. Games and plays are controllable because they are "outside" of the individual. Disturbing thoughts and images arising within the individual are not controlled with equal ease. When play takes on a compelling, obsessive quality, it is no longer play. It becomes a symptom. In this connection, Peller (1954) made the astute observation that an activity ceases to be play when it cannot be stopped at will. In effect, certain types of play may take on an obligatory character and thus, to all intents and purposes, become a symptom. Put in metapsychological terms, one might say that the ego has lost part of its autonomy. The function of the game in defending the ego against anxiety is no longer effective. The game becomes a play that failed.

This brings us to the question of play used to master traumatic experiences, a consideration which has assumed paramount importance in psychoanalytic theories of play. Most authors use as their point of departure Freud's (1920) description of a child's play used to master the pain of separation from his mother. Waelder (1933) suggested one way of looking at the problem by putting play together with the process of mourning and the theory of traumatic neuroses of war. In each instance, the excessive excitation connected with the traumatic event is managed by a process which divides the experience into small quantities repetitively and then assimilates it.

> A painful experience is repeated in play not after it has been overcome and mastered, but before, while it is still unmastered; and it is eventually mastered because of the playful repetition itself.
>
> Thereby, play becomes aligned with assimilative procedures which operate by repetition. . . . This function is not so much the preparation for future activities in adult life as it is the assimilation of the mass of excitations from the outer world, which affect the organism too severely or too suddenly to permit of their immediate disposal [p. 218].

Fenichel (1946) combined economic and defensive functions in his view of play:

> There must be a deep connection between actors acting on the stage and children playing games. The playing of 'parts' certainly also assumes a dominant rôle in children's games. . . . Playing is a process of learning while developing the ability to master the outside world. The primitive game is repetitive. It serves the purpose of achieving a belated mastery of highly

cathected impressions. What was endured passively is done over again in play in an active manner, until the child has become familiar with the qualities and quantities involved. The more highly developed game is anticipatory. It creates tension that *might* occur, but, at a time and in a degree which is determined by the participant himself, and which therefore is under control. Such playing is an antisurprise measure [p. 148].

When the child is overwhelmed by some dangerous, unpleasant reality, and especially when taken by surprise, he may resort to play. He may disavow the reality of his experience or the traumatic perceptions by making it play, not reality.

With these considerations in mind, let us turn to the kind of play that the patients I referred to earlier indulged in during the latency period. A common feature of the play consisted of simulating and repeating unpleasant, frightening, realistic situations, in which the young boys identified themselves with a damaged individual. Many of the forms of play to be described will be quite familiar to most analysts, particularly to child analysts. In several cases, the young boys simulated being blind. One patient said he wanted to know what it was like to be without sight. He decided to act for a predetermined period of time as if he were blind. He would walk a certain distance without opening his eyes. Sometimes he did it in a way that made this pseudoblindness apparent to others. Sometimes he did it only as his own game. Viewed from the surface, it appeared as if the patient were acting out some sort of masochistic fantasy, but this did not necessarily prove to be the case.

Closely related to playing blind is the game of playing cripple. One of the patients would simulate a limp or a dystonic movement, wondering while he did so what effect this motor masquerade would be having on observers. Would they think that he was really crippled or was he fooling them? Another patient did not actually play-act being crippled. Instead he walked along the curb with one foot on the sidewalk and the other in the gutter, in order to create the impression that one leg was shorter than the other. On occasion the patient combined this form of curbside walking with keeping his eyes closed, so he could imagine what it would be like to be blind and crippled at the same time. The patients who played being cripples could trace the beginning of this game to the actual experience of having seen a crippled person. They had been frightened but fascinated at the same time. Part of their response to the unpleasant spectacle was an impulse to follow the cripple, and in some cases they actually did so in an almost compulsive way.

Props in the theatrical sense sometimes became an important feature in the games of playing blind or crippled. Canes or crutches were acquired for purposes of the play. One patient would close his eyes and use the cane to tap out the furniture in his home in order to learn how to navigate his course. The patient who played cripple would lean heavily on a cane, while he would swing a deformed or shortened leg with great effort from behind forward. Most striking of all was the patient who had his mother fashion a pair of crutches out of broomsticks, which he then proceeded to use about the house.

For the most part, these were solitary games. The patients indulged in this form of play by themselves, but, if an appropriate companion could be found, a group of two or more could be formed. An appropriate companion, it turned out, was one who unconsciously shared the same anxieties and the same unconscious defensive fantasies. One form of "damage" play that lent itself to group participation was playing dead. This game took the form of remaining immobile for a long time, while trying to see how long one could hold one's breath. One feature of the game was striking. It involved the element of the leader catching the players by surprise. In the middle of the game, at the command of the leader, the players were ordered to freeze their activity. The players were supposed to maintain their distorted expressions or their corpselike postures until the leader gave permission for the players to relax. Whoever stepped out of his role before the command to relax was eliminated from the game. The one who could keep the position longest was the winner. This form of play sounds similar to a children's game called "statues." In this game each player assumes a pose and is supposed to maintain that pose until released by the command of the leader. Actually, the game of statues did not figure very prominently in the activities of these patients, although they did associate to it when they were thinking of the other games described.

There was another form of play which was acted out in front of the mirror. This consisted of playing stupid, ugly, feeble-minded, or crazy. The little boys would make horrible faces, distort their features, let spittle drool from the corners of their mouths, or jerk their hands around in a grotesque fashion. Here, too, there was frequently a history of having observed people with such difficulties. These games, originally performed in private, not infrequently were acted out in the presence of others, usually the mother or other members of the family. Most often, they had the effect of an aggressive form of clowning. When one of the mothers scolded her son and told him to stop this foolish behavior, his response would be, "You don't have to get angry. I was just playing." Another patient once used this form of play to cause his parents profound embarrassment. While they were entertaining some newfound friends at dinner, in the middle of the meal the patient suddenly began to play out his version of the behavior of a "crazy" person. After the guests were shocked and his parents upset, he resumed his "normal" demeanor and quietly continued with his meal. Recovering their composure, the parents explained to the guests, "He's always playing games."

Other fantasies and forms of play, which appeared somewhat later in the course of development, indicated problems of sexual identity and a tendency toward perversions. The adolescent masturbation fantasies frequently conveyed elements of voyeurism, exhibitionism, transvestism, and fetishism. Some of these ideas were translated into action. One patient, for example, would steal into his mother's closet to smell or fondle items of her clothing. Another, as a camper, used to steal brassieres or panties from the wives of the counselors and bury them in the ground near his tent. Sometimes he would lie in bed and imagine that he was touching these undergarments. Another patient would experience a pleasurable sensation from caressing his cheek with something filmy, something almost transparent, which belonged to a woman.

At one time or another, almost all of these patients had obtained items of women's clothes, usually their mother's, which they donned in front of the mirror. Some of these practices were transformed into "innocent" games performed for the amusement of members of the family. In such games, the patients would amuse their families and friends by putting on women's hats at ridiculous angles, wrapping shawls about their shoulders, or putting on kitchen aprons while mimicking a woman in some activity. If the items of clothing selected for the game were sufficiently removed from the obvious sexual connotations associated with lingerie, garter belts, girdles, and brassieres, such youthful transvestism could pass as a playful prank. However, once the players tried to use dresses or cosmetics, their activities would become suspect to others as well as to themselves, and the play became "too real" for comfort. It would seem that the closer the "playful" transvestite stays to wearing part of the outer clothing used by women, the easier it is for him and his audience to dissimulate awareness of the deeper significance of the behavior. This could not be done when women's undergarments, especially those connected with the genital area, served as the costume for the performance.

But not all of these games were simply amusing in character. Sometimes the game evoked shock and anger from the spectators. The element of surprise was an important component of this version of play. During adolescence, one boy, for example, went into the cubicle of the school bathroom and stuffed toilet tissue about his pelvis in such a way as to make it appear like a menstrual pad. As he emerged into the larger area of the bathroom, intending to see how he looked in the mirror, he wondered what would happen if a schoolmate entered the bathroom at the time. He thought he might be embarrassed, but his schoolmate would probably be horrified.

Play of this kind may easily be transformed into a hoax. One patient, for example, went away for a weekend in the company of several friends and his girlfriend. As he watched his girlfriend putting pink curlers into her hair, he thought he would have some fun. He put the curlers into his own hair and dressed up in her nightgown. Thus attired, he entered a room occupied by some of his friends, sidling in backwards. They thought it was his girlfriend. Suddenly he turned around and faced them fully, while speaking in a deep bass voice. At first, his friends were shocked and then they all laughed. This type of behavior was the model for one of his persistent character traits. He was a practical joker.

The case of another practical joker demonstrated the same dynamics. He would call some persons whom he knew, disguise his voice, and make believe that he was a member of the F.B.I. How surprise contributed an aggressive component to his playing became clear in connection with his behavior toward his mother. Once he put black tissue paper over his front teeth to create the illusion that the teeth were missing. With the paper thus in place, he came home, not saying a word to his mother. Sometime later, she asked him a question. He turned to her suddenly and began to answer. She was horrified when she saw him open his mouth. She had the impression that his three front teeth had been knocked out. At that point the patient, with great delight, removed the black tissue paper, showing his mother that the teeth were intact. In fact, many of these patients found particular delight in frightening their female relatives in this fashion. Like certain exhibitionists, they took particular delight in being able to evoke surprise and fear in those to whom they exposed themselves.

A common feature in the history of all of these patients was a traumatic response to confrontation with a female genital. The mothers of some of them were openly seductive and exposed themselves to their sons in the nude. Others permitted the young boy frequent and intimate contact with the genitalia of female siblings. Still other patients suffered from the effects of early exposure to the realities of female sexual hygiene in the form of menstrual pads, miscarriages, etc. In each case, one method of coping with the traumatic perception of the female genital without a phallus consisted of an attempt to deny the reality of the perception. Some tried to repudiate the reality of the memory of what they had seen. They remained, as it were, perpetually in doubt about the reality of their perception of the female genital. They tried repetitively to get another glimpse of the female genital, but did so always under conditions that made it impossible to gratify their voyeuristic curiosity. In that way, they could maintain indefinitely the illusion that perhaps there was a penis there, if only they could get a good look. Still others developed in the direction toward fetishism. What they saw in reality they denied in fantasy. When threatened by confrontation with the female genital without a phallus, they would conjure up unconsciously a fantasy in which they endowed the woman with a penis.

It was clear from the material, therefore, that playing being damaged or impaired constituted an acted-out representation of what it was like to have a female genital. The meaning of this play became understandable from the analysis of a type of play that all of these patients practiced in front of the mirror during their latency period. They would press their genitals back between their thighs in order to simulate the appearance of the vulva. After a while, they would release the pressure of the thighs, permitting the penis and scrotum to emerge into view once again. As it turned out, it was the reappearance of the penis that was important. It was pleasurably reassuring to be able to demonstrate that what looked like a body without a penis was not really so. In keeping with Freud's earlier observation, the game had created the opposite of reality. The purpose of the play was to render unreal the facts of female anatomy.[1] All the time the little boy was looking at himself in the mirror with his genitals pressed between his thighs, he knew that what he saw was misleading and unreal. All he had to do was to relieve pressure on his thighs and the penis would reappear. Thus, the fun of the game came not from concealing the penis, but from making it reappear and thus bringing the play to an end.[2]

The transvestite, like the practical joker and the child playing the penis game in front of the mirror, presents, shall we say, a

1. In certain patients, on the basis of this dynamic, a character trait developed. They treated the unpleasant aspects of reality the way they treated the female genital. They refused to confront it and looked away at some substitute, reassuring, peripheral perception. The material obtained from these patients served as a striking confirmation of the observation by Lewin (1948) that, in the course of free association, the concept "reality" often appears as an allusion to or a substitute for the female genital.

2. This view is opposite to the one often expressed in the literature, in which the game described above is regarded as a derivative of the wish to be a girl, i.e., to be castrated.

false front. The message reads that what appeared menacing and dangerous was a misperception, no cause for alarm. It is similar to the mechanism which Fenichel (1950) described in connection with *pseudologia fantastica*. The formula for this phenomenon, he said, may be phrased, "If it is possible to make people believe that unreal things are real, it is also possible that real things, the very memory of which is menacing, are unreal" (p. 529).

Certain forms of exhibitionism and transvestism have other elements in common. One is the mechanism of identification with the aggressor. As the little boy was frightened and surprised when exposed to the female genital, in his exhibitionistic play, in his play of being damaged, and in practical jokes, he is the one who perpetrates surprise and arouses anxiety. Very often women, especially the mothers or older sisters, are the prime targets for such activity.

There is a logical progression from fantasy to play to perversion. Most perversions are of the nature of acted-out masturbation fantasies. Some perversions are so elaborately structured that, to all intents and purposes, they come to resemble theater. A very special plot is required and, if other individuals are involved, they are assigned roles and lines and even costumes. There are, as we know, perversions that depend upon a carefully laid out scenario, in which the participants play-act definite roles. In all of these, it is essential that the playful character of the activity be maintained. Nunberg (1954) cited a striking example. A masochistic pervert hired a prostitute, whom he paid to dress up in a very definite style, and who was supposed to beat him with a whip in a fashion which he prescribed. After a while, the prostitute got tired of the game and one day she arranged to surprise the patient. She had her boyfriend secreted in the room and, when the patient assumed the position for his beating, the boyfriend emerged from the closet and administered a more effective beating than the prostitute had been giving. From the nature of the beating, the patient recognized the change of characters. He stopped the game immediately. The pleasure was not in the beating per se. It was connected with a fantasy, which provided the scenario upon which the perversion was based. It was the scenario that had to be acted out, not just the beating. The game has to be played according to the rules and limits set down by the patient.

The repetitiveness of these games and of perverse sexual behavior bears a certain relationship to the traumatic neuroses. Common to all of these conditions is a mastery of a traumatic situation through repetition. There is a difference, however, in the manner in which this mastery is accomplished. In the traumatic neuroses, mastery is supposedly attempted through the piecemeal assimilation of massive quanta of unbearable stimuli by the process of repetition. In the games described above, and in voyeurism, exhibitionism, fetishism, and transvestism, a different set of mechanisms comes into play. A number of significant changes are introduced. First, the patient does not simply reproduce the traumatic situation. It is usually a modified version of the experience and is most often expressed in the derivative form, not a precise reproduction of the events. Second, what the patient had endured passively he now initiates actively. Third, and perhaps most important, each repetition of the game and of the perverse behavior serves the purpose of denying the reality of what was originally traumatic. Fourth, the play or the perverse activity is precisely controlled by the patient. He sets the rules and the limits as to what is to happen. He is in control of the situation and has the power to stop the game at will. A sense of power is restored and the patient has both pleasure and reassurance in being able to feel, "It wasn't real. There was nothing to worry about." And finally, in many instances, through the mechanism of identification with the aggressor, wishes for revenge and retaliation may be gratified.

These measures may or may not succeed in fending off anxiety. In adult life, special forms of play, character traits, or sublimated activity may be required to contain the anxiety connected with the trauma. Less successful resolutions of the conflict may lead to character deformation, sometimes in the form of character perversion—petty liars, practical jokers, unrealistic characters, and swindlers (Arlow, 1971). When the conflict cannot be displaced from the sexual realm, and the playful activities intended to deny reality become the subject of obligatory repetition, perversion may develop. It is the element of mastery and control which differentiates play from the traumatic neuroses and from most of the perversions.

SUMMARY

In this presentation I have tried to describe the connection between trauma, play, and perversion. The connecting link emphasized was the need of the ego to render a traumatic experience unreal through the medium of play. The same elements enter into more highly structured perversions. This is the result of a failure of mastery by the ego. Perversions represent an unsuccessful attempt to solve the unconscious conflicts generated by the traumatic experiences. Perversions resemble a game that has failed in its purpose. When the mechanism of denial in fantasy does not succeed in curbing anxiety, the perverse practice is repeated again and again, but the individual remains unconvinced of his denial of reality, and the game ceases to be a form of play.

BIBLIOGRAPHY

ALEXANDER, F. (1958). A contribution to the theory of play. *Psychoanal. Q.*, 27:175–193.

ARLOW, J. A. (1953). Masturbation and symptom formation. *J. Amer. Psychoanal. Assn.* 1:45–58.

—— (1961). Ego psychology and the study of mythology. *J. Amer. Psychoanal. Assn.*, 9:371–393.

—— (1969). Unconscious fantasy and disturbances of conscious experience. *Psychoanal. Q.*, 38:1–27.

—— (1971). Character perversion. In *Currents in Psychoanalysis*, ed. I. M. Marcus. New York: Int. Univ. Press, pp. 317–336.

FENICHEL, O. (1946). On acting. *Psychoanal. Q.*, 15:144–160.

—— (1950). *The Psychoanalytic Theory of Neurosis*. New York: Norton.

FREUD, A. (1949). Certain types and stages of social maladjustment. *W.*, 4:75–94.

FREUD, S. (1908). Creative writers and day-dreaming. *S.E.*, 9:141–153.

—— (1911) Formulations on the two principles of mental functioning. *S.E.*, 12:213–226.

—— (1920). Beyond the pleasure principle. *S.E.*, 18:3–64.

HARTMANN, H. (1948). The psychoanalytic theory of instinctual drives. *Psychoanal. Q.*, 17:368–388.

LEWIN, B. D. (1948). The nature of reality, the meaning of nothing, with an addendum on concentration. *Psychoanal. Q.*, 17:524–526.

NUNBERG, H. (1954). Personal communication.

PELLER, L. E. (1954). Libidinal phases, ego development, and play. *Psychoanal. Study Child,* 9:178–198.

SACHS, H. (1942). The community of daydreams. In *The Creative Unconscious.* Cambridge: Sci-Art Publishers, pp. 11–54.

WAELDER, R. (1933). The psychoanalytic theory of play. *Psychoanal. Q.*, 2:208–224.

Play and Playfulness in Holocaust Survivors

NANETTE C. AUERHAHN, Ph.D. AND DORI LAUB, M.D.

HOLOCAUST SURVIVORS WHO SPENT YEARS IN NAZI CONCENTRA-
tion camps or hiding out in Nazi-occupied territories, who had
their relatively normal developments broken off and their relatively supportive environments destroyed, have a distinctive attitude toward their own childhoods and those of their children.
We would like to begin a description of this attitude by focusing
on the role of play in the past and present lives of the survivors
whom we have encountered as interviewees at the Video Ar-
chives for Holocaust Testimonies at Yale or as patients in our
practices. Our discussion will unfold through three cases or case
vignettes, but we would like first to set a context for the case
material by presenting what we have come to think of as an
essential traumatic effect of the Holocaust experience.

I

In all situations, people take a certain amount of empathy for
granted. At the most elementary level, they expect some response to messages of need they send out. In the concentration
camps, the sadistic bureaucratic killing of people considered by
their killers to be less than human disproved this basic assump-

Dr. Auerhahn is an assistant professor at the California School of Professional Psychology, Berkeley, and on the clinical faculty of the Department of
Psychiatry, Stanford University Medical School. Dr. Laub is associate clinical
professor of psychiatry, Yale University Medical School, and chairman of the
education committee, Video Archive for Holocaust Testimonies, Yale. The
authors thank Elisabeth Young-Bruehl, Ph.D., for her editorial assistance.

tion for survivors. Furthermore, the empathic response was absent not only from the Nazis, but from fellow citizens and Allies as well, that is, from society at large. When people prove unresponsive or actively malignant on such a massive scale, the survivor retains the memory of a basic deficit; this is felt as a compromise in the very possibility of an empathic dyad. When messages of vital need are not responded to by others, the individual loses the sense that needs will ever be met. Faith in the possibility of communication dies and intrapsychically there may no longer be a matrix of two people—self and resonating other. An essential effect of the trauma inflicted upon the victim of genocide is the victim's felt inability to effect the environment interpersonally, to elicit a sense of mutuality, with the result that there is internally "no longer anyone on whom to count" (Wiesel, 1968, p. 229). The link between self and other is effaced by the failure of empathy.

The development of psychic structure is dependent on the presence of a reliable, responsive human environment. Similarly, the "infant's capacity to develop a belief (a mental concept) in the consistency and constancy of the inanimate object . . . is dependent upon the consistency and constancy of the human object" (K. M. Wolf, quoted in Provence and Lipton, 1962, p. 102), just as such developmental achievements as "memory of the past and anticipation of the future, and the building up of a sense of trust are direct reflections of the adequacy of maternal care" (Provence and Lipton, 1962, p. 83). The wish, the basic structural unit of the mind, is constructed from the interaction of needs with experiences of satisfaction. Ultimately, since maternal figures and other human beings are the only sources of need satisfaction, wishes consist of linked self-other representations (Cohen, 1985). Only when a person has the sense that his or her needs will be responded to do those needs become communicable as wishes.

Psychic structure depends for its maintenance on continuing environmental support throughout life, not just in childhood (Cohen, 1985). Thus, for instance, the capacity to sustain the belief in a benign environment is dependent on continuing satisfactory instinctual gratifications and relative freedom from persecutory anxiety (Winnicott, 1958), while the abilities to remember, structure, associate, and symbolize continue to depend upon the experience of a persisting, positive holding environment. On the other hand, the corruption of the holding environment results in a massive destructuring. Specifically, when people prove unresponsive or actively malignant on a massive scale, the internal representation of the need-mediating context is destroyed and the individual loses the capacity for wish-organized symbolic functioning (Cohen, 1985). Wishes regress to being dangerous biological needs when there is no internal representation of an empathic other.

Recuperative psychological processes such as fantasy, reflection, dreams, artistic productions, and play—our focus in this paper—are compromised when bereft of a reliable interhuman environment, on which they depend. Yet it is precisely the employment of these functions which gives continuity, form, and meaning to a series of disjointed impressions of daily life. The very disruption of these processes in the concentration camps, where every type of human form including that of the human body was under constant assault, created disruptions in survivors' abilities to narrate, symbolize, and integrate abilities that, for children, are manifest in play.

Thus, isn't "death" of the potentially responsive other experienced as a death of the victim? The tenuousness of the victim's interpersonal ties resulted in a sense of internal fragmentation, of being unable to put things together. Metapsychologically, we can speak of destructuring; phenomenologically, the victim experiences a sense of fragmentation. When a memory of his or her camp life intrudes, the survivor experiences a sense of decompensation in his or her capacity to organize and adapt. Experience can be neither absorbed nor organized. Discussing the past is reliving of raw impressions. Formulation would require a sense of contact with a good other who could hold things together and compensate for the disruption in the survivor's ego. (Indeed, when there was an internal other present during the camp experience—as with our case C. below—the traumatic effect followed a different course.)

II

The effects that we have been describing as characteristic of survivors in general can be observed very clearly if attention is focused on the domain of childhood play, which had no place in the world of the concentration camps. The ability of a survivor to play or to be playful is, we will try to show, one important index of the severity of the Holocaust trauma and of the potential for its healing. To be specific about this claim, we turn to our case material.

Search for lost empathy, felt as lost maternal responsiveness and protectiveness, is the recurrent theme of patient A.'s life and dreamlife. He had spent his fifth through seventh years in flight and hiding from the Nazis. During his college and graduate school years and while he was employed after graduate school, he suffered recurrently from panic attacks. When his mother came to stay with him, his affect storms would abate. During the panic attacks, A. was convinced that he was about to be shot, hanged, or electrocuted.

The patient experienced his life as under the threat of death, and his therapy, too, was a continual bargaining with the executioner. When he had panic attacks in therapy, he would plead with the therapist for his life. The treatment contract itself exemplified this bargaining process. He agreed to treatment only after the therapist had first accepted his decision (and the opinion of a consultant) not to seek treatment, that is, only after the therapist had shown, in action, that the patient's plea for a stay of execution had been heard. He was in psychoanalytic psychotherapy for 5 years and then, on his own initiative, returned 3 years later for an analysis of 1½ years duration. During the first 5 years, the patient recalled no dreams and few new childhood memories emerged. But during the analysis, after the 3-year break (which signified to him that the therapist had released him), he dreamed and remembered profusely.

At the point in A.'s analysis that we would like to present, he had considered making certain daring professional decisions. He reported several dreams about changing jobs, moving to another office, feeling very anxious, and having to explain himself to the analyst again and again. These dreams led to a memory of having to write a composition in grade school shortly after emigrating to the United States. He felt that no mistake could be tolerated; that other children might make mistakes, but not he. Another dream followed: "At 10:30 on Wednesday morning, the receptionist was going to be executed. She was very apprehensive. Afterward, she was still alive, working with numbers." He commented, "After what I've been through, nothing comes out right. My brain is scrambled. I have a morbid fear and fascination with executioners, a terrible fear that I will be executed, that I will be electrocuted or hanged." The analyst wondered whether the patient had experienced this threat as he became aware of his wishes to make changes in his professional life. A. followed the analyst's comment with a number of dreams about sexually tempting women with big, sagging breasts that someone was sucking. Dreams of being sent into exile while urinating and feeling unclean came over the next sessions.

After one of these sessions, the analyst had an unscheduled hour and the patient expressed a wish to continue longer. The analyst agreed to an additional hour. The night that followed was a tranquil one, with dreams of a pleasant party. The patient dreamed of gambling in a hotel for a long weekend and of doing well. "I did not want to be interrupted while I was winning. Afterward, I had to spend the night in my house, in an upstairs bedroom. For lack of space, I had to share a bed with my mother. I forgot a business deal and had to reschedule it." The next dream of the same night was a repetition of the execution dream, but with a novel outcome: "I had to go with someone to witness an execution of three people. They were not there. I went alone. The condemned were all chained together. They put them into the electric chair or chamber. The door closed. The iron mask came over their faces. They threw the switch, dispatched them one after the other. Someone played with the switch. It was not so pleasant, but not as bad as I thought. My son was there, maybe he was playing with the switch. I had to come back to witness four more executions. It was not as gruesome as I had thought."

After he reported this dream, A. began to talk about his fascination with executions in the news and about Norman Mailer, whom he envied because, at age 55 with a 35-year-old mistress, he was "getting everything out of life that one could, with gusto." He returned to the topic of executions: "I used to think until quite recently that you should never execute anyone—it's too brutal—on the assumption that everyone wants to live and you cannot deprive someone of all hope. It's a terrible feeling, that no one will come to your rescue. But my attitudes are changing. Some people may not deserve to live."

In the first execution dream, with its interpretation that a wish for freedom led to fear of exile, dirt, and punishment, A.'s fears of imprisonment and death were juxtaposed to his wish for playfulness. In the second one, which came after the analyst had responded to A.'s wish for an extra analytic session, and in the same night with a dream of pleasure, success, and manifest oedipal content, the execution theme was recast in a playful mode. A.'s son appeared as the masterful player, while A. looked on unafraid.

When A.'s dreams of gambling and winning, sharing a bed with his mother, forgetting business appointments, and wishing to live playfully like Norman Mailer no longer led to the once inevitable execution, a dramatic turn had been accomplished. In the second dream, A.'s son playing with the switch served as a model for his own growing ability to take some risks in life without an overbearing sense of guilt and disaster. When A. saw the analyst as a responsive, empathic person, his playfulness (in fantasy, at least) began to break through the barriers of prohibition and punishment.

To indicate the significance of the interrelations apparent here between a transference event (the interpretive, not gratificatory, granting of an extra hour), the playfulness, and the appearance in the second execution dream of A.'s son, we would like to turn to another, later, moment in A.'s analysis. In one hour he brought in several dream segments in which he was skiing downhill as an expert, "wedling." Then he recalled something about a party, a house, fleeing at night. Recently, he said, he had read a series of letters written by an uncle of his who had served with the American army in Italy during the war. The letters casually mentioned furloughs and recreations, but contained not a word about the uncle's family, which had been deported and was eventually executed in gas chambers. The analyst pointed out the parallel between the uncle's and A.'s defensive maneuvers: the light-heartedness in the uncle's letters, the partying and agile skiing in A.'s dreams, which were ways of mastering the sense of danger he had felt in fleeing the

Nazis and the strict discipline of motionlessness and silence he had had to endure in his various hiding places. The patient's immediate response was to talk of his young son. While the boy was coloring in a coloring book, he had repeated to himself, "Have to stay within the lines, have to stay within the lines." A. had felt stunned and asked his son why he had to stay within the lines. The boy said that his grandmother (A.'s mother) had told him to. A. reacted with outrage, urging his son to stay within the lines only if he himself wanted to, explaining that no law or external need governed coloring. The patient realized, as he talked, that staying within the lines had been the condition of his childhood during the years of flight and hiding, and that he felt a frantic need to rectify this condition in the life of his son.

The survivor's wish that his child play is a wish to play through his child. "The pleasure gain associated with playfulness is necessarily linked to the experience of mutuality, whether the interaction occurs with the external object or between internal representation of self and object" (Moran, 1987, p. 28). Play implies an interaction between self and internal other; it "has its origins in the exchanges between mother and infant and derives its stimulus from [that] relationship" (Provence and Lipton, 1962, p. 83). It involves an object relationship as its central theme, be it real, fantasied, or wished for (Peller, 1954). In his dreams and in his reaction to his son, A. was reestablishing the empathic relationships he had lost. In a later session, A. reported a lengthy dream about needing a passport to go "somewhere in Europe. There was no time to get a passport, no time to go to my office or to New York. I thought maybe I'll cancel the whole god-damned trip. I was in a car preparing for the trip. The car had to be repaired. I couldn't even find my photos." His association to the word "passport" was "passing through a door," which brought him a memory, a long forgotten phrase from his childhood: "Voulez vous jouer avec moi, Chantal?" ("Would you play with me, Chantal?") Chantal was a little Christian girl who had lived across the street from A. in a beach town on the French Riviera, one of his hiding places. Snatches of memories of nightclubs, casinos, afternoon card games, strolls on the beach, and summer vacationers were juxtaposed with his terror about being apprehended by the police and deported. The carefree playfulness of Chantal in his memory fragment represented A.'s wish for and link back to his lost childhood play and his prepersecution mother, the only one who guaranteed the safety of his play and tolerated the adventuresomeness that had brought him gratification. For other survivors, the prepersecution sanction comes not from the mother directly but from more general memories of protected places. Hence the great desire in survivors to recapture or re-create the lost past, even though their painful sense of its loss impedes their desire (Auerhahn and Laub, 1984).

We can see the same themes of attempted restoration and attempted healing, woven into a much more conflicted pattern in the case of B., whose loss of maternal or parental protection was more severe. B.'s parents were deported to a concentration camp when he was 4 years old. He then roamed the streets of his hometown passing as a non-Jew. For one period, he was taken in by a Catholic woman who presented him as her grandson. "So I had to do a few things I didn't know how to do, like pray, go to church. The prayers I found I didn't like to do. As primitive as this lady was, she had a sense of what's important and what's not important. I had revealed to her that I had a treasure, a picture of my mother as a young woman. So she agreed that every night before bedtime I would pray to the picture of my mother rather than to the crucifix. I used to take this picture out and pray to God to make this war end and please let my mother come back and get me." B. used the photograph as something like a transitional object, a means of retaining his connection with his mother while he tried to meet the hostile world around him.

B.'s worship also makes clear how the survivor's quest is for the remembered or imagined mother, the idealized mother, not the real one. The latter, like the father, is compromised by the Holocaust. The survivors of the Holocaust, especially those who were children at the time, have, as it were, two sets of parents. The first become almost equated with the persecution that defeated and humiliated them, and the child has a conflicted cathexis of these damaged parents. Being with these parents puts him in danger, so that he may actually wish to escape the real parents to save himself. In the child's mind, it is not this first set of parents who protect him, but the second set, the idealized ones, or the ones from "before."

When B. was actually reunited with his parents, he could not find any way to reconcile them with his imaginary version of them. When he met them, he felt not restored to childhood, but reduced to childhood, to vulnerability and terror. "It was very traumatic. I had the picture of my mother, but of course she didn't resemble my mother at all. They were still dressed in their prison clothes, with the wide stripes. My father was 6 foot 2, and he weighed less than 100 pounds. They were really emaciated, and my father looked terrible. He was tortured, and he had all his teeth hanging out. I just couldn't believe it, that they were my parents. I think that this was the hardest part of all, to accept them again. They were my parents logically, but emotionally I didn't feel anything toward them. For some time, I used to address them by calling them Mister and Missus."

At stake was the magical sense of omnipotence that B. had managed to maintain throughout the war by identification with the fantasized, idealized parents. "This was really the first time that I began to realize what had happened. Until then, I was preoccupied with everyday life. I knew that I could take care of myself. But then I had to become a child again. They came back different. Once I was safe again, I disintegrated. I developed fevers, I couldn't sleep." B. started having repetitive nightmares in which he would be overwhelmed by a feeling of helplessness.

It is not surprising that B.'s attempt at restoration of the empathic bond and positive memories of childhood could not take place directly. There had to be a detour to his children. B. reported the following: "When my first daughter was born, I went on a buying spree, a binge. I bought all kinds of toys that you really don't buy for a newborn—an electric train, a pedal car. I very proudly prepared everything in the room for my daughter, who came home three days later with my wife. My wife looked at all the things and said to me, 'Why did you buy all this?' I said, 'A child needs toys.' She said, 'Yes, but it will be years before she is able to play with them.' It took me a long time to realize what I was doing. I was finally buying toys for myself."

Toys represent the mother's nurturing role. As Provence and Lipton (1962, p. 76) point out, "the infant's satisfaction with toys in general is linked to the emotional relationship with the mother." Toys reevoke the technique of mothering, which is "the thing created by the infant and at the same time provided by the environment" (Winnicott, 1951, p. 241). That is, mother represents a matching between internal self and outer world, between need and response. In B.'s case, the focus was on the toys—which had something of the same function as the photograph of his mother—rather than directly on his child. In other survivors, the focus may be more on the child, who is expected to be exquisitely sensitive to the survivor's needs, to know his mind, to be part of himself. The survivor's wish is to be parented through his child, by his child, in his child.

This need is least apparent in our third case, C., whose need was not to play through his children but to involve them and others in various types of play that all had the theme of triumph over enemies. C. is at the opposite end of a spectrum from B. with regard to the intactness of his empathic bond with his mother. C. spent two years in a concentration camp, but he was with his parents during the whole period and slept between the parents every night. On a number of occasions, his mother showed him her ability to shield him from disaster, and these episodes weighed to a degree against his very keen perception of continuous real danger to his life.

C. recalled the day of the family's deportation. A policeman came to their home while he was riding his tricycle up and down on the sun porch. That night, he found himself with his parents crowded into a cattle car, traveling to an unknown destination. Everyone was crying, and he cried, too, especially for his brass bed at home; his mother consoled him with a promise that a new bed would be bought at their destination. A few days later, the deportees were ferried across a river on a wooden rowboat, and then encamped on a hillside near a railroad track to wait for another transport train. These memories remained vivid to C., but he would remember only a few fragments of his two years in the camp.

When C. returned home, he went immediately to the cupboard where his toys had been stored. It was nearly empty; the tricycle was gone. During the next several years, C. spent most of his time inventing war machines. With boys of his own age (7 to

8), he organized imaginary armies with high military ranks, decorations, and ceremonies. In his fantasies, this army defeated its enemies again and again. Upon entering preadolescence, C. organized one of the many youth gangs in his town, and it, too, had ranks, ceremonies, and preparations for military victories. One of the many motives underlying children's play is, of course, denial (in fantasy, word, act) of painful realities—a kind of empowerment. C. was deprived of this possibility in the camp, but his desire for empowerment was not erased; it reappeared after the war, channeled into imaginary military situations. C.'s military games, with plots and structures typical of latency games (Eifermann, 1987), allowed him creatively to contain the traumatic reality and to invent a different, wished-for, ending.

As C. became an adult, he was fascinated with trains, boats, and camping. He always traveled by train, spent time working on a ship, and bought boats and camping equipment. For his son, C. bought an electric train set with the intention that they would spend hours together playing with it, but this fantasy never materialized; his emphasis stayed on the "grown-up" play of camping and travel. This play was fixed upon the experiences he had on his way to the camp—the last days, so to speak, of the normal world. The content of his play had shifted from military exploits to these precamp experiences, although the theme of it continued to come from his need to master, to win, to triumph over his enemies. We suspect that while C.'s immediate postwar play reflected his need for empowerment by denial of reality, his adult strategy was to build a safe, trauma-free reality by making his play activities central to his gratification in life.

C.'s adult recreational activities were governed, however, by rules not of the play domain. He set rigid schedules, worked against deadlines, moved at a frantic pace, made demands on resources out of proportion to his projects. He left himself none of the time or space necessary for the creative, imaginative processes that are part of play. The train sets he bought, for example, were so complex that they required too much of his time to set them up and their maintenance was a burden. He made it unlikely that his recreational plans would be successful or bring pleasure: his vacations were planned hastily, his vehicles were not properly prepared or checked, safety items were overlooked, and his romantic adventures involved risks to his life or family. Even though his adult toy chest was full, the rules of the labor camp, not those of the playground, governed C.

Different as their Holocaust experiences were, and different as the sustenance available to them from their mothers was, these three survivors had in common a lexicon for the conduct of their adult lives. They all considered life as a game with very strict rules that had no exceptions. They translated—and distorted—the terms of lost childhood play into completely unplayful directives, as though their superegos spoke in the manner of the camp commandant to their instinctual drives. In life's game, they said, one must not make errors or mistakes, for these are irremediable; one must not lose, for there are no return engagements, no future games; one must not break or misplace possessions, for these are irreparable, irreplaceable; one must not show anger or hurt, for they are unforgivable; one must not allow separations, for they are deathly. These rules are usually passed along to the survivor's own children, who hear them as a double message: they are to play freely for their parents as a kind of restoration, while they are also to be constantly vigilant and on guard in a world that is so serious and life-threatening that play has no place in it. For these survivors, the "trying on" or "let's pretend" function of play was missing. Play was serious, not fun. Was it play?

III

We have tried to indicate that the survivor's ability—or lack of it—to recover playfulness is an index both of the severity of his or her traumatic experience and of the potential for healing. The significance of this claim for treatment is that it offers a way to conceptualize the healing process. For the survivor, even the establishment of a treatment constitutes a step in the healing, for the analytic process, with its inherent responsiveness to the patient's intrapsychic experience, is the antithesis to, and an antidote for, the compelling life-rules the survivor obeys and the presence in his memory of the absolutely compelling "universe concentrationaire." The analytic process restores the survivor's faith that the void left by the vanished other can be filled, and it restores his or her belief that the self has the ability to express needs which will be heard, understood, and even responded to.

In the course of an analysis, the survivor is encouraged to give up obsessive preoccupations with the harsh game of daily life and survival by his own sense of being able to elicit an empathic response and by the analyst's attention to the wish to play and endorsement of play in free associations, dreams, and fantasies. The analytic process, with its protected space for stability, neutrality, and freedom, can be felt by the survivor as playful or play-permitting. It is important to let this feeling exist, even if it means postponing the emergence and interpretation of content until the feeling of "free space" and empathic response is established. It is also important to consider that, because the conditions of the survivor's Holocaust experience so drastically exceeded in their lack of empathy any "human" environment, the abstinence of analytic silence may initially exceed what the survivor can tolerate. The analyst's silence may approximate too closely the silences of the survivor's Holocaust world, the absence of any response to his or her messages of need.

For the ambience of play to be reestablished, the analysis will have to pass the survivor's test again and again. In a multitude of different ways, the testing will try to ascertain whether, in the analysis, the rules of the death camps or the rules of childhood play apply. Only after patient A., for example, had tested thoroughly the safety and benignness of the analytic situation did he begin to remember more of his prewar history and of his dreams. The link with the therapist meant for him a relinking with his own inner world, and it was this that allowed the play of his memory and imagination as well as his return to playing. Only then could healing proper begin.

BIBLIOGRAPHY

AUERHAHN, N. C. & LAUB, D. (1984). Annihilation and restoration. *Int. Rev. Psychoanal.*, 11:327–344.
COHEN, J. (1985). Trauma and repression. *Psychoanal. Inquiry*, 5:164–189.
EIFERMANN, R. (1987). Children's games, observed and experienced. *Psychoanal. Study Child*, 42:127–144.

MORAN, G. S. (1987). Some functions of play and playfulness. *Psychoanal. Study Child*, 42:11–29.

PELLER, L. E. (1984). Libidinal phases, ego development, and play. *Psychoanal. Study Child*, 9:178–198.

PROVENCE, S. & LIPTON, R. C. (1962). *Infants in Institutions*. New York: Int. Univ. Press, 1969.

WIESEL, E. (1968). A plea for the dead. In *Legends of Our Time*. New York: Avon, 1970.

WINNICOTT, D. W. (1951). Transitional objects and transitional phenomena. In *Collected Papers*. New York: Basic Books, 1958, pp. 229–242.

_____ (1958). The capacity to be alone. In *The Maturational Processes and the Facilitating Environment*. New York: Int. Univ. Press, 1965, pp. 29–36.

Analytic Discussions with Oedipal Children

DONALD J. COHEN, M.D., STEVEN
MARANS, M.S.W., KIRSTEN DAHL, Ph.D.,
WENDY MARANS, M.S., AND MELVIN
LEWIS, M.B., B.S., F.R.C.Psych., D.C.H.

PLAY ACTIVITIES HAVE BEEN STUDIED FROM A VARIETY OF PERSPEC-
tives in order to achieve greater understanding of the development of cognition, social interaction, language, and imagination
in young children (Piaget, 1945; Gould, 1972; Schwartzman,
1978, 1985; Sutton-Smith, 1979, 1985; Bretherton, 1984; Nelson and Seidman, 1984; Fein, 1981; Rubin and Pepler, 1982).
All of these directions of inquiry have a common basis: the recognition that, for young children, play reflects a dominant mode
both of communicating and of working on tasks that are uppermost in their given phase of development. Child psychoanalysis
from its inception has utilized play to study both the contents
and processes of the inner worlds of children (Erikson, 1940;
Kris, 1955). The child psychoanalyst is guided in his observations of the child's play by a theory of development and of technique which distinguishes the interaction of analyst and child
from other types of social and educational relations between
children and adults and from other methods of clinical investigation. When embedded in a broader therapeutic process, and

The authors are members of the faculty at the Child Study Center, Yale
University, New Haven, Conn.

We appreciate the contributions of Drs. Albert J. Solnit, Peter B. Neubauer,
Samuel Ritvo, Phyllis Cohen, and other members of the study group on the
"Many Meanings of Play in Child Analysis," organized by the Psychoanalytic
Research and Development Fund, and the support of the New-Land
Foundation.

guided by a theory of therapeutic action, the child's play in analytic sessions also serves as a building block in effecting
therapeutic change (A. Freud, 1927; M. Klein, 1932; Winnicott,
1971). In spite of its central role as a source of clinical data, the
analytic method of observing and understanding the play sessions of young children has not received intensive investigation
as an entity in its own right. Moreover, there is no information
about the form and content of analytically oriented play sessions
with "normal" children or those who do not come for diagnosis
or treatment.

Research and Clinical Play Sessions: Methodology

Child analytic sessions provide a setting in which the child and
relatively neutral adult may examine the themes of play, forms
of expression, and patterns of interaction that emerge over time.
The goal of the analyst is to understand the child's internal life,
to relate this to his behavior inside and outside of the analytic
situation, and, if needed, to try to alter inner or outer functioning through helping the child understand his experiences, feelings, thoughts, and the life he is leading. He offers verbalization,
clarification, and interpretation in the context of a relationship
that includes elements of transference, displacement, and therapeutic alliance. In its classic application, the interview proceeds
with minimal preparation of the child about its purposes or
form. The analyst engages as an observer and participant in the
discussion and play which the child leads. The analyst may offer
comments of various types within and about the unfolding action and discussion and may shape the process through his
speech and action in play. The child's responses to the analyst
provide information for understanding, just as do the analyst's
feelings and responses to the child.

Because of the multiplicity and wealth of data that emerge in
child analytic sessions, it becomes difficult rigorously to assess
those specific markers in the child's play which inform the analyst's assumptions about the significance of material presented
by the child. Implicitly and often preconsciously, the analyst
combines his observations of the child's verbal productions,

themes of the play, physical activities, and fluctuations in affects in order to confirm or disconfirm hypotheses about significant aspects of the child's inner world.

In general, observations deriving from play sessions have been studied within the context of the extensive and long-term process of analytic treatment. The analytically oriented play session with the child can, however, be approached from a perspective other than therapeutic. As a model or laboratory setting for the study of functioning of the minds of children, play sessions relatively independent of any clinical intent may provide information about mental processes which are of great interest to analysts and others concerned with development. To pursue this goal, we have initiated a series of studies on the child psychoanalytic method of observing young children.

In the study described in this report, 20 children were engaged in play sessions by psychoanalysts who were completely unfamiliar with any aspects of the children's lives or histories. Without specific information about the child, we hoped that the analyst would be free, or at least less constrained than usual, to follow the child's story wherever it might lead. The setting and play materials remained constant throughout the sessions with all of the children. The child was allowed to present himself in any way he chose—to portray through play and discussion those themes which emerged as uppermost or dominant in the child's mind. The child was engaged for three 45 minute sessions, a sufficient number of encounters to provide a rich base of information and chance to observe changes within the relationship, but too few to foster a relationship which would be felt as a serious loss by the child at the end of the final session. In spite of the limitations in nature and number of sessions, the children revealed themselves to a remarkable degree.

Interviews were videotaped and then transcribed. Tapes and transcriptions were reviewed from multiple points of view, including themes and their variations, the modes of representation through play, discussion, and actions; forms of verbal and nonverbal communication; alterations in language use in different modes; relations with the analyst and use of the analyst; points of transition; associations and disruptions in play, and so on.

The child's and the analyst's latent or manifest responses to being observed and recorded need to be considered in evaluating information derived from recorded research sessions. Children were of course informed that there were observers behind the one-way mirror. Only a few seemed concerned, and then mostly transiently, about the one-way mirror or who was watching. The analysts grew comfortable with the setup, in large part because of the trust developed among the research group. Yet, subtle effects of the method no doubt can be found in the behavior of both children and analysts. From a methodological point of view, such effects need to be balanced against the benefits of videotaping as compared with narrative process notes. The availability of videotaped sessions provides the possibility of meticulous and repeated scrutiny of play sequences and transcriptions of material. The analytic interviewers in this study also made notes about the sessions, to convey their global impressions of content and process. During the course of reviewing the videotapes, the interviewers were always impressed by the richness of what the children and they actually did, the exquisite structure of hours, and the content and phenomena that had eluded their recollection (and often their awareness during the sessions themselves). Videotaping preserved the observable data for independent review by other analysts; approaching the material from different perspectives, collaborators often provided new insights into the meaning of specific episodes and the organization of sessions. In these ways, the videotaping and review of sessions enriched the appreciation of the child psychoanalytic approach by the investigators and their collaborators.

For methodological clarity, it is important to underline how experimental interviews or discussions with children are not the same as psychoanalytic sessions with children in therapy, however similar they may be in global appearance, setting, and guiding interests. In the experimental sessions, the range of information which is needed for diagnostic assessment, usually as provided by parents and others, is absent; nor are these experimental discussions guided by the basic therapeutic concern of psychoanalytic sessions. Most obviously, a session during the second and third years of a child analysis exists within the process of the special analytic relationship, which both reflects and shapes the form of the material. To equate a research interview, then, with a psychoanalytic session would be unfair to the function and goals of either. However, what may be learned from one may be applicable to the other, specifically with regard to making more explicit those levels of observation that are employed by the analyst during an evaluation or during the course of a lengthy treatment.

THE 4- TO 6-YEAR-OLD CHILD: METHODOLOGY

We chose to study children in this age range because of the unique coordination of factors that occurs in this phase of development. For this reason, we thought that this period might generate particularly robust data. The 4- to 6-year-old is attempting to modulate strongly felt aggressive and sexual feelings, centering in general about the parents and the regulation of anxiety associated with attendant conflicts. Increasingly complex mental processes allow the child to represent himself in a variety of fantasy configurations in which he can be both the actor and director. In his play, the 4- to 6-year-old is able to suspend reality in the service of trying on different roles and solutions to problems; he derives pleasure from the relatively uninhibited expression of safely displaced instinctual impulses and trial attempts at their mastery. The rich descriptive capacities for expression—through linguistic and activity modes—facilitate the elaboration of fantasy constructions and their articulation in play. Able to separate from his parents for school and other events, the 4- to 6-year-old child can leave the parent for an interview with a stranger; he can use capacities for socially relating to establish a new relationship patterned on ongoing ones with parents and teachers.

The child's gift for play and his fluid, wide-ranging use of various representations of himself, of others, and of impulses provide a window into those processes which the child employs for mediating his inner world while making sense of the world outside.

The limited number of sessions employed in the current research does not yield the detailed unconscious material that would emerge in the course of psychoanalysis. However, it would appear that, operating under the pressure of powerful urges and fantasies, the oedipal-phase child seems impelled to play, talk, and act in a fashion that reveals manifestations of unconscious configurations and the organizing influences of cognitive processes. His play displays the processes of balancing between sexual and aggressive concerns and the mobilization of various ego functions to modulate their expression—the factors that make this phase of development a crucial staging post for the organization of representational and regulatory capacities.

The children in this study were drawn from day care and nursery school programs. Our approach focused attention on the child's story: what the child thinks and what is currently most compelling to him about his inner world. We deliberately chose a design that did not allow us to answer the question, "Is the child's story confirmed by other informants?" (i.e., parents and teachers). Instead, we wanted to focus on, and learn about, the child's inner world: What is "true" for him? What does he think? How does he experience his inner world at a particular point in time? This study of the child's point of view is preliminary to other studies that will examine the relationship between the child's presentation in initial sessions and what is learned about the child from other informants and how, in the clinical situation, the child's story unfolds over the course of his treatment. The current study represents an attempt to develop a methodology that can be expanded to address these other areas of interest.

THE HOURS OF AN OEDIPAL CHILD

Both the methodology for studying hours and the mind of the oedipal child can be demonstrated best by focusing on one child and one hour. For this purpose, we have selected the third session of Sam, a 5-year-old child. His first statement in his first hour concerned crashing, and during that hour and the next he returned repeatedly to cars crashing and to accidents, as well as to concerns with bodily injury, exciting scenes in which he was involved in crashes with his mother while his father was in other cities, magical fixing, a hungry baby, and his wish for help from the analyst. Alternations between fantasies of omnipotence and fears of injury occurred throughout the first two hours. In his final session, Sam developed these fantasies in two particularly elaborate play themes. We wish to demonstrate how these themes, "The Automobile Accident" and "The Baby Sister," apparently unrelated at the level of manifest content, were expressions of a conflictual, latent configuration about Sam and his mother and father. In reconstructing this latent theme we use two approaches: a psycholinguistic analysis of the spoken "text" of the hour and a psychoanalytic examination of play themes and actions. The use of psycholinguistic tools permits us to specify more precisely the critical moments in the session when derivatives of the latent theme are revealed through variations or changes in Sam's use of language.

The theme of the automobile accident involved both enactments of crashes in imaginative play and narratives about crashes. Of the latter, Sam described what appeared to have been at least one real experience in which he and his mother were in an automobile accident. Similarly, the baby sister theme contained representations in play of caring for a baby, comparative size and strength, and a narrative account of a "real" baby sister named Charlotte. These two themes were joined by Sam's enactment of kissing, hugging, and crashing between parent dolls, between siblings, and various combinations of adults and children.

The facts about Sam's experiences were not known to the analyst until after the completion of the sessions. It was then revealed that Sam had in fact been involved in an auto accident with his mother; second, that Sam was an only child and that Charlotte was a newly created fantasy of the session; and third, that Sam's parents, for deeply felt religious and cultural reasons, did not believe in displays of physical affection between them in Sam's presence.

THE PSYCHOLINGUISTIC PERSPECTIVE

By the age of 5 years, the child's developing cognitive and linguistic skills permit increasing use of verbalization. The child expresses complex ideas and thoughts, engages in successful interactions with other people, and uses language as one means of developing imaginary or fantasy play. The child of 5 moves from the preoperational stage toward concrete operational thought. The processes emerging at this stage, such as reversibility, hierarchical organization, and perception of part-whole relationships (Piaget, 1945) are mirrored in the child's understanding and use of more sophisticated language. The child now is able to be more flexible and can use language out of the context in which it originally occurs. Reporting past events, projecting into the future, and "pretend" play all extend beyond the here and now. At this stage dialogues may have multiple meanings (Westby, 1982), and the child demonstrates an increasing capacity to consider the listener's perspective. The 5-year-old's maturational level has reached a point at which different aspects involved in communicating are coordinated smoothly. Vocabulary, syntax, intonation, stress, and nonverbal cues all contribute to the successful interchanges by which the child discovers more about himself, others, and the world in which he lives.

At the same time the child's sophisticated language can be misleading. While the child is developing an understanding of cause and effect (Westby, 1982) and conservation (Trosberg, 1982), he may not have a complete grasp of the logical relationships implied. This discrepancy was demonstrated verbally by Sam in his confusion as to what happened when he was involved in a car crash "because my Dad was in Boston" and by occasional mixing of temporal and quantitative concepts ("She drinks zillion pounds you know for half an hour").

Sam's sessions revealed several recurring themes characterized by play activities which were closely mirrored by language and affect, the three forming a complex but coordinated pattern. The most prominent themes concerned crashing, comparative measures of size across many dimensions and objects, and the care of a baby. The first theme had a historical context since Sam had been involved in a crash with his mother; however, he dealt quite differently with discussing the real crash and with the "playing out" or pretend crashing. His mood, behavior, and language were subdued when he discussed the crash incident; he was motorically quiet and showed little movement in the room. The analyst engaged Sam in a dialogue in which he asked questions and then offered statements about how Sam might have reacted to or felt about the crash. In contrast, the "play"

crashes—play episodes in which Sam acted out crashing between vehicles and people—were enacted with excited motor
activity, the use of a variety of props, and language punctuated
by lapses into crashing noises. During these games Sam provided
a narrative about what was happening. The analyst, in turn,
adopted a more passive role, acknowledging his continued attention through use of repetitions of Sam's statements or mur-
mers, "mmhmm," but rarely making spontaneous statements or
inquiries. Together, Sam and the analyst developed a tacit
awareness of the complementary style needed to foster their
interactions.

The theme of size and comparative size was mentioned frequently across numerous different play episodes. The use of
action, words, and affect combined to convey a variety of textures. For moments, Sam became a strong "He-man" character,
standing tall and using a deep voice to issue commands and
challenges as he moved around the room. At other times, he
referred directly to his own personal strength, emphasizing
these claims with powerful exclamations, e.g., "Wow, hey, I want
to show you something else, watch. Okay?" His preoccupation
with themes of size was apparent as he contrasted the size of toys
within this small setting with his nursery where everything was
bigger.

Size was also central to the language during the third theme.
The baby sister theme appeared to be prompted by Sam's discovery of a baby bottle during an exploration of toys within the
room, but the elaboration and commitment to the theme suggested that it performed multiple functions for Sam. As Sam
acted out the maternal care of a baby—preparing a meal and
feeding the infant—baby Charlotte became a focus for Sam's
statements about his understanding of growth and the fact that
"the more she ate, the bigger she would become." Later he extended this idea and announced that "the baby was the strongest
person," using a fantasy to resolve this conflict about the issues of
being small and helpless. The rich detail of the play—including
the provision without hesitancy of the baby's name—raised no
doubt about the "reality" of Charlotte or Sam's observations and
involvement in her care. During these episodes Sam's play was
highly organized. Although he stopped the play for moments to

comment or pursue a previous theme, he returned to the point in the baby play at which he had stopped and easily resumed his caregiving.

In the course of the hour Sam departed from the major themes for brief digressions. He commented on his new shoes, mentioned his funny book, and wanted to know whether the analyst knew where he lived. These topics were precipitated by an aspect of reality or an association, e.g., "That's funny. I have a funny book." Comments such as these neither led to an extended interchange nor disrupted the major theme in progress, with one exception which was different in both content and form from anything in Sam's three hours. Sam initiated the episode by stating, "Let's pretend," but as he continued it became unclear as to whether he was pretending or reporting. This was unusual for Sam who generally was explicit when he was pretending. He played out and described some hide-and-seek activity. His language included more complex structures than at any other point in the hour, and he used his longest utterance. Yet, he also became slightly dysfluent (as he did at times when he was in the process of organizing himself for a new game) and made errors in the use of pronouns (using both "they" and "our" in reference to the same characters).

The confusions in this episode (as in the use of pronouns in the baby play) stood in contrast with Sam's capacity for sharply defining self vs. nonself and denoting "the real me" from a role taken in pretend play. This capacity was illustrated best in play episodes when Sam shifted his role, from being the active character to being a "puppeteer" speaking and acting through a doll or playing an assumed role. He marked out these transitions in roles by verbal or nonverbal means, such as "I'm He-man" or introducing a doll by name, through a formal greeting, or by saying, "Now she's the baby again." Sam's style of interaction, voice quality, and manner all changed at these points, revealing his internalized and integrated representation both of himself and of others. This capacity for role-play and for trying on different perspectives—from active crasher to wounded animal, from mothering caregiver to hungry baby—created a rich world of people and events in the analytic interview room.

The analyst and Sam used sophisticated means to maintain

their interactions. Sam's skill at controlling a conversational exchange was seen in his attempts to initiate a new topic. He often used "Hey" as a starter, alerting the adult and attracting his attention. Sometimes he would be less direct but more sophisticated in these efforts, e.g., "I've got an idea," and "Let's pretend." He was aware of the need to keep the listener informed and was careful to set the scene through props and verbal explanations. In addition, he frequently checked back with the analyst about his approval or agreement. This was done by and large through his use of tag-questions, e.g., "Okay?" When playing with the baby Sam became engrossed and his speech was more like a monologue than a conversation. Even then, he maintained a commentary that both accompanied his play and allowed the adult to be included in the activity.

The analyst, in turn, was equally responsive. He wanted to remain involved and to facilitate Sam's play without leading the way. At times when there was less of a call to respond, as with the monologue, the analyst made use of murmured acknowledgments as "turns" indicating his attention and continued involvement. When these were insufficient for Sam or when he clearly wanted an answer, Sam actively drew his partner back into the conversation. He looked at the adult and made direct and indirect attempts via questions, comments, invitations, and calls until he succeeded in getting a response, e.g., "Hey, where did you get this from? From a shop? Hmmm. Hey. Hey, who put this in here? Hey, let's pretend this is a closet to hide in. Okay?" Here Sam appeared to be aware of pragmatic rules which guide conversation such as (1) not asking a question unless you believe the listener knows the answer, or (2) if the listener does not answer right away, assuming that it may be because he has not heard or understood the question.

The analyst made use of partial and complete repetitions of Sam's utterances many times during the hour, a conversational strategy that avoided directing and fostered the continuation of Sam's ideas. Analysis of the context in which the repetitions occurred and the examination of intonational and nonverbal cues revealed that these repetitions served a variety of functions. The analyst used them to acknowledge the previous utterance, offer approval, provide and request clarification, emphasize a point, conspire in a game, or just initiate a conversational turn. Sam rarely interrupted the analyst's comments. When he did, the interrupted comment was always in some way interpretative or explanatory. This was most evident when the analyst commented empathically on Sam's position as a little boy in potential danger. Sam adamantly interrupted and at times indirectly contradicted such assertions. Comments that maintained or complemented Sam's fantasy of himself as powerful and strong were accepted and listened to with some interest.

Errors and linguistic regressions were clues, at times, to both dynamic concerns and the linguistic level of maturity. Sam's errors in grammatical forms, semantic relations, or fluency tended to occur when he was changing from one play episode to another and in the process of organizing his ideas. He also made errors when the material was loaded in its thematic content, such as when he was trying to describe the sequence of events in the crash. Sam's mistakes in his choice of pronouns in the hide-and-seek episode recurred in conjunction with the baby. These variations in reference to the baby were probably related to the confusion as to who the baby was and whose baby it was, "facts" which varied at different points in the play.

Sound effects entered into the play during the crashing games, with Sam at times beginning with speech and then lapsing into vocalizations. This reversion to a less sophisticated communicative form occurred when the issues being played out were most exciting. At these points, language use was inadequate to convey the ideas and feelings or express the excitement, consistent with Katan's (1961) observation that the verbalization of perceptions precedes the verbalization of feelings.

Through his mastery of a whole repertoire of linguistic and communicative skills, Sam was able to sustain imaginative play, comment upon such play, describe his experiences in the real world, invent people and events, establish a relationship with the analyst, comment upon the relationship, respond to explicit and implied queries, and elicit information and responses from the analyst. Moments when his skills broke down—into dysfluency, confusions, or hesitancy—provided further information about affective and cognitive factors. Speech, gesture, and emotion were integrated into recurrent themes, as he played out his inner life by discussion, acting himself and taking on the roles of real and imagined others.

Sam began the third session by directly engaging the analyst with a question and then with the statement that he wanted to make a "giant slide" or "bridge." He returned to this play theme at other points in the session. This opening play occupied three minutes; his bridge was big and exciting, something cars could go very fast on and crash. Although the car crashing was exciting, it led to thoughts of damage. Sam warded off the attendant anxiety about damage with thoughts of rapid, almost magical fixing. When the analyst drew his attention to how dangerous the crashes were, Sam responded with an immediate change of subject which contained a direct denial and reversal of affect, "You know that I have a funny story book?" However, the defensive thought of the funny book did not ward off the underlying anxiety, and Sam turned quickly to the memory of his own accident. He tried to contain his anxiety by returning to the play of powerful racing cars, but again this fantasy involved thoughts of his own crashing. For the first time (5 minutes into the session), Sam explicitly identified himself as the excited crasher, and this was immediately followed by the thought of death—he crashed his car into a cow and it died. There was a marked change in affect at this point as Sam first became quiet and somber and then initiated a new episode with "Hey, I got an idea."

Sam began by substituting a "good little car" for the excited, crashing, powerful race cars. However, the good little car quickly became a crasher too; at the point that it slammed into a baby stroller, Sam began to recall his own accident. The introduction of the stroller represented the first linking of the crashing theme to the baby theme, foreshadowed in Sam's initial session by his statement that during his accident he was riding in "the baby seat." In this first account in session three, Sam did not explicitly identify it as "his" accident: "the little boy" was injured and bloody and the car was thrown away. This narrative led to Sam's somber and detailed recounting of his accident. He first stated that his Dad was away in Boston, apparently as a causal explanation,

"*Because* my Dad was in Boston." With the analyst's help, Sam was able to acknowledge that he "and my Mom too" were very frightened and screamed. This was followed by the introduction of the theme of big and little: his car was so small and the truck seemed very big, although it was only a "middle-size" truck. When the analyst suggested that he and his mother were both hurt, Sam appeared to try to contain his anxiety by minimizing the injuries: the cuts and scrapes received were only "little," "teeny-tiny." However, perhaps because of his association between little and helpless, this minimization appeared not to be effective in containing his anxiety and Sam again became the big, excited crasher. The underlying thought seemed to be: "No, the injury wasn't big, it was little. And I am not little and injured; I am the big crasher."

At this point (10 minutes into the hour), Sam shared with the analyst a funny, apparently incoherent, brief fantasy of one and then two people hiding in a closet. His underlying conflicts, represented in this brief fantasy, were marked on the surface both by the linguistic deterioration (infantile sounds) and pronomial reversals (confusions of "he" and "they," "their" and "our") described earlier in the review of the psycholinguistic properties of the session. In this sequence, Sam offered that somebody was hiding in the closet and then "walking down the stairs with our hands and they're playing hide-and-seek." In the midst of laughter and baby sounds, Sam explained of one of the characters, "He says to the boy, 'We'll close the door again and he can still find him.'" As Sam's excitement (and perhaps anxiety) increased, he again elicited the analyst's involvement with the comments: "Isn't that funny?" and "Hey, hey, that's strange." Immediately following this play, Sam reintroduced the theme of the breaking bridge, crashing cars, and bodily injury.

Although Sam's fantasy about the closet was brief and fleeting, careful analysis suggested that the dynamically central aspects had to do with two people hiding and doing strange things, a boy being shut out, excited crashing feelings, and fear of injury. This sketch of an almost incoherent fantasy ushered in the issues that occupied Sam for the rest of the third session and represented his first developed statement to the analyst concerning his fantasies about the activities of his parents and his wish to be involved in their strange and exciting activities from which he felt excluded.

Sam's fantasy of people hiding in the closet, his wish to intrude, and his anxiety and fear of injury were promptly followed (12 minutes into the session) by a compensatory fantasy of being powerfully strong and the breaker of knives. Sam became He-man, whose magic sword makes him the most powerful figure in the universe; he entered this fantasy by assuming the vocal mannerisms of the famous cartoon character. In addition, the intensity of Sam's wish for omnipotence was expressed by his insistent statement, "This is real."

The analyst interrupted the flow of play with his interpretation of Sam's underlying fear about being hurt in the real car accident with his mother. Sam explicitly rejected this, saying that he had been afraid because he was "sick." However, when the analyst adjusted his interpretation to address primarily Sam's wish that he would have prevented the accident had he been He-man, Sam readily concurred. He began to search his memory for a psychologically acceptable, causal explanation for the accident. His affect changed at this point, and he became somber and sad. The explanation Sam proposed was that the car was old and he was sick. When Sam returned to his play (14 minutes into the session), he seemed to find relief in turning from the passive role of victim to the active role of the mighty "ball kicker" and "ball squasher." He became visibly excited and much more physically active.

As he thought of kicking "high and hard," he reintroduced the theme of "big and little." His activity and excitement centered on determining what was the biggest and the tallest. He was explicit that he was the big crasher knocking down the little ones. However, this denial was apparently not sufficient to reduce Sam's anxiety.

It was at this point of anxiety about danger that the fantasy of the baby made its full-blown appearance (20 minutes into the session)—first through detailed play involving the preparation of a baby bottle and then with the introduction of the hungry baby. Sam hinted at his identification with the baby by making an explicit connection between the baby, Sam's nursery school, and the theme of big (and little). Sam's imaginative play described a magic formula enabling the baby to be transformed into a big powerful housebreaker. He then explicitly equated himself with the baby. When the analyst interpreted the wish, Sam confirmed it both verbally and in action—the baby was the big crasher who could not be hurt. As if to emphasize that the baby was powerful and invulnerable, he again used his He-man voice in speaking for the baby.

This sequence was followed by long, quiet play in which Sam fed the baby (24 minutes into the session). Sam then connected the need for the (magic) food with being sick with a headache, and this was followed by thoughts of nighttime and sleep, a fantasy in which he explicitly engaged the analyst. Sam used his deeper voice to express his wish that the analyst sleep with him, a device which probably allowed him to sustain his fantasy of invulnerability and thereby contain any anxiety generated by such directly expressed longing for the analyst.

As this play continued with Sam's making statements suggesting an equation of himself and the baby, the analyst asked, "Do you have any babies in your family?" (30 minutes into the session). This seemed to be an attempt on the part of the analyst to discover where Sam located himself in this play (was he the baby or the mother?). It is this question that precipitated the introduction of the baby sister fantasy. At first Sam said, "I have one baby"—an ambiguous statement that could be understood to mean he was the one baby, but when the analyst attempted to clarify this, Sam suggested that he and his mother had a baby, Charlotte, and that this was why his mother was no longer with him (as if to say, "I am not a baby; I am big enough to have a baby with my mother"). Sam presented the story of his baby sister with great conviction and convincing detail. Sam repeatedly elicited the analyst's involvement in his imaginative play of nurturing the baby sister Charlotte by his statement, "Let's pretend." Again, it was only after the conclusion of this final session that the analyst learned Sam was an only child.

When the analyst introduced the topic of the conclusion of the sessions (35 minutes into the hour), Sam's affect shifted—he became depressed and momentarily confused. This provided a transitional moment into the last play theme involving the exciting activities of his mother and father. In this explicit fantasy,

Sam orchestrated the parent dolls taking a walk. They kiss and fall down, and then the father becomes bloody. When the analyst queried who could help, Sam replied, "I'll show ya," and then reintroduced the fantasy solution of becoming magically powerful through eating. He readily accepted the analyst's interpretation that Sam wished that he could be big enough so he could take care of everyone and protect them from dangerous car accidents.

Sam then elaborated the theme of kissing, by introducing a brother and sister who kiss, are crashed into, and then run over by a car. He denied the anxiety generated by this fantasy and supplied a compensatory fantasy with references to the He-man theme (the most powerful in the world). He equated the brother and sister with father and mother, suggesting the child taking daddy's place.

This led to excited thoughts of crashing and injuring mother, followed immediately by the small baby theme and its accompanying compensatory fantasy that the baby is the strongest person.

Throughout this final session Sam struggled with the affects of excitement, anxiety, and depression which seemed to be generated by his fantasies about what his mother and father did in his absence, his wish to engage in similar activities with his mother in his father's absence, and his fear that he would be injured or killed as the result of such dangerous activity. Sam tried to resolve his conflicts through the use of a small number of devices: fantasies of omnipotence most dramatically expressed through the He-man persona, denial, joking, requests to the analyst for help and protection, regression ("I'll be a well-nurtured baby again"), and magic. None of these solutions worked for very long, perhaps because of the organizing influence of the actual traumatic experience of the car accident when his father really was absent and Sam and his mother were hurt.

DISCUSSION

THE HOURS OF AN OEDIPAL CHILD

Analysis of the sessions of this 5-year-old boy reveals the successful orchestration of multiple forces within a play interview. Unburdened by any specific information about Sam's current life or past experiences, the analyst followed emerging themes and feelings on the basis of immediately available data and analytic theory about mental functioning. He also took Sam's historical reporting within the context of what was dynamically most salient within the hours. The one or two auto accidents were felt by the analyst to reflect at least one real and serious accident in which Sam was involved. The fact that there was a baby in the family was also accepted as reflecting reality, since it was described by name, cared for realistically, and given as the reason for mother not accompanying Sam to sessions. However, equally clearly, the analyst recognized that the accident was experienced by Sam in relation to his fantasies concerning the power of his aggressive impulses and his need to defend himself from the consequences of these wishes; similarly, the baby was seen as reflecting aspects of Sam's own wish to be cared for and his sense of being a fantasied father of his mother's baby, with the dangers and pleasures this would entail.

The success of Sam's third hour lies in the emergence of these complex, converging fantasies revealed to the analyst through the play activities of the child and through the truly free associations. The analyst was allowed to follow Sam in his struggle to bring together profoundly contradictory aspects of his inner world: his longing for continued and exclusive nurturance and love from his mother, and his wish to grow into a man like his daddy.

Sam was able to experience the contradictions in these wishes because of his new capacity to imagine his parents' relationship without him and his ability to place himself affectively via his imagination in each role of the triad. The analyst not only untangled the complex web of Sam's associations, thereby revealing the underlying, central affectively laden fantasies, but he was able to appreciate and affectively experience these fantasies himself.

Finally, as the analyst could communicate to Sam his affective appreciation of Sam's wish to be the powerful and exciting victor of his mother's heart without incurring injury, damage, or death (loss) for anyone, Sam appeared to realize he had been understood. Sam's deepening relationship with the analyst was conveyed in his open statements toward the end of the hour of his wish for the analyst's loving care in helping Sam to find an internal organization that would permit Sam some measure of confidence and safety in his journey out of, and beyond, the triangle.

During the third session, Sam became able to elaborate with increasing complexity what appeared to be his central and most conflicted fantasy about himself, his mother, and his father. He wished to be the big "crasher" who was both powerful enough to protect his mother and big enough to engage in exciting, bloody crashings and breakings with her as he imagined his father did. However, he was frightened that such excitement would leave him vulnerable to danger and that he would be broken instead of being the destroyer.

Throughout the hour, Sam attempted various solutions to this internal dilemma: through fantasies of magical invulnerability, longing for his father's (or the analyst's) protection, and through intellectually solving the scientific question of big and little. One fascinating attempt at resolution occurred during Sam's longest uninterrupted play sequence, involving "baby sister Charlotte." In this episode, Sam developed the fantasy in which he was both his mother's baby and a maker of babies *with* her.

THE OEDIPAL MIND: PSYCHOANALYTIC AND PSYCHOLINGUISTIC PERSPECTIVES

Interviews with children such as Sam have provided rich data about the psycholinguistic capacities of 4- to 6-year-old oedipal-phase children, and particularly their ability to use language for diverse purposes—reporting past experiences, predicting and projecting about future events, exploring beyond the reality with which they are familiar, making jokes to experiment with possibilities, and creating various types of imaginative play. One can see in such sessions elaborate conversational skills and abilities to take the listener's perspective. At this stage, the child is able to use many levels simultaneously, selecting vocabulary, structures, and appropriate paralinguistic markers, such as intonation, stress, and eye contact, in order successfully to engage with others and follow his own ideas (Chomsky, 1969; Bates, 1976; Bloom and Lahey, 1978; de Villiers and de Villiers, 1978; Olson, 1980).

One might hypothesize that these psycholinguistic capacities are necessary preconditions for social development beyond a certain point, or for entry into the oedipal phase. This hypothesis would find support from studies of children with severe language disorders (developmental aphasia) whose social development remains profoundly impaired (Caparulo and Cohen, 1983; Paul and Cohen, 1984; Cantwell and Baker, 1987). Exploring the linguistic issues in general and their implications for psychopathology is beyond the scope of this paper. However, it is useful to relate these linguistic capacities to some of the critical elements of the oedipal configuration, for example, the child's interest in comparative power and his suspension of disbelief, and what these entail in relation to aggressive and sexual urges and coping with reality.

The comparisons to, and assumption of, attributes of the same-sex parent are highly invested by the oedipal child, who is *convinced* that his or her fantasies of displacing the rival can and *will* be realized if only the object of the longings recognizes his superior worth. How the child defines this worth will differ among children and between the sexes and may be represented in terms of physical power, intellect, abilities at manipulating, seductiveness, cooking skills, friendliness, physical charm, among others. That the conquest of the beloved object's exclusive affection is also predicated on the *elimination* of the rival proves fertile ground for the child's aggressive fantasies and fears of retaliation.

Above all else, the oedipal child is under the pressure of instinctual drives which cannot and will not find immediate gratification in reality. In order to sustain his or her quest, the oedipal child must be capable of suspending disbelief—to deny that he or she is small and cannot enjoy the privileges and pleasures of the grownups (Freud, 1920). However, the child is harassed in his quest by anxieties and real deficiencies which must be denied, lessened, or worked through if his invincibility is to be maintained (Peller, 1954). The little girl must find ways to explain why she does not win an exclusive position in father's life in spite of her attempts to woo him (by baking "special treats" just for daddy, wearing mother's lipstick, sitting on his lap), and his admiring responses. The boy at some level needs to confront his exclusion from the parents' special relationship, even though his mother acknowledges how big, strong, and smart he is. Oedipal children must turn from a passive role in which they might fall prey to dangers and disappointments to an active one in which they are the master of their fate (Freud, 1917). In this task they turn to fantasy and its expression in play.

While the child of this age has an increased capacity for reality testing, his continued facility for magical thinking allows greater access to wishes that do not fall prey to immediate reality-bound repudiation. He is thus protected from the recognition of ultimate frustration. His increased capacity for symbolic representation opens the door to more elaborate forms of binding anxiety and discharging instinctual tension via mentation. The child's advances in cognitive and motor skills both yield functional pleasure and support his central task of minimizing anxieties and compensating for apparent inadequacies when comparing himself to the adults with whom he competes (Peller, 1954).

Perhaps one of the most impressive features in the play of the oedipal children we have studied is the fluid movement through a range of themes whose expression is determined by the urgency of what is uppermost in the child's mind—exciting, pleasurable, or fearful. The child's push toward mastery combines with his curiosity to arrive at solutions in play in which theories may be tested and explored. Do babies come from eating special, magical foods? Do Mommy and Daddy hurt each other when they are in their bed together without me?

The oedipal child's play reflects a plasticity of representations employed in the service of creating and maintaining the illusion of wish fulfillment and invincible mastery. The guiding motif of the child's creativity is contained in the oedipal wish and in his attempts to ward off its attending dangers and disappointing confrontation with reality. The child in this phase of development is able to juggle the inconsistencies he perceives both *within* his fantasies and *between* his fantasies and reality. There is equal flexibility as the constituent themes of the oedipal phase seek expression in fantasy and play. At one moment aggressive competition with the rival may be uppermost as the child assumes the role of the strongest, most attractive, and competent member of the family. The same role may simultaneously give expression to the child's exhibitionistic impulses or wish to protect and care for the object of his longings. The play may easily shift from themes of power and strength to scenarios involving the production and feeding of babies. Repeated crashing of toy cars may at one moment express the child's concerns about aggression and bodily intactness. With additional features and elaboration, the same play may articulate the child's primal scene fantasies. In this latter context, the child's curiosity about the contents and activities behind closed dollhouse doors or in closets and bedrooms may at once give vent both to his sexual excitement and to his disappointment on being excluded from parental activities. Reality events in the child's life—accidents and injuries, as well as surprises and pleasures—are dexterously integrated into his fantasies as they stimulate, organize, and accentuate the specific themes with which he struggles. These issues have been studied intensively by child psychoanalysts, e.g., Bornstein (1949), A. Freud (1951), Fraiberg (1966).

If, in the expression of these specific themes the play itself is unable to maintain an adequate distance from painful, objective reality or anxiety aroused by the fantasy, the child still has a variety of defensive maneuvers at his disposal. He may employ humor or silliness in observing the character he has developed in the play. The role may be elaborated in order to add dimensions that would compensate for the intruding sense of vulnerability. Alternatively, the specific role and theme in the play may be abandoned altogether as the child shifts to ones more congenial to the maintenance of pleasure and the prospect of mastery. This shift might in some instances herald regression to dominant modes of gratification found in earlier phases of development. However, the child might equally turn to an intensification and insistent involvement in the fantasy by pulling further away from referents in reality, even creating in his play fantasied objects such as the baby sister of whom he is the father and who also is he. In these varied ways, the child's play may manifest his search for internal harmony as he moves forward developmentally to higher forms of integration (A. Freud, 1974, 1979a, 1979b).

SUMMARY

In this paper we have described an ongoing research project involving play and communication in 4- to 6-year-olds. The children are seen for three 45 minute play sessions by a child analyst who is presented with no information other than what the child presents in the sessions. The sessions are videotaped and then analyzed from psycholinguistic and psychoanalytic perspectives. The first phase of this research focused on normal children and provided the material for this report; ongoing and future studies include children with various types of developmental difficulties (including anxiety and disruptive disorders).

In spite of these limitations in the nature and number of sessions, the children, like Sam, have revealed themselves to a remarkable degree. We believe that these experimental play sessions, informed by psychoanalytic understanding, may permit us to understand in greater depth the ways in which material emerges during a session and how this material conveys latent structures and fantasy configurations of the child's mind. In addition, we hope that by rigorously analyzing the child's modes of communication, we will be able to make more explicit the methods of observation and data employed by the child analyst in his constructions of the child's mental life.

To a degree that is not possible in the analysis of adults, where action is constrained and language conventionalized, the fantasies in child analysis are presented with an openness and freedom of association and a vitality in presentation. Here, the oedipal fantasy can be studied before it is adulterated. Study of the structure of research hours must not be confused with the understanding of the hours and process of analytic therapy, but the ability to focus on research hours with greater precision because of their experimental simplicity may help increase our understanding both of the structure of hours during the course of clinical psychoanalysis and of the mind of the child.

BIBLIOGRAPHY

Bates, E. (1976). *Language and Context.* New York: Academic Press.
Bloom, L. & Lahey, M. (1978). *Language Development and Language Disorders.* New York: John Wiley.
Bornstein, B. (1949). The analysis of a phobic child. *Psychoanal. Study Child,* 3/4:181–226.

BRETHERTON, I. (1984). Representing the social world in symbolic play. In *Symbolic Play*, ed. I. Bretherton. New York: Academic Press, pp. 3–41.

CANTWELL, D. & BAKER, L. (1987). *Developmental Speech and Language Disorders.* New York: Guilford Publications.

CAPARULO, B. & COHEN, D. J. (1983). Developmental language studies in the neuropsychiatric disorders of childhood. In *Children's Language*, ed. K. E. Nelson. New York: Gardner Press, pp. 423–463.

CHOMSKY, N. (1969). *The Acquisition of Syntax in Children from Five to Ten.* Cambridge: M.I.T. Press.

DE VILLIERS, J. & DE VILLIERS, P. A. (1978). *Language Acquisition.* Cambridge: Harvard Univ. Press.

ERIKSON, E. H. (1940). Studies in interpretation of play. *Genet. Psychol. Monogr.*, 22.

FEIN, G. G. (1981). Pretend play in childhood. *Child Develpm.*, 52:1095–1118.

FRAIBERG, S. (1966). Further considerations of the role of transference in latency. *Psychoanal. Study Child*, 21:213–236.

FREUD, A. (1927). Four lectures on child analysis. *W.*, 1:3–50.

———— (1951). Observations on child development. *W.*, 4:143–162.

———— (1974). Beyond the infantile neurosis. *W.*, 8:75–81.

———— (1979a). Mental health and illness in terms of internal harmony and disharmony. *W.*, 8:110–118.

———— (1979b). Child analysis as the study of mental growth, normal and abnormal. *W.*, 8:119–136.

FREUD, S. (1917). A childhood recollection from *Dichtung und Wahrheit. S.E.*, 17:147–156.

———— (1920). Beyond the pleasure principle. *S.E.*, 18:7–64.

GOULD, R. (1972). *Child Studies through Fantasy.* New York: Quadrangle Books.

KATAN, A. (1961). Some thoughts about the role of verbalization in early childhood. *Psychoanal. Study Child*, 16:184–188.

KLEIN, M. (1932). *The Psychoanalysis of Children.* London: Hogarth Press.

KRIS, E. (1955). Neutralization and sublimation. *Psychoanal. Study Child*, 10:30–46.

NELSON, K. & SEIDMAN, S. (1984). Playing with scripts. In *Symbolic Play*, ed. I. Bretherton. New York: Academic Press, pp. 45–71.

OLSON, D., ed. (1980). *The Social Foundations of Language and Thought.* New York: Norton.

PAUL, R. & COHEN, D. J. (1984). Outcomes of severe disorders of language acquisition. *J. Autism Develpm. Dis.*, 14:405–421.

PELLER, L. E., (1954). Libidinal phases, ego development, and play. *Psychoanal. Study Child*, 9:178–198.

PIAGET, J. (1945). *Play, Dreams, and Imitation in Childhood.* New York: Norton, 1962.

RUBIN, K. & PEPLER, D., eds. (1982). *The Play of Children.* New York: Karger.

SCHWARTZMAN, H. (1978). *Transformations.* New York: Plenum Press.

———— (1985). Child structured play. In *Play Interactions*, ed. C. Brown & A. Gottfried. Gillam, N.J.: Johnson & Johnson Baby Products.

SUTTON-SMITH, B. (1979). *Play and Learning.* New York: Gardner Press.
———— (1985). *Toys as Culture.* New York: Gardner Press.
TROSBERG, A. (1982). Reversibility and the acquisition of complex syntactic structures in 3- to 7-year-old children. *Fluency,* 3:29–54.
WESTBY, C. (1982). Cognitive and linguistic aspects of children's narrative development. *Communicative Disorders,* 7:1–116.
WINNICOTT, D. W. (1971). Playing. In *Playing and Reality.* London: Tavistock Publications, pp. 38–52.

Chimeric Objects and Playthings

MATTHEW COHEN

THEORETICAL OVERVIEW

CHILD PSYCHOANALYSIS HAS LONG BEEN INTERESTED IN PLAY BE-
cause it is not artificial, it is something a child will want to do if
left to his own devices. Play is not experienced as alien or contrived by the child. At the same time, play can reveal the deepest
concerns and emotions of a child (A. Freud, 1965). The observer
of play is confronted by several, often simultaneous phenomena,
including vocalizations, sound effects, imaginative use of the
self, and the use of playthings and toys. These external behaviors are only the outline of a much more complicated event
which includes charged emotions, unconscious wishes and fantasies, as well as scripts revolving around archetypal (or stock)
characters and plot elements, such as the family romance and
the heroic quest. Although it is not possible to assess directly the
creative process which allows for the realization of the internal
constructs in the external play, the child's manipulation and use
of playthings are very relevant to the structure and purpose of
play as a whole. An analysis of this component can serve to
elucidate the development of symbol formation, which has implications far beyond the age when the child ceases to engage in
pure play.

The author is a third year student at Harvard College, Cambridge, Massa-
chusetts.

This paper evolved out of discussions with numerous friends, teachers, and
colleagues, including Professor Jerome Kagan and J. Steven Reznick of Harvard University, and Professor Edward Zigler, Robert M. Hodapp, and Dr.
Albert J. Solnit of Yale University.

The child's symbolic representation and use of the materials incorporated into play are key elements in the definition of play. As Freud (1908) observed, the child "*likes* to link his imagined objects and situations to the tangible and visible things of the real world" (p. 144; my italics). It can be theorized that the desire to link internalized symbols with real-world correlates, following the pleasure principle, might be the major impetus for the child's play, as in most other respects it is indistinguishable from daydreaming and fantasy for its role in the development of the child.

Occasionally the active link between the inner mental world and the external world even determines the content of the play. At the start of a play sequence, the child attempts to externalize fantasies and bring them to life, but, as Erikson (1950) noted, the very process of linking the fantasies to inanimate objects often changes the direction of the play, sometimes in unexpected and disturbing ways. At a certain point, there can be to the child only one predetermined, lawful path to the conclusion of a sequence. The predetermined outcome might be due to the satisfaction of a cultural norm or a more personal, unconscious formulation of values. In a fantasy, the sequence could be dropped at any point, but in play, according to Erikson, the demands of the situation can "seduce" the child, unwillingly and unconsciously, to "anxiety play," which is analogous to the anxiety dream. The arrangement of the play materials next to the child and the momentum of the sequence create a compelling need for the child to finish the sequence which he began, even if it means treading on anxiety-arousing ground.

An understanding of the link between external materials and internal mental processes is important to the understanding of play. Recent work in social cognition has begun the process of a critical examination of the nature of this linkage. Vygotsky's early work (1933) emphasized that an understanding of children's play based on pure logic of the adult conception of cause and effect cannot yield the totality of the meaning and structure of play. Vygotsky theorized that the mental processes involved in play are more than just the cognitive elements; the affective situation and the environmental circumstances, including the materials available for play, are also fundamental to play. Similarly, in his experimental and theoretical work, Piaget (1945) demonstrated that play is guided by a set of rules which have been brought about by the particular circumstances to which they apply.

For example, a 4-year-old child takes a plastic hammer, points it at another child who is playing silently by himself, spreads his legs, and declares, "I'm a hunter." Clearly there are a number of things happening in this sequence. To an adult the substitution of the real hammer for the symbolic gun is not initially obvious. Adult logic dictates that things are viewed primarily in terms of function. From this perspective, there can be no greater gulf than that which exists between the hammer, which is used for construction, and the gun, which can be used only for destruction. But the playing child perceives the object primarily in terms of its form. The real object and its symbolic counterpart are then very similar: both have a long, straight part and a place where they can be held in one hand.

When an object is utilized in a nonliteral fashion, or when certain properties (either particular or relational in quality) have been ascribed to it, the object can be said to have undergone a mental transformation (Fein, 1975). The child does not link the gun to the hammer, it is not a "hammer which can shoot bullets." Within the context of the play, the child believes he has a gun in his hands. The fact that he actually holds a hammer is not important. The mental functions involved in transforming an object are very similar to those used in other domains involving symbol formation, such as in the development of language. The playful, explorational use of words in children's speech is analogous to the use of objects in play. There is some evidence that the type of symbolic representations used in play is derived from the same source as the type used in the manipulation of the symbols of language (Werner and Kaplan, 1963).

Though partially dependent on this internal process, the symbolic representation of the materials used in play is also related to the form and the nature of the external objects which are available to be played with. There are essentially three components of the transformation of materials in play. The first is the pure symbolic component. The child has in mind and visualizes some object or toy which either fits into an ongoing sequence or is itself the initiator of a sequence. The second component is the physical nature of the materials the child has available to him. The child cannot simply imagine a form and have it appear. The playing child works (plays) with the materials available, whether or not they are literal representations of the desired form. The third component is the process of linkage—the child's ability to allow the incorporation of available, external materials into the internal play narrative, the imagined or pretended narrative.

The use of materials in play can be at higher and lower levels of sophistication. The simplest is the nonspecific, as described by Rocissano (1982). A rattle is picked up, shaken back and forth, and then dropped to the ground. The rattle is not associated with any other object, nor is there any investment of energy to allow it to be played with as anything but what its physical properties suggest. At the most advanced level of play, a representation of an object is incorporated into a highly symbolic scheme, involving the complex sort of symbolic representation discussed by Werner and Kaplan (1963). In the course of play, an object might even change its meaning several times, often for quite a dramatic effect. August Strindberg employed this device for the set in *A Dream Play*, perhaps to draw parallels between the symbolism of dreams and the symbolism of the creative imagination. In one scene, an object is a lime tree. In the next, without lowering the curtain, it becomes a hat and coat rack.

When children pretend that an object is something other than what it is, particularly for children under age 4, the physical similarity between a substance and its mental (transformed) representation is of great importance. Most children younger than 4 years will be unable to pretend to brush their teeth with an imaginary toothbrush without a physical correlate (Overton and Jackson, 1973). If he is to succeed at the task, he will need to utilize an object shaped like a toothbrush or substitute a body part for the desired object. The transformation of empty space into the desired form of the toothbrush is beyond the capacity of a 3-year-old. Similarly, although children of 2½ years will be able to understand a task such as "comb your hair," most will be unable to substitute objects dissimilar in form for the desired object (the comb). It is not until age 3½ that children are able to make this transformation when it is requested by an adult (Elder and Pederson, 1978). The child who spontaneously used a hammer as a gun was distinctly a 4-year-old child.

It is not simply a matter of cognitive inability which requires this similarity in form at younger ages. The child must see the object as appropriate for play. In part, this involves many culturally determined norms of the child's role and his relation to his environment which are not dependent on the child's cognitive level. Some types of objects are more supportive of transformations and abstract uses than others. Any object can be characterized by its "carrying capacity," an inherent property which allows for, or blocks, its incorporation into play. The child must conceive of an object as a plaything, which has a definite meaning in relation to his conception of play. If an object is too distal from the represented object, or unlike the types of objects normally incorporated into the young child's conceptual schema of play, the child will not be able to use it in play at all (El'konin, 1966).

A child tends to use a particular individual style of play which is not directly dependent on her level of cognitive functioning (Wolf and Grollman, 1982), though this style is linked to the child's use of symbolic language (Werner and Kaplan, 1963). A child may be mentally capable of sophisticated transformations of materials in play, yet rarely use this ability in a free-play situation. Fein's (1975) study of sequences of transformational tasks showed that easy transformations tended to support more difficult ones. At the end of a sequence of transformations of increasing difficulty, a child can show a degree of abstraction in his transformation which he would not have demonstrated if shown the object without any other transformations leading up to it. On the basis of this finding, Fein proposed that all transformations are anchored by a relatively prototypical context.

This theory is supported by Wolf and Grollman's longitudinal study of 4 girls. They saw that the 3-year-old girls who structured their play on the properties of the objects immediately available to them, using strongly object-dependent transformations, would continue this style of play 1½ years later. This same continuity was apparent in the play of the 3-year-old children who tended to use purely imaginary, invisible objects in their play.

Though few researchers would disagree with Vygotsky's assertion that play involves affective and contextual elements, this is occasionally overlooked in the methodological design of studies of symbolic manipulation in play. Traditional experimental studies ask a child to perform a particular act upon an object or to conform to a certain set of instructions. It is not always possible to generalize the dyadic interaction between the experimenter and the child to solitary symbolic play. In solitary play, certain socially acquired roles and symbols may be applied to particular objects, but the use of materials in play is generally not based on the social modeling. To a child, the experimental "play" situation is often perceived as work instead of play. It might be quite taxing and disturbing, particularly if the child has difficulties in accomplishing the task (Kagan, 1984). It is likely that a different set of cognitive processes are assessed when the child perceives the situation as a task or a test.[1]

The problem of evoking symbolic play to look at the relation between the external objects used in play and internal representations of these objects led to the definition of a class of objects which are particularly open to and actively evoke play transformations. Two groups of 10 individuals were assessed, children from ages 2 through 6 and university students and young adults. In addition to the play with these unfamiliar substances, which I call chimeric objects, the younger children's play with more familiar materials and toys was also observed and coded. In all but 3 cases, the play was observed in a familiar playroom with a wide variety of toys scattered around. The chimeric objects were introduced in this setting. For the college students, the chimeric objects were also introduced in a natural setting. The older indi-

1. Although a child will not incorporate an object into his play in a way he cannot understand, even if he is directly asked (Fein, 1975), a "not-play" environment might create the illusion of (unnaturally) sophisticated play. In the early phase of a study on the play of children with mental retardation (MR), we obtained an unexpectedly high level of symbolic play from a 7-year-old. When reviewing a tape of the experimental session, it became apparent that the child was not actually engaged in free play with the toy soldier. The high receptivity of children with MR to experimental demand characteristics (as shown in the work of Zigler and Hodapp) caused the child to engage in activities which were suggestive of imaginative play but were not self-initiated or reflective of his style of free play.

viduals were presented with the objects and encouraged to talk about them.

The first part of the study looked at the use of toys and other materials in the free play of children. There are two distinct ways of studying children's use of materials in free play. The first method of analysis, the child's choice of playthings, is more properly the subject of a future report, but will be mentioned here so the reader can understand the place of chimeric objects in the larger schema of playthings.

Toys are designed by adults for the sole purpose of children's play and are thus limited in their range of functions in play. Often an instruction booklet or examples of how a toy "ought" to be played with are included with the toy. The child might elaborate upon the overdetermined function, giving a baby doll a name and a personality type, but the representation of these playthings is generally fixed. A second class includes household items, such as hammers and pans, when they are used in the "appropriate" manner for which they were designed. The play defined by this class of plaything is generally imitative and stereotypic. A related class of playthings would be the nonstereotypic use of household items. For example, a pen can actually be a sword in play. Another class of playthings is defined by their physical properties—high malleability and amorphousness. Materials such as string, putty, and play dough allow for a nearly infinite number of possible transformations, but are difficult to incorporate in anything but a supporting, "bit" role, as their shape changes with handling, and it becomes increasingly more difficult to maintain a symbolic representation of it. The last class of playthings, imaginary objects, which includes both chimeric and many transitional objects, will be discussed in the next section.

An object can be used in a connected or nonconnected fashion to other objects, as well as in relation to the sequence of play which the child creates. The deepest meaning and significance of an object are determined both by how it is used and the context in which it is used. An object can undergo the same surface transformation, but be used in two completely different internalized ways. That is, a child can pretend that a plastic container is a vessel containing water and pretend to drink from it; while another child can also transform that same plastic container into a vessel containing water, which he then uses to put out a fire which had been started by the collision of two toy cars. The second involves a much more sophisticated, more abstract symbolic transformation, not by nature of the transformation itself (both transformations of the plastic container center on the property of water containment), but by the relational qualities of the transformed object. In the second transformation, the container is not related directly to the self, but rather is part of a more abstract play sequence with two other objects and an entire narrative behind its use.

The relational quality of a substance used in play is only one type of ascription of meaning which the child can give an object in play. In my work on children's play with toys and other materials, there emerged a hierarchy of such ascriptions and types of transformations. Transformations in play can be analyzed in terms of Werner and Kaplan's concept of abstraction, or distancing, between the physical properties of the referential object and the internalized symbolic interpretation, in individual styles of symbol formation. Contrary to the great continuity in Wolf and Grollman's style of play across development, it must be emphasized that not a single child operated entirely on one level during the course of only one or two play sessions; in fact, the fluctuations in level of play was highest for the 5- and 6-year-olds.

The first level is play which is not symbolic in nature, in effect, zero level play. Nonsymbolic play was more common for the younger children observed. Most 2-year-old children can operate at higher levels of abstraction as well, but tend to spend their playing time in nonsymbolic manipulation of substances. Often this meant simply feeling or sucking an object, or carrying it about, moving it back and forth in one's hands—in essence, exploring the purely physical qualities of an object. A combination of the exploratory play and symbolic transformation was observed on one occasion. A 23-month-old child showed a third level manipulation of a spherical object piece in free play, calling it "cookie," and putting it in her mouth. Such manipulations of objects were observed in older children as well, but for a shorter duration and often while the child was watching someone or looking at something else.

The first level of the symbolic transformations of substances during play involves the simple incorporation of materials into a schema. On this level of play, the child assigns some relational characteristic to an object—one object is associated with another object—but the child does not act to transform the object. A child is observed putting numerous plastic pieces in a box. No special meaning is assigned to the pieces except for the association with the box. The plastic pieces are not the subject of any special attention by the child; they are not considered individually, but rather are gathered for the sole purpose of filling the box. If a child had transformed the pieces, more careful consideration would have been given to each of them, and they would be handled in a more particular style.

The second level is the literal transformation of the objects. A literal, representational object is acted upon so that it behaves as the object it represents. A simple example would be a child moving a toy truck around the room, making engine sounds as he does so. This type of symbolic transformation, when it occurs without relation to a play schema, is determined by cultural stereotypes.

The third level of abstraction is the nonliteral transformation of materials. An object assumes a certain role which is not determined by its environmental or literal features. One example observed was a child handing a hammer to another child, and saying, "Here's a lollipop." Another example of such a transformation would be a series of repeated actions, when a child put a block on his head and pushed it off his head by a quick movement of his neck. In this case, a type of game was created by the child, and the substance must have undergone a mental transformation to be incorporated into the game schema.

The fourth level of transformation is physically oriented, symbolic play. In full symbolic play, the child manipulates a particular object in a connected series of representations, indicating that it has assumed a role and *functions within* a schema. Another type of fourth level play involves more than one object, where the objects concerned are used in both a symbolic and relational, or connected manner. Both the car accident and the "I'm a hunter" sequences are examples of fourth level play transformations.

On the fifth and highest level of play transformations, non-physically oriented play, the child makes only peripheral use of the play material, focusing the sequence on much more internal operations. The particular materials used in such play become less important, in deference to a more rule-oriented approach. What the item represents is not crucial; it is more important how it fits into a symbolic network, which often involves or implies imaginary objects as well. An example of this type of play is a game created or adapted by a child who placed some materials in front of him, sang a lyric from a television show, "one of these things does not belong," and asked a playmate to choose which one is "not like the others." In this highest level of play, one can see the developmental seeds of the adult drama, which as Freud (1908) states, is not only based on, but requires "to be linked to tangible objects and which are capable of representation" (p. 144). At the highest level of play, as well as at the highest level of drama, the symbolic representations take precedence over the availability of tangible objects. In the "poor" theater of Jerzy Grotowski entire worlds of fantasy can be acted out with wheelbarrows, metal pipes, and potato sacks.

CHIMERIC AND OTHER IMAGINARY OBJECTS

The class of playthings which I call imaginary objects does not encounter the problem of undifferentiation which besets the classes of amorphous playthings, while still being free of the overdetermined purposes and functions of toys and household objects. By definition, imaginary objects, both natural and man-made, are open to the investment of personal meaning and thus can be incorporated into play in a large number of ways. These objects are characterized by a high carrying capacity for the investment of the energy of the imagination. Nature is filled with imaginary objects which are readily available for children's play, such as pebbles, which can be used in play as plates, or coins, or missiles. Man-made imaginary objects are also common, an example being a broken piece of a toy, taken out of the context of its original function in the whole toy.

Play with imaginary objects can spring from two paths. In the first path, imaginary objects are introduced into a play narrative already in progress, functioning in a role necessitated by a complex play structure. Imaginary objects, because of their lack of specificity, can serve many roles in a sequence, whenever a tangible object is required to fill a bridge in the internal narrative. A rubber washer can easily be used as a life preserver, or a doughnut, or a hoolahoop, at any time the narrative demands these substances to appear.

In the second path, an imaginary object is found and the child fantasizes and experiments with its possible use or purpose. A true imaginary object, however, does not have a single purpose and can be explained and played with in many ways. In this way, play which starts out as the purely cognitive task of assimilation and differentiation (Piaget, 1945) evolves into fantasy play. Very often, the cognitive process of exploration of the material becomes the starting point for complex play sequences which build into entire narratives.

A special type of imaginary objects are chimeric objects, which are composed of several disparate parts, often familiar to the child, but put together in an unfamiliar order. In my study of play, I constructed two and found one chimeric object. All three objects were brightly colored, visually attractive, and interesting. They also were nonliteral—it was not intended that the whole of the chimeric object could function together to serve a specific purpose. The three chimeric objects were composed of disparate parts, as was the mythical monster, the chimera. The combination of these elements was somewhat whimsical and irrational and, for some individuals, mystifying. It was this whimsicality and bright colors that caused 5 adults independently to call the chimeric objects toys of some sort, yet 10 other adults and college students felt compelled to assign meanings to the objects, some of which were hardly "toylike," but rather seemed to function in terms of their own styles of thinking.

The children were introduced to a sequence of the three chimeric objects. If their interest remained engaged and the child wanted to explore and play with an object following their initial response, they were allowed to do so. In such a way, multiple transformations could be applied to the same object by the same person, changing their symbolic representation of the chimeric object in the process of play.

The first object presented was a bright-red plastic piece, about 2 inches in length, which resembled half a squashed strawberry with a pole sticking out the top if viewed from one side. The other side was hollow and had a clip, an attached strap which could be manipulated fairly easily by the subjects over 33 months, though some of the younger children were not able to clip it back on, and showed some distress at that point, asking me to "fix it." The second object was even more ambiguous in function, though more simple in form. It consisted of a 10 by 5½ inch rectangular piece of thick cardboard with two 6-inch long, brightly colored, wooden poles glued to the longer sides. The third object was a complicated arrangement of two sliding tubes, several wires, a 1-inch plastic block, a small plastic table, a button which squeaked when pressed, a plastic ring, and several pieces of cardboard attached by wires.

In the interactions with children and adults there emerged four levels of increasing sophistication in the interpretation or transformation of chimeric objects.[2] It is worth noting that there was also the zero level of transformation, characterized by a lack of response, an evasion of the question, or naming or identifying a part of the object as an answer to the question of what the entire object meant.

Level one was interpreting the whole from a partial feature of the object. An example of this was calling the first chimeric object a strawberry.

Level two was the conventional use of these nonconventional objects: identifying a chimeric object as a typically encountered toy based merely on one element of similarity. For example, a child might call the third object an erector set because it was complex and had moving parts.

2. In my pilot study of 5 children between age 2 and 5 observed in a day care center, the mean level of symbolic manipulation of objects in free play and the mean level of the transformation of the chimeric objects had a Pearson product-moment correlation coefficient, $r = .98$.

The third level response meant transforming an object into a nonconventional object, which did not quite succeed in uniting most of its parts into a single concept. An example of a level three transformation would be calling the third object a kite. This transformation united the elements of the string and the 90 degree orientation of the two poles in the symbolic formation, but it did not succeed in uniting all the other elements. There was no place in this transformation for the plastic ring, for example.

On the highest level, the transformation made the chimeric object into an entire functional unit, incorporating all the salient features of the object into a united vision. A particularly creative child called the third object a fishing pole. According to this child, you push the button to bring up the fish. The block on the end is a piece of cheese. The handle is at the end opposite the cheese. And the tablelike plastic object is a screen "where you tell if a fish is coming on." This highest level of transformation cannot be called "the most successful," as in a task or problem-solving situation. It is, however, the most highly creative of all response types. Although it might seem that the only people at this highest level of object transformation are those with high verbal aptitudes, most of the transformation of objects was expressed entirely nonverbally, or by nonverbal actions only supported by declarations.

In fact, one of the most striking features of chimeric objects was their ability to evoke touching and manipulating. Even in the adults, the most common reaction to all the chimeric objects was the desire to pick them up, feel them, manipulate them, and rotate them to view them from different perspectives. It was only out of this handling that the high level transformations occurred. Each person attempted to become familiar with them. The children, even though they were rarely asked, would spontaneously begin to play with the chimeric objects upon presentation. There was something greatly concordant in the child's natural desire to play and the chimeric objects; at the same time, the urgency of the initiation of play suggested something greatly discordant in terms of affect.

It is likely that the discordant affect sprang from exactly the same source that made the namesake of the objects a monster for the ancient Greeks, rather than a wonder of nature. The first mention of the Chimera in literature occurs in Book VI of the *Iliad*. Homer described the monster as a lion in its foreparts, a goat in its middle, and a serpent in it hindparts. Though it would seem that this animal could not be particularly powerful, most men could not stand the sight of this mélange, and only Bellerophon could vanquish it. The disparate nature of its parts aroused the curiosity of philosophers—both Plutarch and Virgil subjected the beast to rationalizations, both of which were inventive, but neither of which succeeded in uniting the entirety of the concept of the Chimera.[3]

The Chimera, which lends its name to the class of objects, can be said to be the paradigm for all chimeric objects. The Chimera causes fear because of the arrangement of its parts. Any particular part can be explained and understood. But when put together, the entirety is beyond comprehension. Initial exposure to a chimeric object is essentially an uncanny experience—one sees an element of the familiar within the larger context of the unfamiliar and one cannot understand how it came to be (Freud, 1919). This paradoxical situation causes fear if encountered in a hostile situation, philosophical inquiry if encountered in the intellectual sphere, and play if the chimeric object is encountered in a situation allowing play. In any case, there is an attempt to control the anxiety created by the paradox, to work or play with it so as to place it in the context of known things. The object must be handled, in effect dissected, taken apart piece by piece, to allay the fear that there might be anything supernatural about the object. Thus, both Plutarch's and Virgil's explanations focused on the original separateness of the parts, to make com-

3. Borges and Guerro (1970) summarized these explanations: "The Chimera reappears in the sixth book of the *Aeneid*, 'armed with flame'; Virgil's commentator Servius Honoratus observed that, according to all authorities, the monster was native to Lycia, where there was a volcano bearing its name. The base of this mountain was infested with serpents, higher up on its flanks were meadows and goats, and towards its desolate top, which belched out flames, a pride of lions had its resort. The Chimera would seem to be a metaphor for this strange elevation. Earlier, Plutarch suggested that Chimera was the name of a pirate captain who adorned his ship with the images of a lion, a goat, and a snake."

monplace the truly extraordinary outline presented in the Chimera.

The desire to handle a chimeric object is derived from the desire for mastery and linkage which is seen in free play, but it is strengthened by the anxiety it creates as the individual realizes it is not easily categorized or related to past experiences. The initial reaction of adults and children to the presentation of the first chimeric object was almost always "What is it?" For adults, the initial query was often followed by the request to "look at it." Even if the request was not made, certainly there was a latent desire to "look at it," because if the offer was made, the individual would almost invariably accept. "Looking at it" was in fact a euphemism for manipulating it. Analogous to this secondary reaction of adults and college students was the children's request to "play with it." Their descriptions and explanations of the objects were also very close to the play transformations of the children, and sprang directly from their manipulations and rotations of the objects. For instance, the third object was described as a satanic fetish, a space station, and a carnival game by three adults. This same object was used in play by various children as an airplane, a camera, and a stethoscope—objects which, to a child, are associated with similar types of "supernatural," inexplicable experiences.

The anxiety created by chimeric objects makes them different from transitional objects, which function to alleviate anxiety, but there are many striking parallels in the mechanisms underlying the individual's experience of both types of objects.

The term "object" has many uses within psychoanalysis, including both real, external things and people, on the one hand, and the individual's internal representation of aspects or the whole of things and people, on the other. Winnicott's (1971) conception of transitional objects has played an important role in psychoanalytic conceptions of play. For Winnicott and his followers, a transitional object has both internal and external existence. The transitional object is simultaneously a physical substance with particular characteristics which can be associated with maternal experiences, including tactile and olfactory cues, and a particular type of internal representation, standing between and, in part, mediating veridical perception of the external world and the experience of internal sensations and fantasy. The transitional object, according to Winnicott, is a physical thing invested with personal fantasies and residuals of feelings associated with the primary experience of being mothered. By adopting the earliest transitional objects, children create a mode of experiencing which allows for an understanding of other experiences and objects over development, including music and other cultural experiences.

Both chimeric and transitional objects have a dichotomous existence as both external, manipulable materials and internal symbols invested with personal meaning. In the contact with the transitional objects, internal tension is reduced, although for chimeric objects the cause of the anxiety is often the object itself, while for transitional objects the tension is typically caused by some external force. Neither transitional objects nor chimeric objects outside of this experimental study are designated by the culture or the society (including the child's parents) as "transitional objects" or "chimeric objects." An imaginary object is the creation of the individual who uses them because their true meaning can exist only in the imagination of the user. A parent might give an infant a blanket or a stuffed animal, but it is the child who determines whether this inanimate object is to be a transitional object. Without the act of the imagination a blanket is *just* a blanket. Similarly, a child may see an isolated piece of a toy which is capable of being a chimeric object in play, but rather than picking it up and playing with it, kicks it aside.

There are several important differences between chimeric and transitional objects. The energy invested in transitional objects must be related to the experiences with the mother, while that of chimeric objects comes from the child's desire to play. In addition, transitional objects occupy a more stable symbolic configuration for the child than chimeric objects, whose internal representation is rarely tied to particular associations and meanings. The form of a chimeric can be worked over in one's head.

One individual, a college student, saw the object and commented on it. A week later, she reported that she had been thinking about it and decided it better resembled something else. When incorporated into free play, the chimeric objects rarely received only a single usage. A 4-year-old child started playing with the second object as a bridge, then used it as an overpass, then as a boat within a single play sequence involving vehicles. Transitional objects, because of their ties with a particular type of experience (being mothered), do not tend to have this degree of fluidity. Although the range of interpretations of transitional objects across individuals is very large, for a particular individual a transitional object tends to be capable of a smaller set of meanings, though these meanings can be applied to many situations.

In some cases, the meaning of an imaginary object might not be as clear to the player as to the observer of the play. This is particularly true in adulthood, where play no longer exists in its purest conscious form, as the adult and older child feel compelled to hide the fantasies openly expressed in child's play. Yet play with objects does continue at some level. "Actually, we never give anything up; we only exchange one thing for another. What appears to be a renunciation is really the formation of a substitute or surrogate. In the same way, the growing child, when he stops playing, gives up nothing but the link with real objects; instead of *playing*, he now *phantasies*. He builds castles in the air and creates what are called *day-dreams*" (Freud, 1908, p. 145). Fantasy does become more important to the individual as play ceases. However, this link to real objects is of such importance to the definition of play and the psychic health of the individual that a simple renunciation of the link is not possible. This aspect of play also undergoes a transformation and takes on other forms, only some of which can be called "playful." In a crucial point in Freud's analysis of Dora (1905), he noticed her playing with a small reticule she was wearing at her waist. He characterized her fidgeting as a "symptomatic act."

> I give the name of symptomatic acts to those acts which people perform, as we say, automatically, unconsciously, without attending to them, or as if in a moment of distraction. They are actions to which people would like to deny any significance, and which, if questioned about them, they would explain as being indifferent and accidental. Closer observation, however, will

> show that these actions, about which consciousness knows nothing or wishes to know nothing, in fact give expression to unconscious thoughts and impulses [p. 76].

Thus, while part of the function of play is subsumed under the process of daydreaming (which also exists in childhood), the manipulation of objects which occurs in play can become transformed into adult "playing" with objects. Freud (1905) stated that "there is a great deal of symbolism of this kind in life, but as a rule we pass by it without heeding it" (p. 77).

Play is a unitary process in childhood, with an interval narrative closely related to the sequence of actions directed toward the manipulated objects. In adulthood, there tends to be an increasing differentiation between fantasies (played out in the mind with images and subvocalizations) and externally directed activities. The link between physical reality and internal fantasies and the desire for this linkage can be realized in many types of endeavors and activities, including arranging a collection on a shelf, waxing a car, and idly browsing in an antiquarian bookstore.

The adult "play" with the chimeric objects was similar to the sort of behavior seen in the exploration and appraisal of a work of art, such as a Mayan statuette. Many of the adults found pleasure in manipulating the chimeric objects and performing a transformation upon them. These adults tended to be playful, creative people, including artists and musicians, and their play with the chimeric objects had a playful, whimsical air.

Summary

The symbolic processes underlying the uses of materials in play operates across situations—from free play to chimeric object play. The assessment of the child's use of chimeric objects taps the same processes as use of materials in free play, the very source of creativity. As an approach to seeing how the child works through the ambiguity and searches out meanings, the study of the use of chimeric objects may reveal how free the child or the adult is in using his fantasy life and his or her security in creating new symbols. An adult who was asked what she thought the third chimeric object was answered very impatiently that it had to be a mobile, completely ignoring the ambiguity of the object. Although there was not a visible place to attach it to the ceiling, it had moving parts and string, and therefore, out of necessity, *had* to be a mobile. This fundamental quality of the individual's internal world is related to her earliest experiences, the primary and transitional objects of the first years of life. Rigidity of thinking is less typical of the thinking of children than of many adults. Not all adults recognize, as did a 5-year-old child, that a chimeric object "could be many things."

BIBLIOGRAPHY

BORGES, J. L. & GUERRO, M. (1970). *The Book of Imaginary Beings.* New York: Avon.

ELDER, J. L. & PEDERSON, D. R. (1978). Preschool children's use of objects in symbolic play. *Child Develpm.*, 49:500–504.

EL'KONIN, D. (1966). Symbolics and its functions in the play of children. *Soviet Educ.*, 8:35–41.

ERIKSON, E. H. (1950). *Childhood and Society.* New York: Norton, 1963.

FEIN, G. G. (1975). A transformational analysis of pretending. *Develpm. Psychol.*, 11:291–296.

FREUD, A. (1965). Normality and pathology in childhood. *W.*, 6.

FREUD, S. (1905). Fragments of an analysis of a case of hysteria. *S.E.*, 7:1–122.

———— (1908). Creative writers and day-dreaming. *S.E.*, 9:141–153.

———— (1919). The uncanny. *S.E.*, 17:217–256.

KAGAN, J. (1984). *The Nature of the Child.* New York: Basic Books.

OVERTON, W. F. & JACKSON, J. P. (1973). The representation of imagined objects in action sequences. *Child Develpm.*, 44:309–314.

PIAGET, J. (1945). *Play, Dreams, and Imitation in Childhood.* New York: Norton, 1951.

ROCISSANO, L. (1982). The emergence of social conventional behavior. *Soc. Cognition*, 1:50–69.

VYGOTSKY, L. (1933). Play and its role in the mental development of the child. In *Play*, ed. J. Bruner, A. Jolly, & K. Sylva. New York: Basic Books, 1976, pp. 537–554.

WERNER, H. & KAPLAN, B. (1963). *Symbol Formation.* New York: John Wiley.

WINNICOTT, D. W. (1971). *Playing and Reality.* London: Tavistock.

WOLF, D. & GROLLMAN, S. H. (1982). Ways of playing. In *The Play of Children*, ed. K. Rubin & D. Pepler. New York: Karger, pp. 46–63.

Notes on Play and Guilt in Child Analysis

T. WAYNE DOWNEY, M.D.

SINCE CHILD ANALYTIC TREATMENT SO FREQUENTLY INVOLVES THE medium of play, its technique may give the illusion of change-lessness and timelessness, which are characteristics of the id. In this presentation, which is concerned with the child analyst's use of play, I will consider how there is a never-ending effort to establish an analytic balance between activity and interpretation, play and words, the expression of affect and the acquisition of insight. Then I will focus on the microanalysis of a single session in the analysis of a 5-year-old boy in order to provide an example of these tensions and interactions. The data of this single spec-imen session lead to a discussion of the interactions of play and guilt and a further reconsideration of the role of guilt in psychic functioning.

Freud (1914) described somewhat eliptically the technical di-lemma confronting the analyst of adults as "a perpetual struggle with his patient to keep in the psychical sphere all the impulses which the patient would like to direct into the motor sphere; and he celebrates it as a triumph for the treatment if he can bring it about that something that the patient wishes to discharge in action is disposed of through the work of remembering" (p. 153). In doing so he drew tight technical lines separating action from interpretation in adult analysis. Did this mean that child

Training and supervising analyst at the Western New England Institute for Psychoanalysis; associate clinical professor of pediatrics and psychiatry, Child Study Center, Yale University, New Haven, Ct.

Adapted from the Anna Maenchen lecture presented to the San Francisco Psychoanalytic Institute and Society, January 18, 1986.

analysis was confronted with a quandary? That is, how to integrate the play, action, and words of children into a valid, interpretive, psychoanalytic process. On entering the analytic consulting room, most young children almost immediately turn to action and play to express their inner lives and their conflicts with the outer world unless they are precociously and/or defensively verbal or markedly inhibited in motor or fantasy activities. Children intuitively and aggressively seek action outlets. They turn passive, sullen, and silent, or become openly rageful if such opportunities are denied them. In addition, the younger the child, the more likely is the conflict or memory to be expressed in play rather than words. The earlier in life the memory arises in the older child or the adult, the more likely that it is to be recovered by being made manifest through action or art as an adjunct to words. However, even with all the emphasis on the dominance of play and motor activity, we can identify a child analytic process. Not only does remembering and working through take place, these analytic functions take place *through* the motoric medium of play! Indeed, the playing process in child analysis has become associated in clinical parlance with the process of working through. Such a symmetry is derived from the analogous elements in the play process of thematic repetition with fantasy elaborations tending in the direction of drive sublimation and toward an enhancement of ego functions, while moving away from a prior state of dominance by drive and superego derivatives. Certainly, the theoretical developments in child analysis over the past 80 years reflect this ongoing attempt to adapt Freud's core verbal conceptualization of remembering and working through to the child sphere. In this sphere nonverbal acting out of conflicts *as well as verbal* expression has come to be viewed as not only inevitable but vital to psychic healing and the child analytic process. In an important sense, a goal of analysis with children is to restore through play and verbal reflection the child's capacities for self-knowledge, self-healing, and mastery on both conscious and unconscious levels. Children come to analysis partially deprived of these capacities. They usually have deep feelings of helplessness and impotence engendered by overwhelming frustrations, deprivations, or overexcitations. They are usually filled with an admixture of anxiety and depression. Play is, among other things, a language for communicating about these states of pain and unhappiness. The semantics of play are manifest and latent in the visual-motor imagery which the child creates collaboratively in the presence of the analyst. Playing is to verbalizing as hieroglyphics is to our modern language. It is a primitive, bodily oriented, dramatizing medium stemming from a time before mind was clearly differentiated from body. As adults and analysts we are constantly searching for a Rosetta Stone of play which will allow us more effectively to harness its psychic healing qualities.

HISTORICAL PERSPECTIVE

It *almost* goes without saying that Freud's report of his surrogate analysis of Little Hans (1909) set the standard for the nascent field of child analysis. His technique involved a direct transposition of the verbal-interpretive emphases of adult analysis to the work with the young child. The report of Little Hans's analysis offers the model of children observed in their home environment and (usually by a parent) tactfully questioned about their verbal productions and play activities. They are then offered interpretations couched in a mixture of adult syntax and child vernacular.

In the course of reviewing some of the early writings on child analysis, I was struck not only by how Freud's first report put such a strong emphasis on verbal interventions but also by the many other critical ways in which certain child analytic developmental tensions were struck. For the next 20 years the model of parent as intermediary exerted a particularly powerful effect on the emphases and direction of child analysis. Indeed, the major shift which occurred over this interval involved the liberation of child analysis and the child analyst from the context of the family. Hans's father reported to Freud and acted as Freud's surrogate in the analysis of his son. Freud directed the father's analytic interpretations vis-à-vis his son. This model seems to have been taken consciously or unconsciously by many analysts over the years as one possible model for supervision: i.e., the neophyte analyst as agent for his supervisor's analysis of the patient!

The writings of Hug-Hellmuth (1921), Melanie Klein (1932), and Anna Freud (1926) all seem remarkably similar in tone and emphasis. Great care is taken not to usurp the parents' position as love objects and authority for the child. The analyst remained a peripheral member of the household, observing the child occasionally at home, sometimes looking in on an evening bath or bedtime activities, but mainly working through the parents. Klein propounded meeting the child in a professional office without parents for purposes of analysis.

It is important to note that one aspect of the controversy between Anna Freud (1926) and Melanie Klein (1932) had to do with the question of what was the proper mix of verbalizing and playing in the "true" child analytic process. Anna Freud seems to fault Kleinian play-technique for including too much playing and being both too rigid and too profuse in the use of interpretation. Klein's critique of Freudian child analysis included its lack of as significant an emphasis on play as there was in her technique. Ironically, it was also criticized for an overemphasis on verbal constructs and an underemphasis on interpretation of oedipal dynamics! By their case reports, both Anna Freud and Melanie Klein seem to have started out adopting the model of Little Hans with an intellectual, overly verbal, adult analytical approach using parents as intermediaries. They both observed and analyzed play activities to some degree. Their main focus remained on exploring the verbal productions of their young patients as manifest through dreams, daydreams, storytelling, and wishes. Drawing was occasionally included. By 1945 both approaches seem to have come into close synchrony in terms of the proper balance between playing and talking in the ongoing process of child analysis (A. Freud, 1945).

In the interval between 1926 and 1946 Waelder (1932) took Freud's (1920) conceptualizations regarding the nature of play and placed them on more orderly theoretical ground. In doing so he legitimized play as an internalizing, psychologically assimilating, healing process in its own right. It was seen as an important aspect of the child's ongoing quest for mastery and self-assertion in the face of the eternal conflict between wish psychology and the pleasure principle and guilt psychology bound to the reality principle.[1] He delineated the multiple functions of

1. For the preoedipal and early oedipal child this formulation requires modification which puts the emphasis on the child's fear of drives overwhelming the ego through the medium of magical thinking.

play as follows: "instinct of mastery; wish fulfillment; assimilation of overpowering experiences according to the mechanism of the repetition compulsion; transformation from passivity to activity; leave of absence from reality and from the super-ego; fantasies about real objects" (p. 224). In terms of child analytic technique, Waelder's paper offers an implied rationale for the acceptance of the motoric nonverbal aspects of playing in the child analytic setting as potentially *expressive* and *ego organizing* rather than solely or mainly defensive and ego regressive.

Berta Bornstein (1949) provided a matchless synthesis of id and ego psychology which prepared the way for the contemporary emphasis on the vicissitudes of drives and object relations in child analysis.

Winnicott (1971) subsequently expanded on the existing play characterizations by locating play and playing in an intermediate "transitional" area between inner and outer realities. He located play activities in a realm which owes most of its existence to intrinsic intrapsychic rather than to extrapsychic processes. This conceptualization has served to reinforce the notion of play originating in the earliest pictographic preverbal realms of ego formation. It also seems to raise the same questions of technique that have been present since the beginnings of child analysis. Are we relying enough on the health-promoting aspects of play? Paradoxically, to what extent does an overly verbal, interpretive approach become repressive and thwart the child's development of true self-knowledge, self-control, and understanding of self vis-à-vis the world of love objects and others? Winnicott's final words on the subject suggest that in adult as well as child work we may err in the direction of talking too much in order to undo defense rather than respecting the power of the unfolding, relatively undefended, transitional play process, whether manifest in child's action or adult's words.

MICROANALYSIS OF A CHILD ANALYTIC SESSION

This session was selected for several reasons. One, it seemed particularly illustrative of the ebb and flow of play and verbalization in the opening phase of a child analysis. Secondly, the session seemed to be quite vivid in its depiction of the guilt experienced by so many children entering analysis. This guilty reaction is a common part of our everyday analytic endeavors, but it is my impression that it seldom finds its way into print. Finally, in this session we can apprehend the preliminary phase of the reconstruction of a frequent childhood traumatic situation.

BACKGROUND

Jared was an almost 5-year-old boy when he was referred for child analysis some years ago. His parents, the Kellys, had reluctantly and gradually become aware that he was "different" from their other two children, Zack, 2 years older, and Nora, 2 years younger than Jared. They had attributed his "headstrong" and "unpredictable" moods to external sources. They thought he had either an allergy or a dietary excess or lack. Possibly there was some instrumental problem in their manner of disciplining him. Grandparents and extended family members continually referred to Jared as "spoiled." This contributed greatly to the guilt, frustration, rage, and despair which his two well-educated parents felt for him. Through their pediatrician the Kellys were referred to a child psychiatrist who in turn recommended analysis.

Jared's parents were alternately relieved and bewildered. They had been externalizing Jared's difficulties, looking for physical causes and educational solutions for their son's problem. With support and repeated, detailed, psychodynamic descriptions of their son, they allowed their denial of Jared's psychological problems to lapse. They replaced it with a clearer vision of his developmental difficulties. At the outset the Kellys were sparse historians. The few emerging historical data indicated that a marked change in Jared had occurred about one year of age. At that time he shifted from being a quiet, easily satisfied, passive baby to a cranky, irritable, incessantly demanding toddler. This coincided with his mother becoming pregnant for the third time. Mrs. Kelly also became significantly, albeit subclinically, depressed. Mr. Kelly had to change his employment. The pregnancy had not been planned. Jared's mother became physically ill on top of it. She had to quit her job, which added to her distress.

The Kellys anxiously remarked on the most obvious aspect of their middle child's disrupted interpersonal and object relations. He rarely met people and life with direct eye contact or direct action. Since his second year he had glanced at the world out of the corner of his eye. At the same time he had regressed. He began experiencing extreme difficulty letting his mother out of his oblique line of sight. He clung to her. He refused to eat or dress himself without her help. What he had attained of stable relationships in the first year of his life were eroded and compromised in his fitful attempts to dominate and possess his mother. He regressed significantly. As a measure of her frustration and helplessness in dealing with his plight Mrs. Kelly waxed in return from excessively sweet overcontrol of Jared to uncontrolled outbursts of rageful shouting and slapping. Often these outbursts ended with her exiling Jared to his room for their mutual protection. She felt much guilt and remorse over her behavior and his. Through all this turmoil Jared became more and more attached to his transitional object, a small stuffed teddy bear. He would venture nowhere without it. He required it to fall asleep. If he awoke at night or in the morning and he could not find his bear, he would erupt in ear-splitting rage which often continued for hours even after his parents had restored his transitional object to him! The Kellys finally devised the solution of pinning Jared's stuffed animal to his pajamas. This successfully addressed his need for the illusion of inseparability and benign love toward his cherished inanimate mother substitute.

Matters became compounded toward the end of Jared's second year when his mother gave birth to Nora. Within a few weeks thereafter she left precipitously with her newborn daughter to attend a family funeral on the west coast. During the 10 days she was gone Jared was cared for by a baby-sitter during the day and by his father at night. He was inconsolable in his despair and depression. Finally, in his wife's absence, Jared's father took time off from work to be his disorganized and despairing son's full-time caretaker. Jared responded more positively to his father's presence, but he still remained quite upset. When his mother returned, he alternately ignored her, clung to her, and otherwise battled her around comings and goings and accepting or rejecting her love.

As they initially explored Jared's life from a psychological perspective, it seemed to the Kellys that Jared had shown some slight improvement in his mood between 2 and 3½. He had been toilet trained without great distress. After this period his object relations generally worsened. His solitude and isolation had deepened. When he finally let go of his mother at nursery school, he would only play by himself. He seldom acknowledged, let alone followed, his teacher's directions. At home he was obsessed with seeing a particular TV program. He insisted on watching it at every opportunity. Otherwise he spent endless hours in solitary repetitive play, listening to tape recordings of songs and committing them to memory. While Jared enjoyed music and singing, he was hypersensitive to noise. He became easily upset and disorganized by unfamiliar sounds or excessive noise other than his own. He also began collecting alphabet books. He would obsessively read and copy from them as long as his mother would permit.

HOUR 15

Jared presents a kaleidoscopic style of play and engagement sometimes encountered in young children with high levels of emotional turmoil fueled by anxiety and guilt. His play is further sustained and supported by a good intelligence. Instead of one central depiction he presents brief vignettes on the themes of drive control, separation, and object loss. To make the session more cogent and easier to track, I have separated it according to these vignettes. I have followed each one with my commentary and speculations—the play of a child analyst's mind, if you will, on the play of the child. What is perhaps most salient about these observations is how little is voiced relative to what the child's activity evokes!

Jared arrived for his 15th analytic session attired in his "Steelers" football jacket, worn brown corduroy pants, and faded blue sneakers. He was a slender boy of average size for his age. His brown hair was tousled. He greeted me with his usual tentative side-long brown-eyed glance. He did not remove his jacket throughout the session. Hesitantly he showed me the two hand puppets he was wearing as mittens. He left his mother easily for this session.

As soon as he entered the consulting room, Jared's mien changed. He moved quickly and precisely. He appeared to be suddenly infused with aggressive energies. He looked directly at me as he introduced for the first time his two puppets "Monster" on his left (nondominant) hand and "Lizard" on his right hand. Jared was usually accompanied by one of his stuffed animals or by his favorite teddy bear. Two sessions prior to this one he had changed his mode of physical contact with me. Instead of apparently casual or accidental brushing and light touching, he insinuated himself onto my lap while presenting me with one of his alphabet books to be read. In the 14th session he again initiated more direct, sustained, albeit squirming, physical contact. He directly asked to sit on my lap. He had also selected specific children's books of mine which he asked me to read. In the 13th session Jared had used the bathroom for the first time. As he emerged he pointedly exhibited his genitalia and bottom as he was struggling to readjust trousers which were still tightly buckled and belted. Toward the end of the 14th session he blurted out a nonsequitur "going poop in the pants." I will present this session in the present tense. I will also intersperse the verbatim process of the session with my conjectures about the material.

> Jared initiated "pretend play" immediately. J.: "Pretend you don't know I came in yet." P.: "Okay." Jared runs over to the couch and disappears under it. The two puppets pop back out from under its fringe. He commences his dramatic play direction to me as his audience. J.: "Lizard's the good guy. He's going to beat up Monster who's bad." Jared then performs several play sequences in which Monster threatens the world. Then Lizard comes along and attacks and subdues Monster, biting off its long blonde braids. Monster cries out with hurt and rage. Monster surrenders.

Jared introduces his version of a medieval morality play. It is Jared's preoccupation with the intertwined themes of guilt, punishment, attack, and retribution which give this session its singular prototypical quality. The puppeting sequence with the "good" Lizard and the "bad" menacing Monster dramatizes his primitive intrapsychic morality and drive conflicts. In play we may speculate that he dramatizes an object relations version of his battle with his mother.

After 10 minutes of this play Jared proclaims, as he emerges from under the couch, "Okay. No more pretend." P.: "Oh, Jared, where have you been?" J.: "No! That's pretend! Noooo [in a very whiney tone]. I said *no more pretend!*" He gives me another side-long look, this time of anger rather than guilt. It is clear that I am supposed to feel guilty for violating his direction of the action in the session. J.: "Okay." P.: "Okay. You got pretty mad at me when I didn't understand that you wanted everything to be real again." J.: "I'm not mad. I'm just frustrated! You made me frustrated when you kept pretending." P.: "I guess being frustrated is a smaller kind of anger." J.: "Yes, okay." This was Jared's characteristic response to a reasonably correct comment or interpretation.

In this sequence I attempted to extend the fantasy ("Jared, where have you been?") as Jared is attempting to close it off. His angry reaction highlights his transference expectations of me. I must respond *precisely* to his wishes and commands as the ideal parent with precise empathic attunement. In earlier sessions he had wanted me to move exactly as he did and he had expressed the wish that we be identical friends. In general, I follow Jared's directions, within the limits of safety and propriety. I do this in the interest of facilitating his sense of the analytic space as transitional "free" space. My intent is that the analytic space will support a medium in which he can freely move, play, associate, and respond in the service of reconstruction, recovery, and psychological growth. I am aiding him in playing out his restitutive fantasy of a time when he and his love object, most likely his mother in this instance, existed in a harmonious union which he experienced as under his omnipotent control. My activity threatens this fantasy by making my differentiation more apparent and Jared's anger ensues. I am testing the limits of "Pretend," which is Jared's shorthand way of communicating that we are relating on a different level of ego organization. We are relating on a level where the reality principle is in a more formally acknowledged state of suspension than is usually the case in an analytic session with a child his age. Identifying Jared's emotion and quantifying it are my fundamental attempts to replace his damaged expectation of fusion with a higher level of emotional relatedness closer to more mature empathy.

Jared continues: "Let's play something else. Let's play that baby gets taken away from his mother. No, let's play that mother goes away and baby gets put in jail by Monster and Flower." Flower is a cushion shaped like a smiling sun. P.: "What do you want me to do?" J.: "You be Monster and Flower; the bad guys. I'll be baby and Lizard and policeman." Policeman is a small stuffed rabbit. J.: "We play that while mother is gone [to the very farthest end of the room from where we are located], Monster and Flower put baby in 'jail' in a covered toy basket. Then Lizard and policeman come to the rescue of baby. They *turn the tables* on the villains and put Monster and Flower in jail. Now we'll tape their mouths shut so they can't scream and cry." With great delight Jared puts layer upon layer of tape over their mouths. He instructs me to make cries of alarm and fear. He also tells me to make the cries more and more muffled as the tape builds up. Finally he pauses, obviously delighted and satisfied that the villains have been silenced and punished. During the pause I change the tone of my voice to signal that I am stepping outside the play. P.: "Have you ever had your mouth taped like that, Jared?" J.: "No." He responds in a quick and matter-of-fact manner.

Jared's anger with my attempt to extend the previous "pretend" play becomes woven into a scenario in which a mother leaves a baby unprotected and villains are silenced. The maternal transference is confirmed. An attempt is made at absolution of abandoning mothers. The play converts mother's actual abandonments from *activity* (she did it) into *passivity* (it just happened while she was gone), the reverse of the way this defense usually works. In reworking his short personal history, Jared attempts to absolve his mother and himself of their guilt-ridden conflictual relationship. Mother is not actively abandoning baby. Both mother and baby are victimized by the villains.

Jared's emotional intensity grew greater and greater as the play progressed toward its mouth-taping crescendo. Such a strong emotional mix of pleasure and aggression led me to suspect that the kernel of a real event might lie at the center of this segment. It seemed likely that a "real" passive traumatic experience was being revived in mirror form in the play; possibly a guilt-evoking passive experience was being exuberantly transformed into an active fantasy experience. Hence my question about his real experiences which he denied with easy, but not necessarily convincing aplomb.

Just as dreams vary in a night and yet generally build toward or away from a final vivid one in which a most parsimonious compromise between wishes and disguise is achieved, so Jared's play moved more vividly and precisely into the area of unmastered personal experience and memory. Through the lense of analysis we can condense and focus both baby's fear and despair at being put in jail and the similar feelings of the jailed villains with their bound mouths. In such a condensation we may catch sight of an alive emotional representation of times when Jared felt physically and emotionally immobilized, imprisoned, and abandoned.

I was reminded that drawings of people "in jail" had preoccupied Jared. I thought Jared was referring to early traumas, now in the process of being played out and worked through in his analysis; the times when his angry, helpless mother had isolated him emotionally and physically in his kitchen chair or his room. Jared is attempting to master in small bits (Waelder, 1932) the accumulated times when he was left feeling helpless, terrified, angry, and guilty by the actions of his parents. There are two villains, one male and one female, after all, not one.

Furthermore, the play suggests Jared's perception that it is his parents together rather than his mother alone who gang up on him, a significant block in the area of object relations to his oedipal advance. It may also reflect more current events in the family. At the time of this session the parents were striving to be more fair, firm, and consistent in their reactions to their son. Finally, a scenario which had emerged in bits and pieces earlier in this opening phase of Jared's analysis comes more clearly into focus. That is Jared's transference fantasy that he is being left with me by his mother for punishment of his misdeeds as he experienced his protective father's early absences. The mouth-taping play suggests making too much noise, being too loud, making too many demands as one area where he has been "bad."

> After the pause during which Jared denied ever having his mouth taped, he introduces a play variation. J.: "Let's play it again. This time it is the bad mother who puts the baby in jail. Then father comes and gets baby and punishes the bad mother

and puts her in jail. He takes baby to work with him and they have a good time."

This segment introduces a progression in which it is not the primitive, impersonal policeman who deals out justice; it is a loving, beloved, and protective father who rescues his son from his "bad mother." The transference at this point seems to shift 180 degrees, changing my valence from "bad" to "good." In fantasy Jared comes to me each day for protection from his "bad mother," just as in play he goes to work with his father.

> J.: "When we play, make sure you don't say sorry. That makes me angry and I want to go home and tell my mother that I never want to see you again. But if you say Rabbit, Rabbit, Rabbit, Rabbit [holding up 4 fingers in sequence], then I'll want to come here and stay with you all day. I know you can't see me Thursdays because you have to go to work. I don't care, though. I watch TV." P.: "If you want me to say Rabbit, Rabbit, Rabbit, Rabbit so you can stay with me all day, then maybe you are wishing that you could see me Thursdays and every other day too?" J.: "Yess, I do!"

Unlike his father whom he sees daily, he sees me only four days a week. As a novel object I possess important maternal and transitional object qualities which will serve to allay the agony and distress of primary object separations. He looks for magic solutions, through an incantation. In my early sessions with Jared, I would say, "I am sorry to interrupt, but it's time to stop." He seemingly accepted this intervention without emotion. Now, as he accepts the constancy and neutrality of his analyst and the analytic setting, he directly voices his perturbation at having to interrupt his pleasurable play in the interests of reality.

> J.: "Let's play what I said before. Who will be the bad mother? How about Flower and we'll have Mrs. Squirrel [a stuffed animal skunk, actually] be the good mother. See, baby is put in jail by the bad mother and here comes my good mother with the policeman to rescue baby. The policeman is small, but he can beat the bad mother with his stiff pointy ears [aligns the ears forward together like a unicorn's horn]. Now they put the bad mother in jail. She cries! She's very upset! [he says delightedly]. Now they tape her mouth shut so nobody can hear her yell and cry." He pauses as though to shift the play activity. P.: "You

know, Jared, I think you like coming to see me very much now."
J.: "Yes, I do." P.: "When you first came, I think you were afraid
of me and afraid you were going to be punished and put in jail
here by me because your mother was mad at you for something
you'd done and maybe you thought you were going to be
punished by me because you were mad at her too. I think you
were afraid she'd leave you here and not come back to get you."
J.: "I don't feel that way now. You're nice. We play and my
mother comes and picks me up at 3:30."

Here, Jared's play is followed by my interpretation and his
acknowledgment. There is a partial resolution of his earliest,
repressed transference dynamic. Through play it emerges from
repression and is available for interpretation. Analysis was perceived as his mother's ultimate punishment, abandonment, and
rejection. It is his punishment for his anger and for something
he did to her which remains repressed. The good father-bad
mother oedipal theme regressed to a preoedipal theme involving a split good mother-bad mother. It is obviously a good Jared-
bad Jared split as well. In the regression it seems likely that
positive, loving, paternal identifications are displaced onto the
image of the good mother to shore up that positive maternal
image. This would be counter to the usual developmental thrust
in which positive identifications with the maternal love object
invest the child's "discovery" of the loving father. It is an encouraging prognostic sign that the good mother wins out. In real life
she will come at a prescribed time to pick him up at the end of
sessions. This is partially wish fulfillment since Mrs. Kelly is
rarely on time. As a measure of her unpredictability and difficulties ordering her own life, she is usually early or late. She is
always overextended. She is always in a hurry. In her comings
and goings from Jared's sessions she afforded a symptomatic
physical expression of the psychological inconstancy which has
plagued her son. As the analysis went on, the temporal structure
which it afforded Mrs. Kelly contributed to her developing a
more regular rhythm to her own life.

J.: "Is it time to go?" P.: "See for yourself." J.: "It's three one
five. I leave at three two five, right?" P.: "That's right." J.: "I
want to make another star to take home then I'll have five, how
old I am." He draws a star. J.: "Look, didn't I do that good? and

fast too! [Whines:] Help me find the scissors! There they are. Help me cut. No, I can do it. Look, a beauty! Give me a long piece of tape to stick it up with. [He pulls a piece off the roll himself.] Too short! [He gets another one.] This is long enough. Good. 3:25?" P.: "Yes." J.: "Good-by, I'll see you Monday." He picks up hand puppets and star and leaves.

In this final segment of the session Jared prepares to leave. He has devoted 25 minutes to displaying the panoply of his transference developments. He has played himself into a partial reconstruction of the earliest part of his brief analysis as well as an attempted construction of a nodal traumatic event. He completes his major fantasy thrust 20 minutes before the session ends. He clearly articulates his perception that sessions are finite. He shows an *apparent* acceptance of the time for ending; possibly a cognitive manifestation of subtle oedipal development. He ties it to his mother's reappearance. It is significant that he is active at the end of the session in announcing when time is up rather than passively awaiting my statement. It is another way in which he takes charge of the session. Bringing the hand puppets was another. Directing the play was a third. His stars add up to his age and also to the number of people in his family. Jared defensively uses an early, repetitive, cognitive-intellectual exercise to absorb any unpleasure about departing. He takes something of mine (paper) with him. Through his creative energies it has been modeled into a star. Many aspects of separation anxiety and object constancy have been addressed and played at. Jared leaves in an unusually relaxed and accepting mental state. Guilt, anxiety, and depression have been decreased. He has become once again more "innocent."

WORKING THROUGH OF HOUR 15

In subsequent sessions Jared withdrew. His play became less obviously metaphorical. He retreated into copying the alphabet. He became fastidious and perfectionistic about getting any letter in the alphabet or whatever he was drawing exactly right. At the same time he was irritably, fussily, but emphatically using sheet after sheet of drawing paper in the pursuit of perfect letters. And yet in his determination to get his letters "just right" there was strong evidence of a pleasure in messing and wasting paper.

I was reminded of his anal concerns in the preceding sessions. Much of his play emphasized coming and going and disappearing and reappearing.

About two weeks after the specimen session I met with Mrs. Kelly. I asked her whether she knew of Jared ever having his mouth taped shut. She did not. Her associations, however, went to an episode and symptom group she had not previously mentioned. After a long period (12 to 18 months) during which Jared had been responsible for his own toileting, he began to wet his pants during the day and to insist that his mother wipe his bottom after every bowel movement. This regression was subsequent to Mrs. Kelly losing control and striking Jared hard after he had stopped up the toilet once again with the voluminous amounts of toilet paper he used to clean himself. Following his mother's outburst and assault Jared only went to the bathroom as a last resort. He wet during the day and held his bowel movement until the last tolerable moment. Interestingly enough, Mrs. Kelly reported that over the past several weeks Jared had begun to wipe himself again!

The taped mouth of the dolls in what I had suspected was a traumatic re-creation turned out to be a displacement upward from the toilet-paper trauma associated with his mother. In the play sessions his spoken wish to make a mess and his reaction formations to do everything "right" took on historical meaning. So did his compulsive need to mess up and throw out sheet after sheet *after* sheet of drawing paper—all this amidst questions directed at me as to whether I minded his making a mess and whether it made me angry. It did not, and I encouraged him to think about why he derived so much pleasure as well from spilling paint and scattering it over the play platform. When I interpreted the traumatic situation he was attempting to rectify and attached it to his conflict about anal messing, or its reaction formation, being perfect with me, Jared looked interested. He first said, "I don't memember that." He paused thoughtfully. He gazed out the window. Then he said, "Now I do memember that." He knew the word "remember." I took his use of "memember" as confirmation from the unconscious of my interpretation. "Memember" might also refer to the phallic component of his activity vis-à-vis his mother! Over the following months he continued to play out his toilet-paper trauma with increasingly easy acknowledgment of its derivations. He also continued to use my bathroom toilet for practicing his re-acquired toileting autonomy.

DISCUSSION

Taking the brief selective survey of developments in child analysis with which this paper opened and adding the clinical material of Jared's 15th analytic session stimulate a number of more general statements. There is now a greater *theoretical* synchrony between play and interpretation as essential elements of the therapeutic process in child analysis. Play drives the analytic process of the younger child. In and of itself it *partially* shapes and refines emerging ego and superego functions. However, play functions in this fashion in an object relations context. While the young child directs his play in the analysis, the analyst articulates and informs the treatment process through interpretation. In undertaking this function the analyst becomes a novel object for the child. As Ritvo (in Panel, 1980) emphasized, this "identification with the role of the analyst is one of the long-lasting effects of analysis in childhood" (p. 174). At the same time the contemporary analyst may consult with the parents to gather timely information for the analysis. The analyst also consults to facilitate the establishment of an analytically supportive home environment wherein the child's analysis neither dominates nor is minimized.

As a more sophisticated object relations theory has clarified the role and function of the child analyst, we are able to glean from the treatment process more information about transference issues and transference illness in children. Certainly, Jared's transference developed immediately, as it does with most children. It was then largely repressed only to reemerge in quite obvious form very early in his analysis.

There is another important point which Jared brings us back to; that is the need to reconsider the role of guilt in child development and child's play; for guilt continued to occupy a central position in his analysis. Yet guilt seems so much a part of the fabric of psychoanalytic thought and clinical psychoanalysis as to defy reformulation. The material which Jared presents presses for a reevaluation of this elusive affect. Guilt seems at times a bit like a greased pig. While it is obviously right there, it is difficult to get a hold of!

Our conceptualization of guilt also may have become overly restricted. Do we read Anna Freud (1970) too narrowly if we conceptualize guilt as *only* immanent at the pinnacle of superego formation in the oedipal phase where "the advance from anxiety to *guilt* is made as the crowning step in this chronology of infantile fears" (p. 32)? A conceptualization of Jared's guilt calls for a schema similar to the one which Edgcumbe and Burgner (1975) used to differentiate preoedipal and oedipal aspects of phallic development. As shown by his play material, indicators of oedipal-phase strivings are scant and transitory in Jared's case. Yet he is obviously a very guilty as well as very disturbed little boy. His guilt is well developed. It permeates his whole existence. He is either acting under its sway or reacting to it. In addition to its allusion to armor, "Steelers," the name on his jacket, plays on the word "stealer" emblematic of the preoedipal aspects of his crime against his mother—that is, to steal her, against her wishes, to make her his possession!

The vicissitudes of Jared's play develop a quality of guilt which seems developmentally close to that embodied in Ferenczi's (1925) term "sphincter morality." The same kind of guilt underlying the "semiphysiological . . . morality [which] forms the essential groundwork of later purely mental morality" (p. 267). In Jared's instance the feeling of his guilt, its harshness, its stark polarization of "good" and "bad," its rampant "semi-physiological" anal-phase drive conflicts seem more conducive to a conceptualization along "preconscience" lines. His is primarily guilt before castration anxiety has crystallized the citadel of conscience proper. Its drive representations closely parallel bodily functions. Jared's guilt shares sphincter qualities. It contracts his ego. It limits his expressivity vis-à-vis the world to retentive isolation alternating with explosive rage. Further, he shrinks from human contact.

Such characterizations of guilt, so closely derived from physical experience,[2] suggest some more speculative possibilities.

---

2. As the guilt associated with castration anxiety certainly is.

The physical experience of guilt at its most conscious and most intense has a primitive visceral quality which is analogous to nausea. It is a commonplace experience to be "wracked" with guilt; to suffer the "pangs" of conscience! I am reminded that the internal experience of guilt is never far from external action. The antidote to guilt is in undoing damage, atonement. Atonement often involves physical acts such as fasting and genuflecting. Scourging one's body and transcending it are important to expiation in adulthood, as play is in childhood.

Guilt is central to the individual's sense of personal responsibility for his actions (using action in the broadest sense). With the increasing emphasis on the origin of object relations in earliest infancy coupled with the notion of the infant as aggressive and assertive in his own right, the possibility of constructs like responsibility and guilt arising much earlier in life than we have imagined must be considered. Apart from the excesses of her idiomatic view of infancy and the quirks of her developmental time table, perhaps Klein (1937) was quite on the mark in her insistence on the infantile origins of guilt! This would provide a proper prestage to Ferenczi's overworked concept. Certainly, the infant's sense of being intermittently out of synchrony with his mother must be vivid, universal, and inevitable. To the extent that such a dysjunction in the mother-infant unit is accompanied by glares, growls, and harsher handling on the part of the mother, the infant may quickly translate feeling bad into being bad. In the sense of feeling bad and becoming bad, guilt is the inevitable residual of the processes involved in internalization and individuation.

Another enduring attribute of infantile sexuality seems to be infantile masturbation guilt. The durability and persistence of this particular aspect of guilt imply an origin relatively disconnected from educational and social forces. To a significant extent this aspect of guilt may emanate from the child's sense, enhanced by the environment, that he has done grave damage to his relationship with his mother by turning to his own body for libidinal pleasure.[3] Hence the guilty sense of body damage accompanying masturbation may antedate castration anxiety. It becomes a symbolic replication of the partial rupture of the

3. Even though masturbatory activity inevitably includes an object relation.

libidinal relation of child to mother. In this context the "play" associated with infantile masturbation takes on an ironic connotation since this erotic "play" intensifies rather than diminishes the guilt subsequent to the fantasied damage to a loved one!

This discussion brings me back to an idea elicited and confirmed by Jared's session. Guilt is central to both play and normal development. It is not just a neurotic abreaction. In addition to play functioning for aggressive drive discharge (Downey, 1984), it also serves the expiation of guilt. This complements Loewald's (1979) conceptualization that in later development guilt is one of the central organizing forces in psychic growth.

SUMMARY

A brief historical review of the tension between play and interpretation reveals that a technical and theoretical balance has been struck between play and interpretation in child analysis. An unusual child analytic session is presented in detail in an attempt to elucidate new directions. It was not a typical session but a summary session of the same sort as the "good," reconstructive, interpretive hour in adult analysis. Microanalysis of the session suggests that given the recent gains in ego psychology and object relation theory, further development in child analysis will involve a review of the developmental model for affects. The hypothesis that the dysphoric affect guilt occupies an early and central position in the functions of play and in psychic development is formulated.

BIBLIOGRAPHY

BORNSTEIN, B. (1949). The analysis of a phobic child. *Psychoanal. Study Child*, 3/4:181–226.

DOWNEY, T. W. (1984). Within the pleasure principle. *Psychoanal. Study Child*, 39:101–136.

EDGCUMBE, R. & BURGNER, M. (1975). The phallic-narcissistic phase. *Psychoanal. Study Child*, 25:161–180.

FERENCZI, S. (1925). Psycho-analysis of sexual habits. In *Further Contributions to the Theory and Technique of Psycho-analysis*. London: Hogarth Press, 1950, pp. 259–296.

FREUD, A. (1926). Four lectures on child analysis. *W.*, 1:3–69.

———— (1945). Indications for child analysis. *W.*, 4:3–38.

———— (1970). The symptomatology of childhood. *Psychoanal. Study Child*, 25:19–41.

FREUD, S. (1909). Analysis of a phobia in a five-year-old boy. *S.E.*, 10:3–149.

———— (1914). Remembering, repeating and working-through. *S.E.*, 12:147–156.

———— (1920). Beyond the pleasure principle. *S.E.*, 18:3–64.

HUG-HELLMUTH, H. V. (1921). On the technique of child analysis. *Int. J. Psychoanal.*, 2:287–305.

KLEIN, M. (1932). *The Psychoanalysis of Children.* New York: Delacorte Press/ Seymour Lawrence, 1975.

———— (1937). Love, guilt, and reparation. In *Love, Hate and Reparation.* London: Hogarth Press, pp. 306–343.

LOEWALD, H. W. (1979). The waning of the oedipus complex. In *Papers on Psychoanalysis.* New Haven & London: Yale Univ. Press, 1980, pp. 384–404.

PANEL (1980). Conceptualizing the nature of the therapeutic action of child analysis. L. M. Sabot, reporter. *J. Amer. Psychoanal. Assn.*, 28:161–179.

WAELDER, R. (1932). The psychoanalytic theory of play. *Psychoanal. Q.*, 2:208–224, 1933.

WINNICOTT, D. W. (1971). *Playing and Reality.* New York: Penguin, 1980.

Children's Games, Observed and Experienced

RIVKA R. EIFERMANN, Ph.D.

IN SHARP CONTRAST WITH THE FREE PLAY OF YOUNG CHILDREN, THE
rule-governed game play of older children has raised little interest
among psychoanalysts (Stokes, 1956; Philips, 1960; Golding,
1978). The one exception is a paper by Peller (1954), who compares play as an aspect of libidinal and ego development with
game-playing in the postoedipal stage. While Peller regards children's games as essentially social and competitive (which they
not necessarily are) and also as "primarily a pastime of boys"
(which is simply not true), she offers some interesting ideas,
derived from the psychoanalytic theory of development.

I shall try to examine games mainly in relation to how their
distinguishing characteristics, their framework of fixed rules,
may function in unconscious conflicts and fantasies expressed in
games and creative expression in games. I am aware that my
selection of unconscious fantasies and creativity as the special
foci of my exploration of *games* may seem provocative. For it is
precisely with regard to their differences in these two areas that
play has been again and again distinguished from games. *Free*
play, as it is often termed, is generally described as "unre-
stricted" and "spontaneous," and therefore as providing optimal
conditions for the nurture of fantasy, imagination, and creativ-

Psychology department, Hebrew University, Jerusalem.

Presented at the International Symposium on "A Psychoanalytic View of
Play and Trauma," Jerusalem, March 1986.

The preparation of this paper was made possible with the aid of a grant from
the Sturman Center for Human Development of the Hebrew University of
Jerusalem.

ity. In contrast, games, governed as they are by "strict rules," are said to allow for little or no such freedom.

I shall begin with just a few words about my past games research (1970, 1971a, 1971b, 1973a, 1973b, 1978). By referring to that research, I hope to illustrate, in shorthand terms, the benefits to be derived from combining the normative data and findings based on the systematic *observation* of children's games and players with my present work, based as it is on *reported experience* and the analysis of the child within the adult, as he or she replays in the mind and associates to his or her childhood games.

My past research was a huge operation that engaged my attention for about 10 years in the 1960s to 1970s. The observations were conducted by 150 observers, on 7,000 children, in 14 schools during recess, and in the streets of two neighborhood areas, once a week for a period of 14 months. The records of play participants over this extensive period of observations amounted to a cumulative total of over 100,000 players. The observations were conducted with the aid of a record sheet designed for the purpose, and observers were positioned in such a way that every play group (as well as a sample of solitary players) was recorded. In addition, there were coordinators whose task it was to deal with various emergencies and prevent multiple recordings of moving players. Besides such information as the sex and age of the players, the name of the game was also recorded. "Free," unstructured play (such as "Balancing on a plank, in a row," or "Staging a demonstration") was described by the observers. Descriptions of formal, rule-governed games were obtained separately, through interviews and demonstrations. Altogether some 2,000 detailed descriptions of the variants of different formal games and some 3,000 brief descriptions of free play were collected.

My wide sample of children—which included both Jews and Arabs as well as those living in villages, towns, and cities, kibbutzim, moshavim, and development towns—and the extensive period of observation allowed cultural differences as well as phenomena not affected by such differences to be identified and defined. The wide age range of children—any age in the streets, 6 to 14 in schools—allowed developmental trends to be clearly traced as well. Hence whenever I refer to that research, as in my statement above that games are not necessarily "primarily a pas-time of boys," this is based on solid grounding in our records.

GAMES AND UNCONSCIOUS FANTASIES

I find it rather surprising that psychoanalysts have left the rich world of children's games almost untouched. For, as the Opies (1969), English folklorists who wrote a charming and quite ex-tensive book on street games, say, such games "have been tested by generations of children, who have passed them on, as chil-dren continue to do, without reference to print, parliament, or adult propriety!" (p. i). Peller (1954) acknowledges this fact when she says, "'games' are not personal creations but tradi-tional forms which are passed on from group to individual and from group to group" (p. 193). The parallel cases of fairy tales and myths, which have also passed the test of generations, have attracted considerable attention among psychoanalysts. Indeed, many tales and myths have been interpreted in terms of their communal unconscious fantasies. Peller discusses fantasies com-mon to game players, but only in reference to general fantasies, which she regards as typical of all team games. For example, she proposes that one fantasy underlying all such games is "sibling rivalry." I know of only one attempt (by Philips, 1960) to in-terpret games in terms of specific fantasies, and this attempt is limited to two games.

This neglect of games and game-playing is perhaps even more surprising when one considers that street games, unlike fairy tales, are transmitted by children almost to the complete exclu-sion of adults, and as such may be considered a "pure form" of child culture. But precisely this may be why it is so difficult to investigate games. For, while fairy tales are directly accessible to adults and are often shared with children, latency games are not. Besides, when we read a fairy tale, we have direct, experiential contact with the material of our study, and this is certainly far from being the case when we read a description of how a specific game is played. In fact, the description of common games like Tic-Tac-Toe or Hopscotch makes tedious reading, as they con-tain neither plot nor narrative, but only a series of instructions and regulations.

Such material does not provide a basis for unraveling communal fantasies which may underlie these games. Even the description of games with such inspiring names as Shalom, My Lord the King, Fist and Black Hand, or Old Hag, or of those which have a plot and narrative as elaborate as Sign Posts,[1] do not provide the "liveliness" one feels while reading a tale or myth. The dryness of this material may have caused analysts to be far more reluctant in attempting its interpretation than Bettelheim (1976) has been in his extensive interpretation of the Grimms' tales. Yet his interpretation of tales remains problematic, since it does not explicitly rely on children's actual responses to the tales. Interpretations of games arrived at in a similar manner to Bettelheim's on tales, when the depth of associations has not been obtained from the players of a game, can at best be considered hypothetical.[2] For, if the players themselves are not taken into account, the analyst's interpretation of that game, in terms of its underlying conflicts or fantasies, will express his own fantasies. While the interpretation may be of interest in *that* sense, it does not offer a basis for generalizing.[3] This is the case with Philips's rather ingenious explanation of how he concluded that the communal fantasy underlying the game of Tag (Catch, in England) is "contamination."

Philips (1960) compares Tag with Drop the Handkerchief, a game played by younger children. In that game, he says, a stigma is represented in a concrete object, the handkerchief, and each player must try to get rid of the "stigma." In Tag, the child tries to avoid, or attempts to dispose of, contamination resulting from the physical contact involved in being "tagged." One of Philips's conclusions from his comparison of Tag and Drop the Handkerchief is that—since fear of contamination is not uncommon even in adulthood—it is the amorphous, unknown nature of what is transmitted in Tag which allows it to be played over a broader span of years than any of the other games. While our

1. In which one group of players goes in search of another group, which leaves various signs, tracks, and instructions on its path.
2. In a recent paper (Eifermann, 1987a), I have attempted to test one such hypothesis with regard to *Little Red Riding Hood*.
3. I have argued this with regard to fairy tales (Eifermann, 1987a, 1987b, 1987c).

data on Tag confirm that its life-span is outstanding relative to other street and playground games (Eifermann, 1973a), Philips's interpretation of the game's underlying meaning must be considered private and idiosyncratic, unless proven otherwise.

Although the question of communal fantasies remains open, even the simplest game of Tag can be experienced very differently by different individuals. This is even apparent in how the game is described. Let us look at three such descriptions:

> The rules are very simple, if you are ticked on any part of the body, you are a man. But that's when the trouble starts. Some players deny that they were took, and a fight starts.

This description, quoted from a boy in the Opies book (1969), is very different in spirit from the following student's observation:

> Ovadia was king in driving crazy. He was not a fast runner, but he could never be caught. Three, four, around Ovadia and Ovadia moves his belly as in a belly dance, turns his bum, and laughs at everyone. And it is impossible to touch him. It was also difficult to catch Doodi, who ran very fast by comparison. But Ovadia was the king in driving crazy.

I shall not go into a comparison of these two descriptions, except to say that the same game rule, of being "took," or touched, is approached very differently by the two players quoted. The intensity of underlying meaning is made more explicit in the following description, obtained from a female student:

> The children run and the catcher (the *it* in Hebrew) has to run after them and touch them. When he succeeds in touching one of the children, they turn into catchers themselves. *The way to stop this* is *"to scream* Poos," but I don't remember who has to say that—it's logical that it should be the *"pursued/persecuted"* [one and the same word in Hebrew; but the word commonly used for this role is "escaper"] who has to say "Poos" *in order to stop*, but I think it is the opposite. Gradually all turn into catchers. [No italics in the original.]

After the urgent emphasis in this description on how "to stop this," and the choice of "to scream" and "pursued/persecuted," whether intentional or not, it may come as no surprise that this student went on to comment:

> The game is for me associated with the fact that I run very slowly, and very clumsily: as a matter of fact, I can hardly run, something that caused me much embarrassment in childhood.

Even these brief descriptions suggest that a wealth of experiences and related unconscious conflicts and fantasies may lie behind each one. I therefore find it hard to accept Peller's view (1954) that the fantasy underlying games is necessarily "impersonal and conventional" (p. 193) and "carries but little emotional cathexis." Even though she remarks that "with this leitmotif fantasy [e.g., "sibling rivalry"] other fantasies may coexist" (p. 191), she comments, "The goals of latency play [games] are more reality-adapted for two reasons: the older child has greater abilities and *he aims at far more modest targets in his play fantasies*" (p. 191; my italics).

Therapists who have had the experience of playing games with older children may share my surprise at the second statement: it seems to be a *non sequitur*. The wildest and most passionate of fantasies may hide behind even the simplest and most restricted game. Whether or not this is the case is a matter for investigation.

What underlies this idea for Peller is her own differentiation between oedipal play and postoedipal games. She describes oedipal play actions as "confabulated on the spot" (p. 193), and as having "the greatest leeway for his [the child's] fantasies; his play activities are colorful and imaginative" (p. 188). In contrast, "Strict rules are the backbone of games" (p. 191), and, by comparsion with free play, "games have little leeway for their actions, the plot follows a traditional pattern, it runs on tracks, unforeseen developments are limited to a narrow margin" (p. 192)—that is, *if there is any plot*. Although the above is more or less the case, the extensive analysis of different categories of game-rules shows that there are some types of instructions, regulations, and metarules, which, rather than being strict, allow players considerable flexibility (Eifermann, 1973b).

Yet the formal confines of games, their restricting rules, may also *serve* older children to hide and disguise their conflicts and fantasies, from both themselves and others, to an extent that the younger child feels no need to do. Peller states that "the latency child feels ashamed of his daydreams and keeps them secret," whereas "The young child neither exhibits his play nor has any intention of hiding it (Freud, 1908)" (p. 195). It therefore seems that much more effort is required, on the part of both analyst and child, if we are to reach the meanings and fantasies that underlie games.

My Game, Experienced

I have attempted such an analysis in the reconstructive experience of myself playing a game at about age 11. In presenting aspects of this self-analysis here, I propose to demonstrate how the reactivation of the playing child within me has enabled me to reach preliminary, tentative hypotheses concerning the functions that rules have in games—aside from their social regulatory function that apply when the game is a social activity. This social factor has been isolated as I played my game by myself. In addition, the presentation may help me illustrate the intensity of the conflicts and fantasies that may be hidden behind a relatively simple game. I tend to believe that regardless of the accuracy of such a reconstruction-in-mind in terms of past "reality," it is highly productive for illustrative purposes and in particular as a means of reaching fruitful hypotheses. I have elsewhere (Eifermann, 1987c) discussed some of the problems and the special merits of this method.

My game was a simple one, primarily of physical activity, and although I used to play it on my own, it can be played, as variants of it are, by two or more children taking turns. One can often see children playing a variant of this game, in which you throw your ball, the size of a small basketball, at a wall, and must catch it on the rebound. You count every catch, but once the ball is dropped, you must start counting all over again if you play alone, or you lose your turn to the next player if more than one is playing. Easy throws do not count. Just like Jumprope, Jacks, Head Ball, and many other games, when played alone, this game may serve as practice for social play. In my variant of the game, I had to call out something while the ball was in the air—or have to start counting all over, as in a variant similar to a game called Ball to the Wall in Israel, which is usually played with a tennis ball or a ball about that size.

In my games research this game would be categorized as one of physical activity coordinated with some mental activity. It would be categorized similarly by researchers such as Sutton-Smith (1972), Roberts and Sutton-Smith (1962), Avedon (1971), and also by Piaget (1945). But, for me, my game was also an intensive play on my own emotions.

When I read over the following spontaneous description of my experience of the game, I realized that I had already condensed in the first sentences a great deal of what the game turned out to be all about for me. At the same time, I had left out one essential aspect of the experience, most difficult to put into words, which I could therefore reach only at a very late stage in my analysis. I shall reach it here when I discuss creativity in games. This is what I wrote:

> Whenever I think of children's games, the obsbasic [a slip condensing "obsessive" and "basic"; *obsisi* in Hebrew, the language in which I wrote] game of ball exchange/messages [*mesirot*] with the wall occurs to me—the intensity/might/force [*otsma*], the fear—that the ball will, after all, inevitably fall in the end. Some kind of fear that "I shall be caught" . . . that Ya'acov [my brother] will come from around the corner [of the house] . . . that I shall be disturbed—that I shall be caught red-handed—that it is forbidden, impossible, under any circumstances to stop, that it will be terrible if I am stopped! There remains something here that is unclear.

(I would like to stress right away that although on the face of it this description emphasizes a compulsive element in my game, this is not in itself a focus of my analysis in the paper.) Later on, I added:

> *Chimoomim* [hot hits/shots/messages], I had not described the experience of the *chimoom:* to throw with all one's strength/ might.

It did not take too long in my associations to reach the rage and aggression which I was expressing, with each *chimoom* toward my own "house/home" [one and the same word in Hebrew], and against which I was playing. Yet, it also occurred to me, the wall of my house/home stood there, perhaps indifferent to my rage, but in any case allowing me to express it freely, indeed, in compliance with the rule of my game, and at the same time confirming with each *chimoom* that it could withstand my attacks. Besides, it occurred to me, I got back from the wall precisely as hard as I hit—tit-for-tat, so that my guilt at my (unconscious) destructive feelings toward home was thus reduced. I also realized that the shots were loaded not only with rage, but also with a message of "hot" love, of *chimoomim,* and that the *ball* as object was similarly embraced, rejected, hit, only to be reembraced. It was, of course, the ball that was at the center of much of my attention—for the most important thing was not to lose it on its return to me. The urgency with which I felt this need was quite alive, as in my mind I entered into playing this game from my childhood. I could feel the flow which I almost desperately sought in playing the game: the fear that I would be stopped, the rising anxiety lest the ball not land in my hands. But no less alive was the tremendous feeling of exuberance, excitement, and elation that went with throwing the ball in different ways—up and down against the wall, looking in one direction but throwing it at the opposite side of the wall—and still catching it on the rebound. This is how it came to mind:

> I would make it hard for myself by catching a ball that flew high over my head [of course, it was I who threw it at the wall so that it would be high on the rebound]. The success—the feeling of omnipotence—that I can catch *every* ball! And with one hand! And with the right hand [I am left-handed]! And the special know-how [involved in such achievements, for example, with the high balls]: first, by blocking the force [of the flying ball], then by hitting the rebounding ball high [and only then catching it as it falls], and so on—there isn't a ball that can't be caught.

But, as I was caught up by these tremendous feelings of know-all and do-all, I found myself writing, in the same sweeping stream: "*All or nothing.* If not all, then everything is *lost.*"

As I was reliving these complex feelings in my mind—of anxiety, indeed, of a sinking feeling of desperation and a loss of heart as the ball eventually flew right into the hedge so I missed catching it or even touching it, but yet picking it up again quickly with renewed good feelings of excitement, mastery and control, fulfillment, even beauty and grace—associations began to come, bit by bit at first and then in streams. These memories, thoughts, and reflections were all connected with my engrossing game either directly or indirectly.

Before summarizing some of my associations, I should like to describe the verbal activity I required of myself in this game; it had a secretive element to it, which I did not recall at first. As the full reconstruction of this part of my game took some days, I can only present here an incomplete version of my recorded notes, which may provide some idea of how difficult a path it was: I resisted, reached some painful revelations, regressed, and then saw some more, until the way was eventually paved for me to recognize and fully face my elusive rule.

In my first reexperiencing of the game, I was vaguely aware that, "There remains something here that is unclear." Later came the thought that "I also had to call out something while the ball was in the air," so I added a note in parentheses in which I tried out different calls. My note said: "('Hard!' 'Again?' Did I count? Was [I] as-if turning to someone?)." My thoughts were drawn to this rule again still later in my associations, when I wrote:

> What was it that I was calling out? 'Curses,' occurs to me. 'Ass!', 'Scoundrel!' (*M'nooval*), 'Fool!' . . . I remember that I never had a large enough stock of 'curses'—so I used to repeat the same ones.

In reexperiencing, I distinctly recalled how I used to get stuck— holding up the flow of my game, because of this unfortunate limitation. When I went over these notes on the following day, I wrote next to "Ass" and "*M'nooval*," a matter-of-fact comment saying (quite correctly, yet thereby undermining its significance): "not curses[ing]—it is [just] calling names." It was not until days later that I finally had it: "*Yimach shimcha!*" (May your name be wiped out!); later "*Lech la'aza'zel!*" (Go to hell!) came to my mind, both of which I found most awesome and fearful. For, although these curses are the most common in use by both children and adults, they acquired and, for the child within me in the context of that game, still possessed a very special, concrete meaning. Yet, in accord with the rules of my game, I could not help but pronounce these words aloud repeatedly.

The intensity with which I was reliving the feeling of the possible destructive power of these curses (which I experienced consciously as general anxiety) may have already been unconsciously condensed, as I wrote the original description of my game, when I had not yet recalled having cursed. I had written, "Some kind of fear . . . that I would be caught red-handed," which does sound pretty criminal. The Hebrew idiom I used was that I would be caught *be'kalkalati,* spoiling or damaging. When I went over these notes, I could not help but be struck by the affinity between *le'kalel,* to curse, and *le'kalkel,* to damage. Further, as I was reporting on this "disgrace," while writing my rough draft of this paper in English, I had a "slip of the pen" in which I dropped the *s* from "cursing," so that I would have been "curing" the "damage" instead of causing it.

Though, on its own, such evidence may represent the worst kind of retrospective thinking, it does tally with the memories and related fantasies that came to my mind as I kept reliving this game. For me, it is evident that a game of this kind may have and, as I have discovered in my associations, did have many layers of meanings. One predominant preoccupation which kept returning in all sorts of ways had to do with a trauma of loss and the threat of further loss, with attempts to undo the loss and overcome the threat and attempts to prevent them by having full control, by constantly perfecting my ability through making it hard for myself to retrieve the ball. (The case of the little boy described by Freud [1920], who continuously "sent away" and then "retrieved" a toy representing his "gone" mother, comes to mind.) Above all, there were feelings of hopelessness and helplessness, and attempts to deny these feelings through becoming, in fantasy, both the wilful cause and the angry avenger of my loss.

UNCONSCIOUS FUNCTIONS OF A RULE STRUCTURE

How did the specific rule structure of this particular game *serve* the complex unconscious contents of its player? My ambivalent feelings and fantasies were expressed in many and differing ways in my game; in the act of rejecting and embracing, and in hitting hard, "hot"; in making my throws so difficult for myself that it was hard to catch the ball, and, at the same time, making it my business to "save" them all by the threat of the heavy penalty of losing everything and having to start all over again if I failed. Thus, my desperate efforts to perfect my performance in accordance with the explicit and implicit demands of my rules, so that I could "save," "not lose," every ball, as well as the sinking feeling that came with each failure, are in themselves evidence of this persistent intent (and although it seems that I tried my best, I could not destroy the wall). But my efforts with the ball, to make certain that *every ball must hit and then be caught,* were countered unconsciously by the rule that I must curse, that my curse must have a content the meaning of which was total destruction and loss. There was no way for me to "soften" or "undo" *that* blow. The curses "could not be helped," as they were required by rule. And they remained, loud, clear, and undenied, "hanging in the air."

In my childhood, I did not, of course, understand the meanings of or recognize the fantasies that went with this rule (or of any other rule, for that matter). However, in my analysis I discovered alongside my fear of being caught in this "damaging" act, the wish that someone (my brother) would appear and either put an end to it or share my secret act with me. This wish was, of course, greatly facilitated by my rule to the effect that I must shout the curses out, and not just say them quietly, "in my heart." Thus, it was *the rules of my game, repeatedly counterbalancing one another,* which made possible the unconscious expression of my contradictory feelings, anxieties, and wishes. In fact, I must emphasize that, for me, the rules of the game were what dictated my actions, and not vice versa. In this sense, my taking it upon myself to adhere to these rules fits in with the spirit of Peller's explanation of how rules function in children's games.

Peller states, "players recognize them [rules] as absolute for the duration of the game. Their meticulous observance gives independence from external superego figures" (p. 191). What she is saying here is that, because the rules of games represent a freely chosen and accepted code, one strictly adhered to although not imposed by an external authority, the capacity to play according to this code is indicative of the growth of an inner authority, independent of externally imposed demands. Although this is, indeed, a *freedom* that younger children do not possess, it seems to me that following the rules of a game may just as well "free" the child from feeling responsibility for actions taken while playing. Thus, my strict adherence to my "cursing" rule, since it was within the confines of my game, allowed me "time out" from the full responsibility I would otherwise have felt for my behavior. In the sense that I was telling my conscience, "I can't help it, rules must be followed," playing the game gave me the freedom to relax the standards of behavior which I applied outside of that special game situation. In other words, I would not, other than in the game situation, stand on our lawn screaming out aloud, *"Yimach shimcha"* or *"Lech La'aza'zel."* This leads me to the somewhat paradoxical conclusion that playing games with rules provides an opportunity for two contradictory freedoms, that of taking both greater and lesser responsibility for one's actions.

The extent to which rules that free from responsibility are common in children's games can be investigated by systematically examining the game descriptions in our collection. A quick glance through some of them indicates that they are probably not unusual. There are rules that require mocking, hitting with a ball or a fist, insulting, or even imposing some degree of torture. There are also rules that call for behavior unacceptable outside the game, for example, boy kissing girl. The line between this category of rules and those that require players to act "silly" or outright "ridiculous" may sometimes be hard to draw. But in all such games children "must," according to their self-imposed rules, relax their inner standards of behavior. What I would like to stress here, without elaborating, is that the child who acts in accord with the dictates of the rules of his game is different from the younger child who "just pretends" when he plays such "as if" games as doctor or bus. (Such play behavior may at times also be observed in older children or even adults, and is utilized in all sorts of ways [Arlow, 1971].)

Additional intensive, individual analyses would be needed in order to investigate other kinds of conflicts and unconscious fantasies that may lie behind performing according to rules of this kind. Such investigations might also lead to further explorations of my finding with regard to my own game: that its rules counterbalance one another in a way that made it possible for me to express contradictory emotions, fantasies, and wishes.

CREATIVITY IN PLAYING GAMES

My focus on the anxieties, tensions, and unconscious contents involved in my game has led me to neglect, far into my analysis, the basic and crucial fact that I *loved* playing it. This focus overshadowed to some extent the good feelings I mentioned above of excitement, of mastery and control, fulfillment, as well as my constant undercurrent feeling even of beauty and grace.

But when I then tried to conceptualize the quality of that experience, in terms of the extant explanatory concepts applied to play, my attempts did not satisfy me. Such rather vague, descriptive concepts as "need for mastery" or "pleasure in being the cause" seemed not fully to account for what I was directly enjoying while playing the game; nor did explanations in terms of a gradual reduction in the effect of traumatic experiences, gradual assimilation of anxiety, or practice of skills and enhancement in ego development.

I found myself partially in agreement, but nevertheless completely dissatisfied, with those distinctions between play and games that have led psychoanalysts and others to connect "playing"—but not the playing of games—with "creativity."[4] Peller (1954), for example, says that games "lack the quality of spontaneity which seems one of the essentials of play" (p. 193), and that the oedipal child's play activities "are colorful and imaginative," in contrast with the activities engaged in while playing the postoedipal child's games (p. 188). Although some kinds of earlier play are associated with the compulsion to repeat, many other forms are discussed with reference to such concepts as novelty, curiosity, exploration (Berlyne, 1969), and creative imagination (Greenacre, 1959). Indeed, the slow, repetitive, step-by-step advances typical of such popular street games as

---

4. Winnicott (1971) must be excluded from this generalization.

Hopscotch or Jacks (Five Stones), Tops, Elastic, Hand-Clapping games, Heads (Batting), Chewing Gums, Leapfrog or Marbles may very well lead people to conclude that they are neither inspired nor inspiring. Yet children play them with the utmost dedication and concentration—to the point where they often have great difficulty in tearing away from them when they must. This type of game, the so-called "seasonal" game, is often called a "craze," because such games often spread like wildfire in the playground.

I tended and still tend to think—and this, as I have said, still awaits investigation—that unconscious fantasies, conflicts, and anxieties may very well underlie a great deal of children's intensive engagement in games. Still, I remained puzzled why I always recalled the direct enjoyment involved in playing my own game, and some of these other games, when their descriptions and the actions involved in playing them seemed so boring.

It was only as I returned to the child within—throwing my ball at the wall once again, to the left, to the center, up and left, hard—that the words "virtuosity," "flow," "harmony," and then "master *performance!*" jumped into my mind. This proclamation, however immodest, provided the solution to my puzzlement: What I was experiencing and enjoying in playing my game was precisely my ability to create an endless flow of variations *within* its strict rules. In this sense I was *performing* creatively! The distinction I am making is analogous to that between creating a new piece of music and performing it. As does any performing artist, I practiced a great deal, intent on constantly improving my performance. Is there not a similarity between, say, the musical performer and the player of many games, whether he or she plays alone, one part in a duet, or in an orchestra? The great performer *creates* the piece of music as he plays. Although his performance is defined by the *very strict rules* of the composer's music, his special way of performing that music is unique.

As I was reflecting on my game-playing, and that of others, I began to recall some of the great game "performers" among the children I had known: Naomi at Jacks, Moishe with Marbles, and even Ovadia, the boy my student described as evading being tagged by moving sinuously like a belly dancer. These thoughts led me to believe that children play so many of the games in which they have to wait their turn not only because these games satisfy their need strictly to observe that the others play according to rules; these games are also played because they afford the players an opportunity to evaluate and compare the performances of different players with a subtlety that is the exclusive province of the interested expert. Children appreciate great performances when they see them, although such performances are usually entirely lost on the adult onlooker. This may partly explain why our games research showed child onlookers as a constant feature in the playground. But, just as the subtleties that add up to make a great artistic performance are lost on the uninitiated, much of the quality and special characteristics of children's performance in games is lost on the remote adult.

Once I moved away from my own position of remoteness, by opening myself up to the child within, I could better understand how difficult it is to reach the "creativity" perspective on games "from the outside." It was only through the process of reexperiencing my own performance while at the same time observing it that I could—once I laid aside my (dynamically) unconscious *content*—put another facet of my *experience* into words. I had had great difficulty all along in describing my performance in words. Saying "left," "right," etc., and talking clumsily about the various "tricks" I performed came nowhere near to describing what actually went on. I now realized that this was a great barrier to conceptualizing this contentless facet of game-playing. It is the very difficulty of articulating the details of the experience that makes it even more difficult to reach the general concept that will describe precisely what it is. This is the reason why children can be of only limited help in our attempts to understand their experience in playing games. For children cannot experience what is happening and at the same time observe themselves, attempt to verbalize their observations, and then go back to reflect upon the experience. This can only be done by adults when they open themselves up to, and "cooperate with," the child within. For me this additional perspective is one of the great benefits of using the method of investigation which I propose. Reaching the playing child within may offer us yet further insights that are difficult to reach "from the outside."

I have not actually attempted to replay my game, with a real ball. As it is the child within that I must turn to, this is best done in mind. Even in mind, however, I had considerable difficulty in repeating my childhood feat of shouting out curses, in "harmony" with the other actions required by my rules. Obviously I am out of practice! But this makes it evident that the form of exploration I have used can only be applied in those cases and with those games that either still live or can be reawakened within.

I would like to conclude with a brief comment on my conception of the child within (Freud, 1905, p. 226; Sandler, 1985). I have used the concept as a metaphor implying continuity in our self-experience and an ability to retrieve and construct various aspects of our past in the present. There can be no certainty that such experiencing in fantasy corresponds to the original experience. As I have tried to show, such reliving in the present can nonetheless broaden our perspective on and understanding of the experiencing child.

BIBLIOGRAPHY

ARLOW, J. A. (1971). A type of play observed in boys during the latency period. In *Separation-Individuation*, ed. J. B. McDevitt & C. F. Settlage. New York: Int. Univ. Press, pp. 157–170.

AVEDON, E. M. (1971). The structural elements of games. In *The Study of Games*, ed. E. M. Avedon & B. Sutton-Smith. New York: Wiley, pp. 419–428.

BERLYNE, D. E. (1969). Laughter, humor and play. In *The Handbook of Social Psychology*, ed. G. Lindzey & E. Aronson. Reading, Mass: Addison-Wesley, 3:795–852.

BETTELHEIM, B. (1976). *The Uses of Enchantment*. New York: Knopf.

EIFERMANN, R. R. (1970). Cooperativeness and egalitarianism in kibbutz children's games. *Human Relations*, 6:579–587.

_____ (1971a). *Determinants of Children's Game Styles*. Jerusalem: Israel Academy of Sciences and Humanities.

_____ (1971b). Social play in childhood. In *Child's Play*, ed. R. E. Heron & B. Sutton-Smith. New York: Wiley, pp. 270–297.

_____ (1973a). It's child's play. In *Games in Education and Development*, ed. E. Bower & L. M. Shears. Springfield: Thomas, pp. 75–102.

_____ (1973b). Rules in games. In *Artificial and Human Thinking*, ed. A. Elithorn & P. Jones. Amsterdam: Elsevier, pp. 147–161.

_____ (1978). Games of physical activity. In *Physical Activity and Human Well-Being*, ed. F. Landry & W. A. R. Orban. Miami: Symposia Specialists, pp. 741–752.

—— (1984). Teaching psychoanalysis to nonanalytical students through work on their own dreams. *Psychoanalysis in Europe*, 22:38–45.

—— (1987a). Fairy tales—a royal road to the child within the adult. *Scand. Rev. Psychoanal.* (in press). Märchen. In *Das Märchen—Ein Märchen?* ed. J. Stork. Stuttgard-Bad Canstatt: Frommann-Holzboog (in press).

—— (1987b). Varieties of denial. In *Denial*, ed. E. Edelstein. New York: Plenum, pp. 38–55.

—— (1987c). Interaction between textual analysis and related self analysis. In *Discourse in Psychoanalysis and Literature*, ed. S. Rimmon-Keynan. London: Methuen (in press).

—— (1987d). "Germany" and "the Germans." *Int. Rev. Psychoanal.*, 14 (in press).

FREUD, S. (1905). Jokes and their relation to the unconscious. *S.E.*, 8.

—— (1908). Creative writers and day-dreaming. *S.E.*, 9:141–153.

—— (1920). Beyond the pleasure principle. *S.E.*, 18:3–64.

GOLDINGS, H. J. (1978). Jump-rope rhymes and the rhythm of latency development in girls. *Psychoanal. Study Child*, 29:431–450.

GREENACRE, P. (1959). Play in relation to creative imagination. *Annu. Psychoanal.*, 14:61–80.

OPIE, P. & OPIE, I. (1969). *Children's Games in Street and Playground*. Oxford: Clarendon Press.

PELLER, L. E. (1952). Models of children's play. *Ment. Hyg.* 36:66–83.

—— (1954). Libidinal phases, ego development, and play. *Psychoanal. Study Child*, 9:178–198.

PHILIPS, R. H. (1960). The nature and function of children's formal games. *Psychoanal. Q.*, 29:200–207.

PIAGET, J. (1945). *Play, Dreams and Imitation in Childhood*. London: Routledge & Kegan Paul, 1951.

ROBERTS, J. M. & SUTTON-SMITH, B. (1962). Child training and game involvement. *Ethnology*, 1:166–185.

SANDLER, J. (1985). The id—or the child within? Inaugural lecture, University of London, at University College, London.

STOKES, A. (1956). Psycho-analytic reflections on the development of ball games, particularly cricket. *Int. J. Psychoanal.*, 37:85–192.

SUTTON-SMITH, B. (1972). *The Folkgames of Children*. Austin: Univ. Texas Press.

WINNICOTT, D. W. (1971). *Playing and Reality*. London: Tavistock.

Treatment of an Atypical Boy

AUDREY GAVSHON

AS THIS STORY UNFOLDS, IT WILL BE SEEN HOW FROM INFANCY onward Martin's development lagged at all levels. His archaic fears could not be met by normal support and comfort. His odd behavior was becoming bizarre; he rocked intensely and did not listen. He showed an almost complete inability to relate to other children.

At home he showed obsessional activities, panic reactions, and fear of loud noises. His father wrote, "On top is his unwillingness to communicate, difficulties in understanding the spoken word, and refusal to participate in group activities; he has been behaving in a disturbed way, e.g., throwing food about (until firmly rebuked) and making bizarre body movements and gesticulations. He has become the object of derision and revulsion among the children at school, which only makes matters worse."

By the second year of life Martin's erratic development was compounded by periods of deafness and general ill-health lasting until he was 5 years old. His defenses against confusion and annihilation resulted in a libidinal withdrawal from his objects, who in turn withdrew from him.

Martin's speech did not develop normally, and the process of reciprocal communication was interfered with from infancy. This influenced ego functions such as synthesis, reality testing, and secondary process thinking. The problems were intensified by the parents' lack of psychological understanding and their

Member of the Anna Freud Centre, London, which is at present supported by the G. G. Bunzl Charitable Foundation, London; The Freud Centenary Fund, London; The Anna Freud Foundation, New York; The New-Land Foundation, Inc., New York; The Leo Oppenheimer and Flora Oppenheimer Haas Trust, New York; and a number of private supporters.

inability to give structured meaning to his feeling states. Language for Martin did not serve as a means to an end and could not be used for discharge of tension. This created behavioral difficulties at home and at school. Martin had not been able to use speech as a communication to express his affects, impulses, or other inner experiences; nor could he use words to influence his objects and so promote the gratification of his needs. He was unable to verbalize his feelings to bring about a delay action which would allow him to judge the situation. Without speech as a vehicle for discharge, tempers and strange, uncontrolled body behavior were his motor affective outlets for chaotic drive derivatives and affects. The rising instinctual wish, and the behavior aimed at its fulfillment, could not be checked by reasoning.

One of the earliest aims of treatment was to find ways of communicating with this 8-year-old inarticulate boy. These would not be primarily dependent on verbal rapport but would involve "playing" with him on a preverbal level.

BACKGROUND

Martin was the youngest of three children. His brother Paul was 3 years older and his sister Claudia was 19 months older. His parents came from prestigious academic families, both went to boarding school, and neither was a product of a warm family life. Yet they were physically affectionate toward each other as well as toward the children. They were unequivocal in their expectation that the children would achieve academically and become self-reliant, an attitude which both hindered and helped Martin's development. Mother and father were indifferent to the fact that none of the children was interested in any form of sport, but they were passionate hikers, and all holidays were spent walking for many hours.

The mother was attractive, articulate, and energetic, a MENSA candidate who worked hard and, on weekends and holidays, played hard. She prided herself on her time and motion efficiency. She knew that many members of her family had had problems in making relationships. After she had been an eccentric, difficult child who did not get on with her peers, she pulled herself together and arrived at a happy marriage. She therefore dismissed her daughter's withdrawn and "immature" social behavior as something she would outgrow, as she herself did. The mother did not return to work until Martin was 5 years old and then, without conflict, went back to her highly esteemed full-time job. Martin was a constant source of interruption to her carefully planned organization, particularly when the journey to his school was long and complicated and he needed to be escorted. She was without psychological awareness and interviews with her were as unusual as her son's treatment. However, through identifying with my feeling that Martin was worthwhile, endearing and commendably motivated to mastery, she was able to revalue him, and there were times when she showed tenderness and compassion. Unlike her husband, she warned the children before she got angry.

The father was a soft-spoken, apparently gentle, sensitive man. Martin was very much like his father as a little boy; and he certainly resembled him physically. The father, too, was without insight and only very recently could he be shown the sort of support Martin needed from him. His sense of doom about his son's future alternated with his critical view that a boy of 10 should not behave like a baby. His anxiety caused him to complain, with disgust, about Martin's table manners and regressive collapses. While the mother reported Martin's improvements, in a way which strengthened her denial and perhaps added fuel to her omnipotent wish that inherent defects would disappear, the father had to be encouraged to say anything positive. His unexpected shouting was a major problem for Martin. However, despite their unalterable disturbances, they were conscientious parents who grew to respect and trust the help Martin received.

Neither mother nor father seemed to have an appropriate appraisal of affects outside of their own relationship which was close. For instance, it took a long time and included a joint interview for them to realize that Paul's teasing was excessive and sadistic. The mother said cheerfully, "but he teases me too," and the father insisted it was normal for the eldest child to tease his siblings, denying the quality and intent of Paul's banter and Martin's inarticulate helplessness in dealing with it. Through regular meetings with the parents I experienced not only Martin's frustration at their psychological insensitivity but also their impatience and pain over his present and future predicament. Their personality disturbances made active support of our work difficult.

The pregnancy was planned. In her second month the mother suffered a virulent 'flu. Martin was born face upward after a short and painful labor. The father was present at this birth and the mother felt that it had drawn him especially close to his third child and, at the same time, intensified his sadness and disappointment at Martin's slow progress. The parents kept a book of their children's milestones, a record which included their achievements, the identity of their christening robes, their birthday presents. It omitted anything which could have caused them anxiety such as Martin's fevers and hospitalizations; but the detailed notes of his development were laced with a thread of despair. Martin presented such a strange picture that I described his early history in some detail. Both said that Martin was a "solemn baby." They recorded that he smiled at 5 weeks. At 10 weeks he "*at last* dropped the 2 A.M. feed." When Martin was 7 months he "at last" was able to drink milk from the cup; and at 8 months had begun saying "dadada" constantly and proudly; Martin crawled at 11 months, somewhat "laboriously"; he seemed "to be either pushing with both knees simultaneously or lying on one side and pushing with the other foot." At 12 months the mother noted, "He appears to say mamama with meaning, to attract my attention or when I come into the room. He adores being in the bath. He still cannot sit up except in the tripod position." At 14 months Martin was able "at last" to get into a sitting position with his hands off the floor. At 18 months she wrote, "Martin can now feed himself with a spoon and has taken two unsupported steps. He loves climbing onto furniture. He can drink unaided from a two-handled baby mug without its spout lid (which he refuses to use)." At 20 months he took four unaided steps.

Shortly before his second birthday the mother was convinced that Martin was deaf; he did not look up when a low-flying aeroplane passed by. The family doctor was dismissive, regarding her as an overanxious mother; but she persisted and was finally seen at the Royal National Ear Nose and Throat Hospital where "secretory otitis media was diagnosed. Removal of the adenoids and bilateral grommets were at once recommended. The hospital reported a history of several upper respiratory tract infections. He may well also have had otalgia. He had wax in his ears. An impedance test gave a flat response on both sides, suggesting fluid still in the middle ear. It was impossible to do an audiogram as Martin refused to co-operate." But on the day of the operation Martin had a temperature of 102. When postponment was decided upon, the mother expressed impatience, saying if the hospital was to wait for Martin to be well, there would never be a suitable time because he invariably had colds or fevers. (He was almost 3 when, ultimately, the operation was performed.)

At nearly 5 the mother again became concerned about Martin's hearing. She again was treated dismissively but persisted until an appointment was fixed. It was discovered that the grommets had coated up and for some time could not have been serving any purpose. While undergoing the operation for the removal of the grommets, Martin's tonsils also were taken out without preparation. In the aftermath Martin developed a very healthy appetite and had "an enormous" growth spurt. The mother stayed with Martin in the hospital for 3½ days.

When Martin was 2 years old, the mother wrote, "Although he can hardly talk, Martin can sing more than one tune." According to his father, Martin had developed an extensive vocabulary by the time he was 2½, but was unable to join his words into meaningful sentences. At 4 he was described as speaking like a 3-year-old despite his large vocabulary, but he could not yet narrate a sequence of events, was not asking how-and-why questions, could not follow simple stories, and had a very short attention span. During this period, he had two speech therapists, but he did not improve.

At 2½, the record says, Martin was "at last somewhat erratically using the potty, but is far from trained." He became adequately trained for bowel and bladder by age 4, although he occasionally continued to wet his bed until he was 10.

When he turned 3, Martin joined a playgroup; he settled down well, put jigsaws together with great dexterity, but did not relate to other children. When he was 4, he attended the nursery class at his local primary school. The teacher reported that Mar-

tin was "miles behind" the other children and suggested that his
parents should seek the advice of the Tavistock Clinic and place
him in a private school.

The parents eventually accepted this advice. Martin was
placed in a small private school in Hampstead when he was 5.
The family was seen at the Tavistock Clinic and therapy was
recommended for Martin. The mother turned down the recommendation: she felt criticized and infantilized by the Tavistock
approach, and she resented the close-circuit television setting. In
addition, because they lived on the other side of London, she felt
unable to cope with the complications of getting Martin to appointments. Later, the father expressed regret at that decision,
reasoning if treatment had started earlier Martin could have
progressed sooner.

Mr. Moran tested M. when he was 7. On the WISC his verbal
IQ was 137, his performance was 104, and his full-scale IQ 123.
His reading age was that of a 10-year-old. Mr. Moran reported,
"The discrepancy between verbal and non-verbal measures of
intelligence is not indicative of learning disability. He may have
been poorly motivated on the picture completion sub-test. His
low score on the Picture Arrangement sub-test is consistent with
his low level of awareness of social/personal relationships." In
October 1986, Martin was again tested by Mrs. Davids. This time
his verbal IQ was 113, performance 104, and full-scale 112. He
scored 17 for arithmetic and 6 for comprehension. Martin's attitude toward the test could be viewed as changes which have
taken place during his analysis. Mrs. Davids said, "Throughout I
was struck by M.'s strong desire to do well and his perseverence
in the face of difficulty. The lowered scores on the non-verbal
scale must be viewed in terms of M.'s high anxiety and his slow
work tempo accompanying a tendency towards meticulousness
and need for perfection. Attainment on the Information and
Vocabulary sub-tests indicate a substantial range of information
and long-term memory. The lowered score on Comprehension
together with a low average score on the Picture Arrangement
suggests difficulties in social judgement."

Martin was put in Category 5 on the Diagnostic Profile; i.e.,
there were primary deficiencies of an organic nature, or early

deprivations, which distorted development and structuralization and produced retarded, defective, and nontypical personalities.

It was agreed that Martin should have analytic treatment on the condition that the parents send him to a school which catered to children with special needs. The parents, especially the mother, at first resisted the recommendation. Martin stayed at this most caring and supportive school for 2½ years. Then he was able to go to a small local school from where he could walk to his sessions. The family by then had moved house to North London.

Martin was a very tall, thin boy with longish, fair hair and large, dark eyes. Despite his often pale and unwell appearance, he never missed a session through illness. During treatment he was prescribed glasses. He was pleased about this because his father and brother also wore spectacles. His gait was awkward. He presented a picture which ranged from appearing somewhat strange and uncoordinated to looking spastic. His feet turned inward and his legs were more or less floppy. Invariably his shoe laces were undone. Martin had an exceptionally long tongue, which could touch the tip of his nose. He drank his orange juice in a peculiar way, putting the glass over his face so that the rim touched his glasses. It was as though his lips knew no boundaries. His teeth protruded slightly and seemed to sink into the liquid; when he dribbled or had a streaming nose, he would never wipe away the moisture, as though he did not feel it. (And yet, there were times when he was relaxed, and I was struck by his lovely head and sensitive good looks.)

TREATMENT

This report will focus on Martin's struggle to attain and sustain mastery of his anxiety reactions through educational, developmental, and analytic help. The initial phase of treatment was essentially a period of tuning in to each other. Martin's defective synthetic function, his inability to verbalize, and his narcissistic vulnerability made it necessary for us to seek unusual ways of connecting. Throughout treatment his wish to participate and respond made the uphill journey possible. His capacity for self-observation was greater than that of many children whose ability to integrate was unimpaired. And perhaps it was this strength which so highlighted his immovable frailties.

Martin started treatment when he was 7 years and 4 months old. In our first sessions he became so frustrated when I did not understand him, and so denigrated when I asked him to repeat a word, that many of my earliest responses were a hit-or-miss. His speech when it was comprehensible was laborious and came after long silences. Because his finger movements were rigidly tense, I showed him a finger game, "This is the church, here is the steeple, open the door, and see all the people." He tried to copy the action, not resisting my touching his hands to position them, and this led to a game of fingers walking on the desk. It was this action which put the seal on our union: our fingers did the talking. As he arrived for his session, he would silently clasp his hands, showing his wish for me to make the church, and then after a while would say, "Run on the desk again," or "Tell me another story with your fingers." I asked him for an idea and he replied, "They go to Italy for a holiday." He would not associate, but was captivated by the action of the boy running, the aeroplane flying. With infantile pleasure, he smiled as each story ended with children putting their hands against their cheeks as they went to sleep. On one occasion my fingers enacted a little boy crying because he could not run as fast as his brother and after a long silence, while Martin mustered the words, he said, "Tell him the reason why he is crying." From then on it was possible to interpret his fear of failure and ridicule if he could not understand or make himself understood, and his despair at the thought that he would never be as clever, as fast, as strong, or as good a speaker as his brother. Without these attributes neither his parents nor his therapist could love and value him, and his main recourse would be to run into the corner and cry like a baby or stamp his feet. The significance of this interaction was that our first meaningful communication was preverbal and perhaps reflected a short time in Martin's life when he felt safe enough to receive and to respond.

This game was replaced by a family of dolls. Again Martin was intrigued by the action of the dolls walking, swimming, jumping, but it did not help him to volunteer information about relationships at home. As his single activity at weekends was his involvement with a Sinclair computer, Sinclair joined the family. This inanimate object became the vehicle for verbalizing emotions, an experience he had not had with his parents. He thought it very funny when I said, "Sinclair can't be a real friend because he can't say, 'I want your crisps.' He can't laugh or cry, feel angry or sad, or say, 'It isn't fair.'" Martin would then repeat my words. He never forgot Sinclair's role, and later in treatment he said, "I have three friends—Mrs. Gavshon, Sinclair, and myself. Do you think I mind not having more friends?" During a game when the father doll went to the telephone and waited for Martin to say "hello," he looked at me pleadingly and finally said, "Please let's not do the telephone." It was possible to interpret his fear of the uncontrollable unknown, his bewilderment of voices with no faces, and the threat to his object constancy. But sometimes he completely collapsed, as in a game when he went shopping and I asked mother to unwrap the biscuits. "How can we unwrap the biscuits," he shouted. "We've got nothing for biscuits." This time he would not accept a symbol and his panicked screaming left me as helpless as he felt.

Through games of hangman Martin was introduced to associations. At first his words were clever and random (as his father had described his original unconnected vocabulary); e.g., radiator, symbol, tradition, but eventually he identified that I was linking words and he imitated the style. After a weekend in the country, we had a sequence using his description—cottage, flowers, hedgehog, trees, birds, and then, apparently irrelevantly, Martin said, "Jam." He was agitated when I asked how that fitted in. After interpreting the injury and rejection I had caused by not understanding his thoughts, he explained very slowly, with lots of long pauses, that the bird sat on the bush and grandmother made jam-berry bush jam. Throughout treatment his parents complained about his inappropriate comments, and this exchange shed some light on their origin. What objectively appeared disconnected and fragmented had a logic for Martin. The mother and Martin, for example, went on a picnic hike together, but the treat turned into a trial for Martin because it rained. He was silent during most of the walk and did not respond to mother's jolly comments about the surroundings. Suddenly he announced, "We have 24 meat knives, 24 meat forks, 24 fish knives, but only 23 fish forks." Mother felt despair at what she thought was her son's madness and rejection of her communication and responded impatiently, thereby rejecting him. The explanation was that around this time Martin, unasked, had delighted and surprised his mother by laying the table for a large lunch party. He was proud of his achievement and was much praised because he had remembered everything. It was possible to show Martin how he could not express his disappointment at the failed outing and that he had tried to compensate for feared reprisals by recalling and repeating an event which had given mutual satisfaction. Similarly, his father accusingly reported that while the family were engaged in intelligent conversation, Martin who had not participated said, out of the blue, "Everyone loves strawberries." The father sometimes responded critically to Martin's non sequiturs and this reduced Martin to helpless rage or silence. In treatment Martin talked about how his difficulty in speaking fluently made him feel excluded. He dealt with his anxiety by searching for a route to common ground in the family constellation. If his aim was to gain pride not punishment, he would have to recognize his frustration and contain himself so that he could become socially apt, because his parents and siblings were not therapists and couldn't understand his inappropriate comments. Martin welcomed the interpretations and clarifications and both he and his parents maintained that he now joined in and "held forth," but he could not sustain a line of thought if he was interrupted; he had to begin each sentence over again instead of continuing from where he had halted.

It became clear in the early stage of treatment that M. would have to be taught most things that other children acquire naturally. He had to learn to speak more intelligibly; to have eye-to-eye contact; master a tie knot; play pretend games as well as board games, dominoes, and pelmanism; and familiarize himself with kinship terminology, such as father's brother is an uncle. It was through his response to educational processes that he gained understanding of his defenses (notably regression, projection, and denial), his omnipotent thinking, his castration concerns, his low self-esteem. By the fifth week of treatment we had found the formula for the analysis. M. readily accepted that "little M." was the uncontrolled, infantile, diffusely anxious part of himself and he was able through this displacement to ally himself with me in the therapeutic work and to observe his disorganization and aspire toward gaining ego strengths.

Martin soon expressed his anger when I interrupted his comic reading in the waiting room. He sat hunched in a chair with his back to me, sulkily refusing to speak. He could accept interpretations about "little M." who was so cross that he would not speak and that if he did he would say such awful things that I would reject him. So he talked with his body instead and he did the same thing at home and at school. His fear that his words might be explosive and bring retaliation brought about Martin's fantasy: "I'm frightened if I shoot them with a bow and arrow; they will shoot me. It would stick in their throats and then Paul and the children couldn't tease and you couldn't say, "Martin, put your comic down.'" With encouragement he mimed a bow and arrow, using flamboyant, disconnected arm movements, shooting the invisible weapon into the waiting room, at me, his brother, and the children at school. We had endless stories about "little M." who felt stupid because he did not speak well and thought the only solution was to sit in a corner and pretend he did not hear. If he pretended to be deaf, maybe he magically wouldn't hear the sadistic teases or adult reprimands and in that way he could protect himself from attack. But he knew that he couldn't erase these worries by using tippex, as he said he could make mistakes disappear on Claudia's typewriter. "When worries get smaller, little M. will grow as big as big M.," he said. He told me that when he was a little boy, he could not say the "Fl" sound and pronounced "flowers" as "clowers." He enjoyed a joke about candy-closs and then, knowing that his father was an enthusiastic gardener, a story about little M. who asked his father for some clowers and father did not understand. Martin collapsed into uncontrolled body language. He wanted to identify with daddy and share his love, but was spurned and denigrated because he wasn't clever enough to say the word properly. Now his worry about getting things wrong had become so big that he wouldn't try because it meant risking humiliation and rejection. "That's how little M. felt. Big M. knew his daddy loved him even if he couldn't speak properly," he replied. "How long will it take little M. to catch up with big M.?" Martin's admiration and esteem for his father, except when he shouted suddenly, were constant throughout. When (unnoticed) I have observed them together, the father was patient and gentle.

After many sessions of practice, Martin was able to hear the difference between C and P, G, and B, and with delight exhibited his mastery. "I can say cry, I don't say pry. I can say grass, not brass." The Th sound posed a greater difficulty. In a game in which we blew paper across the desk, it was clear that he had trouble exhaling. Trying to learn this sound made him roll his tongue around inside and outside his mouth, at first nervously. He asked if it was a sausage, and this introduced (displaced) castration themes—how, when he was small, he thought his teeth might bite his tongue; interpretations were extended to other parts of his body that he had to protect. When his fear of uncontrolled anger was linked with castration, he finally responded, "It was simple for little M. to hide his secret [i.e., anger], he went just like this." He showed tight lips, a concealed, nonspeaking, safe tongue. At the same time he covered his penis, "Little M. thought daddy might want his willie because he wanted daddy's flowers," he said.

Oral accomplishments remained a source of great narcissistic pleasure for M. He successfully struggled to use correct pronunciation and to extend his vocabulary. In treatment it was possible to recharge his flagging motivation by imbuing him with phallic assertive language. If I suggested that he would triumph, be victorious, conquer little M., his observing ego was resuscitated and I praised him for courage and his heroic struggle.

After 5 months of treatment Martin's change of school propelled us prematurely into material before he had had time to stand firmly in the small steps he had taken. He was in the same class as a psychotic child, Lucy. On his first day at school the teacher told Martin that if he continued to do silly things, she would become angry with him. We talked about his regressive resort to crazy movements when he felt threatened, frustrated, and stupid. He asked for more and more stories about his behavior at his previous school. But interpretations of his fear of humiliation and loss of control accelerated his anxiety and he responded by performing actions, flailing his limbs, and making facial grimaces. He was, however, proud to tell me the names of some of the children, acknowledging that at his former school after 2 years he had only known the name of one boy. Martin said, "Lucy doesn't talk, she just grunts and cries like a baby." He complained fiercely that she messed up his work and he had told her to go away, but she didn't listen. He wondered whether she was deaf and insisted that when she was older, she would be able to speak. He allowed me to tell him about little M. who feared his identification with Lucy and to define again his real (otitis media) hearing problems which a doctor had made better and over which he had no control and his pretend ones which protected and isolated him from the world and which he could change himself. But the sessions were bombarded by his incessantly talking about Lucy: "Now talk about why Lucy can't hear. Now talk about why Lucy can't listen." He demonstrated (with some gratification) how Lucy behaved. He imitated what he called her animal noises and described with outrage how "she eats every minute, not every second." He asked, "Will Lucy one day say when I was little I couldn't speak and felt very sad."

When his class was taken to the Tate Gallery Lucy did not go and on the bus the teacher told him that Lucy did not talk at home either. Martin said, "She doesn't talk at home, she doesn't talk at school, and she doesn't talk to herself either—and don't ask me how I know." Attempts to show him the difference between him and Lucy were met with "Talk about the Tate. Don't talk about Lucy." By referring to little M., I could interpret how his whiney, infantile behavior at the Tate expressed his anger and frustration at being on this boring outing and his wish and fear to be as uncontrolled as Lucy and stay at the school. "Did I feel so angry I thought a bow and arrow would go into the teacher's throat and she would send one into mine?" he asked. He came for a session defiantly repeating, "Don't know, don't care," copying a character in a comic. He initiated a game of teacher and pupil and allowed me to say, "Don't know and pretend I don't care." It was possible to show him how he imitated people he admired (the cheeky comic boy) and feared, and how by turning passive into active he hoped to control himself as he tried to control Lucy by grabbing and pushing her. To test my patience he provacatively tried to blow bubbles, swamping his mouth and chin with saliva, and finally announced, "I think you must be queen of the people who don't get cross when I'm naughty."

The father reported that at home Martin had been destructive, swinging his toy frog and was told to stop. Martin then punished the frog by hanging him in his cupboard. "Kermit has been punished. He has to stay in prison for one months," and he wrote 30 lines "I must be sensible—I must be sensible," revealing his primitive superego. Lucy invaded his thoughts, and his sessions were deluged with accounts of her behavior. When they were both standing on the hot pipe, Martin said, "If you are cold, go inside. If you aren't cold, get off the pipe." Lucy did not move, so "I grabbed her right arm and I grabbed her left arm and took her inside, simple. Now talk about that." But talking about Martin's fear of Lucy's strange behavior only excited him and he clutched his penis, squeezed his eyes, and put his fingers over his face. Finally I told Martin that we would have to stop talking about Lucy because it was not helping our work together. "You mean about little M." he asked. That was Martin's recognition that he could distance himself in order to regain some mastery over his anxious excitation and discharge, and he proceeded to say that Claudia knew a boy who couldn't talk, whose name was Dibs. He calmed down considerably and we talked about his fears of hearing and not hearing, of communicating and not communicating, and his concern that he would never be able to control himself or his speech. With much embarrassment he was then able to tell me how he was being victimized at school. Boys had thrown a stick at him, "but I was too shy to throw it back." We could then talk about his past and present dread of his aggression which he turned against himself and his fantasies about the destructive violence of his family and peers. "I might be so angry, I would fall down like the Leaning Tower of Pisa. I might be so angry, I would crash like a crane—jump to the ceiling and hurt my head." He wanted me to repeat stories of when he was a baby and mother could not understand him. He asked for more and more until she became so angry, she smacked him. He feared her wrath had damaged his tongue, his ears, "and my willie and arms and legs." For months he continued to bring bulletins about Lucy in a way that was therapeutically useful—how she did or didn't put her shoes on, how the teachers helped or became angry with her. He accepted that Lucy did all sorts of things with her shoes, arms, legs, and eyes, because she could not speak. "Why does Lucy do this with her arms?" he asked, wiggling his; in response to my comment that she used her arms instead of her tongue to express her feelings, Martin asked, "Like a tongue twister?" Martin wondered if Lucy didn't speak because she was frightened of something invisible. He explained that "invisible" was something you couldn't see, but you could feel, whereas vanished meant you couldn't see it or feel it. He could accept interpretations of his archaic fears of annihilation and abandonment, and we recalled his dread of the faceless telephone, and the days at his nursery school where his mother had left him and he feared she would never return.

Martin said he would never sit like Lucy in a crouched position. He made it easy to relate Lucy's muddy mess to his prolonged toilet training and his fear that mother's rage would suddenly crack down on him like the circus whip. He had had a memorable panic attack when he was unwillingly taken to the circus at age 4. Much later in treatment Martin arrived for his sessions having defecated in his trousers, but it was a long time before he could talk about it. He would not use the school lavatories because they did not have locks on the door and he was frightened someone would come in and see him. His sister advised him to shout, "I'm here," but in a situation of tension Martin could not rely on the words being effective. His shame at being seen superseded the disgust of walking around smelling. Martin thoughtfully refuted many anal interpretations which were linked to the pleasure and pain of losing control in the past and present. Finally, I suggested that his mother might have unexpectedly come into his unlocked bedroom while he was masturbating and that his shame at being seen by other children in the unbolted lavatory belonged to the shame of his exposure of sexual pleasures. Martin responded, "Now you're talking sense," and could express his surprise that I had not rejected him because of his smelly pants and actions.

While Martin was spending the best part of 2 years regaling me with Lucy's psychotic behavior his tendency for obsessive perseveration reached an almost unendurable peak. At the time of referral his parents had proudly reported his knowledge about the Beaufort Wind Scale. In treatment this started with Martin calculating the mileage to and from the Lake District, Brittany, the Channel from his house, from the motorway to his school and to the Clinic, subtracting, adding, and measuring. When he learned to tell the time on his eighth birthday, he would spend much more of the session relating the time to the second, watching the second hand, formulating complicated sums. He wanted to know the meaning of the phrase "Time passes quickly" when you were having a nice time, badgered me for an explanation but didn't hear the answer, just repeated the question. While his activities could be related to anxiety about separation, or wanting to be "chief of the time," Martin persisted, "If mummy and daddy go to bed at 11 and I go to bed at 8 and it's 3:40 now, I'll be in bed by. . . ." Any comment from me was license for another permutation, and when that was over he would start another subject. Accumulated knowledge about the planets took over—the earth is 80 times bigger than the moon. It would take a billion hours to get there if you walk, go by spaceship, aeroplane, etc. Endlessly he told me about the French words he had learned, spelling them phonetically and in French, the listings in the Guinness Book of Records, the English Dictionary which he was learning from the letter A. Next he started on height, weight, and birthdays—daddy is 6'3", Paul is, Claudia is, the mother's help is, mummy is—then how everyone's age and birthday related to each other and how much everyone weighed in relation to their height and to each other. Martin said he was very pleased he was a boy of 4'8", and that he thought Claudia would like to be as tall as he was and have a willie, but she couldn't. He only wished he could be older than Paul. Being so proud of 4'8" led us to his 2'6" Lucy behavior, when he couldn't wait for more ice cream, made a fuss, and was sent to the kitchen in disgrace to finish his dinner. Growing tall "inside" was the ego-strengthening concept he understood and it was a spur for his passionate wish to be strong emotionally and physically.

This tendency has recently taken a new form in his letter writing to people who sent him gifts. The contents were detailed, endless, and boring, resembling an autoerotic quality. His parents' approval that his information was clever enhanced his persistence, and the mass of useless information became libidinized. They even gave him complicated sums and then checked his answer with their calculator, for instance, in converting miles into kilometers. With pleasure they brought me xeroxed copies of intricate maps he had drawn from memory and letters to godparents he hardly knew. It was more as a result of my bland disinterest, rather than anything verbalized, that they finally understood this was a symptom, which alarmed rather than pleased me, and was not to be encouraged. In contrast, I expressed my relief when Martin gave up encyclopaedic reading and became engrossed in Roald Dahl and Enid Blyton books. In our sessions I constantly interpreted Martin's feeling that he would win love and approval only if he was clever and that I too would value him for his knowledge and not for himself. "But little M. is getting taller inside," he said. When I suggested that he thought clever equalled love, he replied, "Did little M. think stupid equalled hate?"

Martin overwhelmed me with his information as concerns about Lucy flooded him. In an attempt to change gear, I suggested we play a game. It was exhausting to try and make some inroad into his world. Although he sometimes listened and even tried to use interpretations to master his "loony" behavior, I did not feel he was with me, or rather it was too taxing to try to keep him connected. Martin agreed on snakes and ladders, the first board game we played. He had no idea about counters, how to throw a dice, which color to move. His bewilderment verged on panic which he tried to control by shouting, "I know, I know, I know." He settled down after responding to interpretations that when he did not know something he got so worried that he was stupid (and unworthy), that he did and said silly things to hide his fear of not knowing. If he wasn't as clever and controlled as his siblings and couldn't be included when they played together, he excluded himself by doing little M. things, such as disrupting their game. Martin was joyous when he finally conquered the game and it became the springboard for work on his omnipotent wishes and fears. Shaking the dice frenetically he would plead, "Abracadabra, please give me a 6." But shaking the dice noisily did not bring the magic number, nor could abracadabra imme-

diately gratify his wishes. He joined in comments about how nice
it would be if we could say abracadabra "make me as big as Paul,
take away the noisy washing machine worry, make me stop gig-
gling when I look at Lucy, make me say the 'th' sound, make me
4'6" inside." Martin also began to understand that destructive
wishes could not come true; that he could not annihilate his
brother or parents when he was angry with them; and since they
had no magic either, they could not shatter him. Martin later in
treatment said, "I wish I could say abracadabra and I was 4 again
and could hear and speak." We talked about his despair that he
could never magically go back and undo those difficulties, but he
was doing something about them now, and the recognition of his
control was rewarding and endorsed his pleasure in mastery. He
no longer believed that regressive baby behavior would result in
gratification of his wishes and resolve his frustration.

During the months of playing snakes and ladders, Ludo and
dominoes, Martin gained some insight into what was acceptable
in treatment but unacceptable elsewhere. His brother had accused him of cheating in a game. I explained that he moved his
counter in a way that looked like cheating and that he had to
abide by his brother's rules. Martin became wild, feeling I had
criticized him as his father did. He yelled, "I didn't cheat, I didn't
cheat." He calmed down when I observed that little M. was very
worried about his inadequacies and again we talked about his
need to repeat himself when he felt denigrated, linking this to
his earliest years when he felt no one understood him or his
speech. When he desperately shouted, he drowned my voice,
and also big M.'s voice. Babies couldn't play Ludo and boys of 8
only repeated themselves when they were worried. "Do you
mean I can do what I like with Mrs. Gavshon, because she's
Queen of the people who don't get cross, but I can't do what I
like with Paul and Claudia?"

In Martin's case the developmental line from play to work was
reversed. He had to learn how to play. Although his pleasure in
task completion and problem solving may have been clouded by
his obsessive tenacity, once he had overcome his fear of failure
he enjoyed working, even practicing the piano. He also gained
gratification from his mastery of bodily activities. From being an
adventurous tree climber, he learned how to excel at walking on

a Pogo stick, ride a bicycle responsibly and exploratively, and swim well. While he justifiably baulked at the family marathon walks, he loved climbing challenging mountains and going in chair lifts. He was happy roller skating until even strangers, astounded by his clumsiness, stopped him on the pavement and told him he was not doing it the right way. He was pleased to report that at his new school he climbed with other children, whereas in the beginning he had climbed a parallel tree. It was paradoxical that Martin's strange, awkward body should have become so highly cathected, although his earliest milestones highlighted his pleasure in physical exploration despite his awkward movements.

Martin's fear that his body as well as his mind were damaged made him vehemently deny the smallest ailment. If I commented that he had a cold, he would shout, "I haven't, I haven't," as though I had attacked his very being.

Just before the summer holidays, his mother succumbed, despite her realistic anxiety, to Martin's incessant pleas to let him travel to school alone like his siblings. The journey involved three changes and after many rehearsals he was finally allowed to go alone. He arrived for his session triumphant: "Guess what, the train carried on and I was only a little bit frightened, I had to get off and go back a station." That he had made a mistake, kept his wits together, and mastered the error was as important for Martin as his new-found travel freedom. It also reinforced his belief in therapy.

Like his parents he had fluctuated between apprehension and denial of his problem, but with his sense of self more established he was able to ask the question he had most dreaded: "What is the difference between very handicapped like Lucy, and a little bit handicapped." Martin said very mentally handicapped meant you couldn't read, write, or talk, and he agreed with the suggestion that a little bit handicapped meant you couldn't talk very well but could learn, and we listed the things he had accomplished since therapy started. "When I was 7, little M. was much more than I was. He was everywhere, now he's hardly here at all. He's only there when daddy shouts suddenly. Little Lucy is around a lot of the time; you can see she never had therapy. I think she must have millions of worries."

At this time Martin's right foot had been turning inward and his gait, never good, was extremely lopsided. His parents were concerned that he would spoil their summer walking holiday. They sent him to their physician who, to their consternation, referred them to a neurological department. He was given a series of physical tests (no scan), advised to wear different shoes, and was cheerfully dismissed by the consultant as having "Two left feet."

In treatment when I first noticed it, Martin angrily denied there was anything wrong with his foot. But eventually after repeated interpretations about his omnipotent negation, he was able to say it hurt a little and he sometimes rubbed it. I insisted that he couldn't rub out the worry by pretending nothing was wrong, like he couldn't rub out the worry with a magic eraser about daddy shouting. Facing the problem had helped him get rid of the fear of balloons bursting, the washing machine, circus whip noises, and trying new things. Painful confrontation had also helped him with his speech. Martin confirmed this in characteristic style: "I'm only 9 and tall for my age and I only got a little bit nervous when the train carried me on." Finally he said, "Little M. thinks if he says his foot isn't sore, it will go away. He also thinks if he says it often enough, Mrs. Gavshon will believe him, but he is wrong on both things." His driving wish to appear perfect, strong, and integrated in every way produced great efforts in him to adapt to physical pain in order to sustain his longed-for image of a masculine boy, intact and as good as, if not better than, everyone else.

He reported after the hospital appointment, in a very superior tone, that he had been right, there was nothing wrong with his foot. His father had told the doctor that he came to the Clinic for worries and when the doctor asked Martin what they were, he replied, "About being shy, and not making friends. I didn't tell him the worry about daddy's sudden shouting because that's a secret." When his foot was pronounced "undamaged," Martin was able to understand more about his denial and fear that his therapist, family, and school children would think of him as he thought of himself and reject the wobbly, inadequate boy.

It was far more complicated to help Martin on the developmental line from egocentricity to companionship. He knew that

I regarded his failure to make friends as a serious disturbance. While this helped him to question his ego-syntonic solitary state, it could not produce a genuine wish or need for companionship. The decrease of primary narcissism, selfishness, and ego-centricity was the necessary step for the line toward peer relationships and for Martin the smallest moves were momentous occasions, e.g., the first time he lifted his eyes from his comic when he heard my footsteps across the hall; the first time he said "Hello" to Mary; the first time he said with excited pleasure, "Oh, I forgot to show Anneta my conkers." Martin said he now had only two worries. "The one about daddy shouting unexpectedly, the other being shy to talk to other people." The latter reflected his identification with my attitude, but it did not contain a natural or convincing longing. He listed his infantile definitions of friendship: "A friend is someone who says hello and good-by; a friend is someone who gives you a crisp; a friend is someone who sits next to you." In the course of trying to fathom this incomprehensible concept, Martin became preoccupied with who kissed whom and why, who smiled at whom and why. Once Claudia had been in the back of the car and two ladies in the car behind waved at her; why, he wondered, did they do that? If an old lady asked him to help her across the road, he would refuse because she might smile at him. He didn't like kissing anyone except his parents, but Claudia liked it. "Mummy told me that in the olden days grown-ups kissed all the children on both cheeks, I'm glad I don't live in those days." I reminded him of the time he left the session to go to the lavatory and forgot to return, and of the time when I met him in the street and he treated me like someone he had never seen. Did he think I was only his friend inside the room? What would happen if he saw me on Saturday or Sunday; would he not smile in case I smiled back, tried to touch or kiss him? "Next time I see you in the street I will say hello," he resolved and he did. To show me how hard he was trying, he announced, "I told May about my Easter holiday and that started a conversation. A conversation is different from a chat." When I inquired whether he asked May about her holiday, he replied, "I didn't think of doing that."

The family cat became a barometer of Martin's attempts to risk physical contact. Only in the past months was Martin able to stroke him, and he regarded this as a major achievement which he now extended to stroking other cats. Some happy dreams were about pigeons and mice, who were so tame they ate out of his hand.

He never showed any concern about separations from me. He explained, "I was too busy to think about you." When pressed, he added, "But I did think of things to tell you." I asked whether he knew what missing meant and he said, "Missing means wanting to be with someone who isn't with you."

Before the summer holidays when we were talking about friends, he said, "Saying you want a friend doesn't make it happen. It isn't abracadabra. I'll send you a post card when I go away," and he remembered to do so. But this term when unexpectedly I had to be away for two weeks, he showed no interest or disappointment, and arrived for his first session after my absence happy to give me his news, as though he had seen me the day before. His parents were pleased to report that there had been no collapse during this time.

Recently the analysis has been centered on Martin's conflict over aggressive and sadistic impulses. To be like the big brother he tried so hard to emulate, he had to tease cruelly. However, he was learning from the model I represented that I did not support this "big boy" accomplishment. In a session in which I reminded him that he was worried that I felt about him the way he felt about himself, he thoughtfully replied, "But you don't like me when I tease Lucy or am nasty to Adam and tell him he is stupid," thus showing some awareness of the feelings of others. He has just begun to know the appropriate use of the word "sorry" and to barter a sip of Lucozade for a square of chocolate, but it seems unrealistic to hope this dawning will develop into empathy, consideration, and reciprocity. Perhaps Martin will be able to reach a level of superficial socialization (Weil 1970) despite his deficient personality structure.

The analytic setting was crucial for Martin's progress. It provided a shelter where divergent stimuli were reduced to a minimum. It gave him a framework which even the most caring parents would find difficult to maneuver in a family situation. He never doubted his one-to-one relationship with me, and once he had established I was queen of the people who never got

cross, he "borrowed" my secondary process ideas and used me as
a vehicle for getting stronger. He showed no curiosity about my
life, the lockers in the room, or other patients. He was disin-
terested when occasionally the session was interrupted. He
moved from asking whether I had "children related" to me to
saying, "You must have teen-age children," but these comments
were in connection with a calculation about ages. He trusted our
time together was a secret and had no concern about my interviews with his parents.

There were times when I was swamped and fatigued by his
confusion and also struggled to find a way through the fog.
Therefore I could appreciate the exasperation and helplessness
of his parents, and this was useful in understanding and interpreting the earliest interaction between this atypical child and
the parents' incapacity to make his path easier.

Understanding Martin's material was not a major problem,
but finding a meaningful way to communicate this understanding was. It involved creating a language that would engage him
long enough to make sense. To keep Martin connected I had to
concentrate for us both, think for us both, and speak for us both;
if my investment was not absolute, I would lose him. My intact
psychic apparatus was at his disposal until he was capable of
replacing id processes by ego processes, and could manage without auxiliary ego support. This required inordinate patience.
Having depleted me, he would demand more replenishment to
satisfy his urgent wish to help him grow strong and tall inside.
He taught me to speak slowly, very slowly, in short sentences, as
when he desperately shouted after an interpretation, "Now say
that again, but don't say so much." Interchange was also impeded by his attention span and his slow laborious speech, and during one phase of treatment a severe stammer. It took a long time
for me to know when he was silent whether he was daydreaming,
thinking, or preparing to speak. A pulsating in his neck was
usually the prelude to a sentence. He often said after a painstak-
ingly constructed interpretation, "What did you say, what did
you say?" In addition, Martin's incapacity to make the shift from
concrete to metaphoric thinking hindered the continuity of our
exchanges. Since there was no balance between synthesis and
fragmentation, abstract thinking could not develop. On one oc-

casion when I was relating his speech improvement in the present to the past, I commented that at his nursery school he had not "opened his mouth." Martin said, "But I did open my mouth to eat and drink." It took a long time to explain what I meant and when he finally understood the idiom and was able to use it appropriately, he was proud of his skill. But it did not resolve the inherent problem. When a boy at school admiringly told him he climbed a tree like a monkey, he felt narcissistically abused and it was some time before he accepted that it was a compliment. "My mummy said I swim like a dolphin," he acknowledged with a smile.

Martin's growing strengths, born of his recognition that he could contain his anxiety and was not mad, and only a little bit handicapped, partly influenced but did not resolve his weaknesses. There were times when I found Martin endearing in his struggle to achieve ego control and age-appropriate behavior. This must have been transmitted and understood as approval, thereby enhancing his self-esteem. But my gratification when he had satisfactorily reached a goal matched my despair in the areas where he seemed inaccessible to progress. It is interesting that Martin comprehended the therapeutic process early and formed a treatment alliance despite the fact that object relatedness remained his most significant problem. One cannot predict what changes will occur in adolescence, but the inhibited, isolated child who first came to the Centre 3 years ago is at present a relatively happy boy with a fighting spirit and wider, enriching interests.

DISCUSSION

Martin was a child with ego deficits and a high level of intellectual potential. The combination made his therapy both taxing and rewarding. His lagging ability to integrate and to verbalize could, in part, have been the result of his hearing loss and abnormal speech development which limited communication between himself and his objects. He was unable to identify and label his affects, and this led to a discrepancy between the strength and complexity of his feelings and his modes of expression (A. Katan, 1961).

Since verbalization was not available for the harnessing and mastery of feelings, his ego was repeatedly overwhelmed; his despair and frustration produced regression to primitive behavior which, in turn, brought him into conflict with himself and his environment.

A necessary condition for structural development is the acquisition of language. Martin did not have the equipment to control discharge of affects through thought and verbal expression. The disturbance in his synthetic function, whatever its causes, impeded the interaction between the developing internal agencies both with each other and the external world. His ego was flooded with primitive drive derivatives, and he could not reduce bewilderment and panic to the adaptive form of signal anxiety (Yorke et al., 1980). This left him with a sense of defeat, painful inadequacy, and narcissistic depletion.

The safety of the analytic setting and his use of special opportunities provided by the therapist enabled Martin to learn and practice what he learned. This was coupled with the development of his speech and his capacity to respond to clarification and interpretation. Structuralization was thereby facilitated and led to a broader range of adaptive defenses.

Therapy also provided Martin with a new benign object who took an active role in playing and inventing games. The earliest therapeutic communications were silent, preverbal activities in which the therapist had to guess Martin's feelings reminiscent of the way that parents guess at their child's wishes when they are too young to verbalize them. Martin felt accepted and understood the trial-and-error investment as an indication of being worthwhile. This counteracted his sense of despair both in relation to himself and to the object. Interpretation focused on his fears of humiliation, making it possible for him to experiment with verbalization. By imitating and gradually identifying with the therapist's actions, Martin slowly learned to "act" in play and eventually was able to comprehend the labeling of affects accompanying the activity. Verbalizing perceptions of the external world preceded verbalizing the content of his internal world and this promoted reality testing and ego control over the id impulses (Anna Freud, 1965).

Martin's experience of reciprocity in play—of receiving and

responding, then of mutual giving and taking of actions and ideas—paved the way toward genuine conversation and meaningful interpretation. His capacity to differentiate between self and object was strengthened in his games with the therapist. By learning to take turns he understood who was who, who had what, and what was and was not permitted. It then became possible to try to help him to understand why he was "different" and in this context to define the therapeutic aims.

Verbalization increased for the ego the possibility of distinguishing between wishes and fantasies on the one hand and reality on the other hand. But since Martin did not have this facility, he could not initiate, or respond to, fantasy play as this would threaten his reality appraisal and result in bewilderment and panic. Reality testing could not contradict existing fantasies or his belief in the power of his magic wishes and (annihilating) fears. His inability to form linguistic symbols and metaphors was analogous to his inability to "pretend."

As he was able gradually to master his anxiety, reality testing improved; and finally he was able spontaneously to build a village out of bricks, introduce characters, tell a story, and say with delight, "It's only pretend."

SUMMARY

Martin was a child who, from infancy, lagged in all his developmental milestones. Those difficulties were compounded by intermittent hearing loss and poor speech. His defective synthetic function, his inability to verbalize, and his narcissistic vulnerability made it necessary for his therapist to find preverbal ways of connecting with him in their exclusive one-to-one relationship. While he was easily overwhelmed with anxiety, he also was highly motivated to succeed. He recognized that therapy was a process which could help him reduce tension and strengthen his ego and improve his performance. He had to learn how to master anxiety and to understand his sense of humiliation in order to improve his speech.

As verbalization improved and his practical skills became autonomous, he became less dependent on his therapist for auxiliary ego support. Improvement in reality testing paved the way toward a life enriched by participation with objects and growing pleasure in play.

BIBLIOGRAPHY

EDGCUMBE, R. M. (1981). Toward a developmental line for the acquisition of language. *Psychoanal. Study Child*, 36:71–104.

FREUD, A. (1965). Normality and pathology in childhood. *W.*, 6.

KATAN, A. (1961). Some thoughts about the role of verbalization in early childhood. *Psychoanal. Study Child*, 16:184–188.

GIOVACCHINI, P. L. (1972). Regressed states, timelessness, and ego synthesis. *Psychoanal. Forum*, 4:294–332.

WEIL, A. P. (1953). Certain severe disturbances of ego development in childhood. *Psychoanal. Study Child*, 8:271–287.

———— (1970). The basic core. *Psychoanal. Study Child*, 25:442–460.

YORKE, C., KENNEDY, H., & WISEBERG, S. (1980). Some clinical and theoretical aspects of two developmental lines. In *The Course of Life*, 1:619–637. Washington: U.S. Department of Health and Human Services.

Therapeutic Play in Space and Time

ELIZABETH L. LOEWALD, M.D.

AS WE TREAT YOUNG CHILDREN FOR THEIR PRESENTING SYMPTOMS, a part of their improvement is often a better "location" in time and space. Their movements oftentimes grow more sure, vigorous, and accurately aimed. The size and relative positions of objects and people seem clearer to them; there is less missing and colliding. As to time, there is less sense that it is "too fast" or "too slow" for them as it passes. It loses some capricious and depriving qualities. They know more of what has happened and will happen to them, and when: they are proud of that. How does this happen? By and large we have not focused upon it. Therapist and child have interacted, largely, each in his own time-and-space frame. The adult therapist has his own, habitual, orientational stands. The 2½-year-old patient, for example, has an entirely different method of orienting himself in space, by physical and psychological sightings of his mother. These must be remade at intervals within a certain time frame. The child does not understand our ways of being in time and space. We have only occasional empathic access to his. Still we manage, as parents and educators and children have always coexisted, in this way. The adult therapist may actively teach the child patient something about our accepted time frames. But in large part, the child simply catches up spontaneously, in successful therapy, on the time/space developmental line, as he does on others. As to space, the child's own actively expanding use of space in therapy is vividly apparent.

From the Yale Child Study Center, New Haven, Conn.

Various time/space orientations are characteristic of growing children in a certain sequence, at certain ages and stages of development, as part of the inherent possibilities of the normal child. In the most disturbed young child patients we may see a recapitulation, during treatment, of this entire developmental line. Even in less disturbed children, there is a constant flow of progression and regression in time/space orientation, as various conflicts and arrests are confronted.

What is being recapitulated? A baby begins by sensing, exploring, manipulating the spatial relations of his body to others, and parts of his body to each other. The infant progressively explores space from what is near to him to what is more distant. He discovers his own body from cranial to caudad, face and fingers to belly to toes. Then comes exploration from the seen to what is unseen or remembered; and eventually, from the concretely present to imagined and conceptualized objects in space. As new stages are attained, old methods are also retained and used.

Piaget (1969) has clarified for us the child's developing sense of the sequence of events. The baby's "ideas" of this are at first somatic, evolving from the recurrences of natural rhythms of sleep, hunger, and earlier fetal rhythmic experiences. Gradually, environmental responses and stimuli and experience of delays become included in the apprehension of "time." Sequences and clusters of happenings are noticed, and their different durations. Piaget has shown us how egocentric the child's sense of time remains for several years. The child measures duration by his own sensations of how quickly he is acting, or how long he feels he is staying still. At 4 or 5, he notices the cycles of morning and evening, yesterday and tomorrow. He knows how old he is. But only by 7 or 8, with the attainment of "operational thinking," can he estimate the *relative* ages of two or more people.

Like other developmental lines, the child's unfolding orientation in time and space is heavily influenced by familial and societal orientations. Cultural influence on this line is particularly strong. Our human placement in space and time has always been understood as central to our human functioning and identity. Philosophers, religious leaders, and scientists throughout history have been preoccupied with defining or explaining temporality, and placing us in this universe. Likewise, the impact of a psychotic person's disorientation upon us is particularly, powerfully, disturbing. Though the way stations of development have the same nature and order of succession in every human child, the goal of adult "normality" and comfort in time and space is set differently in different cultures. For example, the Hopi Indian child enters a societal group in which much of what we call "future" is regarded as predestined and unchangeable. That is not "future" as we know it. The language he learns "contains no words, grammatical forms, constructions, or expressions that refer to time or any of its aspects" (Whitrow, 1979, p. 2). His adult "location" in time will be far different from ours in our twentieth-century Western urban life. The duration, importance, and, as it were, the "space taken up" by past cultural and familial events, present endeavors, and future possibilities have a very different cast.

In these statements, the concepts "space" and "time" have already mingled. In ontogeny, they differentiate only gradually from each other in the child's mind. The baby who can now play by bringing his foot to his mouth, moving in space, begins to sense that it "takes time" to bring it there. (And not only the sensations of contracting muscle groups, and visual and tactile sensations, enter into the "time it takes." Also included are his sense of intention, the strength of his satisfaction, and many other things. Many cognitive and emotional factors already interweave with the time/space orientation.) An older child is not only perfecting his logic but disentangling the concepts of space and time when he progresses from believing at age 4 that bigger persons and things are necessarily older, to understanding at age 8 that this is not necessarily so. (Bar, 8 years: "The big ones may be older, but that's not certain because big trees can be old or young. So? We have to know when they were planted.") (Piaget, 1969, p. 236).

We can notice our child patient's "catching up" on many of these time and space differentiations, as treatment progresses. Also reenacted, in condensed form, in therapy, is the extraordinary ongoing perfusion of time/space perceptions into physical and psychological functioning and vice versa. As one function changes, so do the others. The *quality* of conceptualizing and executing motor acts, for example, is greatly affected by our perception of the space in which we operate. Activity level, motility in space, flow and coordination of movement are influenced. Body image is partly determined by what we understand of our place in space, and the distance from us of other important persons. Conversely, developmental stresses for a child may alter temporarily or permanently his sense of time and space. The 2-year-old suddenly separated from parents—thrust out into vast, lonely, and malignant space—is one cogent example.

What we may consider, as therapists, is how we might foster the child's efforts to "locate" himself. Can his "therapeutic play in space" with us be better understood, as a major tool of child therapy? Can the structuring, mastering value of his improving time-and-space placement be encouraged, to help break through impediments on other developmental lines?

Some ideas on this subject have crystallized, for me, around a line of thought developed in other connections by the French philosopher, Gaston Bachelard (1884–1962). I will summarize briefly some of his concepts. Then I will consider the course of one 4-year-old child's therapy, with special attention to his use of time and space.

Gaston Bachelard was a professor of natural sciences, then a professor of philosophy, in the universities of France. Though he retained a primary interest in the philosophy of science and art, he was well versed in the psychoanalytic theory of his time. His book, *The Psychoanalysis of Fire* (1964), first sets out his ideas of the prime importance of imagination in human psychological life. Then in the *Poetics of Space* (1969), he pursues the study of the "phenomenology of the imagination." He sees "image making," revery, as a "major power of human nature"; not simply as sublimated product. "By the swiftness of its actions, the imagination separates us from the past as well as from reality; it faces the future. To the *function of reality,* wise in experience of the past, as it is defined by traditional psychology, should be added a *function of unreality,* which is equally positive . . . any weakness in the function of unreality will hamper the productive psyche. If we cannot imagine, we cannot foresee" (p. xxx).

The exercise of this function, Bachelard believes, occurs in a "felicitous space"—one we've found to be safe and comfortable for its exercise. That is a "space that may be grasped, that may be defended against adverse forces, the space we love" (p. xxxi). It *cannot* be a hostile space. Not only is this safe place necessary to allow the flowering of useful thoughts; but the intimately known space is "seized upon by the imagination" (p. xxxii) and assumes imagined values which enrich and enlarge the person within. This is true whether the felicitous space is the corner of a child's room; a house; a meditation, while studying something; or one's own soul, "as an abode." We need the space to house our memories, and the "things we have forgotten." It can stimulate us to new images.

Many psychoanalytic concepts resonate to Bachelard's approach. We may think of the mother's breast as the first "space that may be grasped." We may translate his words into our language as ideas of omnipotence and its loss, splitting, incorporation, object constancy, separation-individuation, sublimation, and many more.

But I continue with Bachelard's thoughts, which are immediately evocative of common uses children make of the room and of the therapist, in play sessions. Bachelard's ideas might help us to revitalize our concepts and to use them better.

1. People, and animals, have a *primary function of inhabiting*. Feeling comfortable and safe in a space of our own gives us an "immediate sense of well-being." We love that space. As we live our lives, "images of felicitous space" in our minds are necessary to our comfort. We need a "domain of intimacy"; without threat or repellence. Our dreams of defense and aggression come only afterward, as we begin to make contact with the outside world.

2. The house—be it mansion or hut (or, indeed, dollhouse)— shelters our "daydreams." By this word, Bachelard designates our image-making fantasies, by means of which we turn again to the outside and the future. (Our pejorative use of that same word refers more often to the failure we experience in returning to the "outside" with our dream.) The daydreaming is the mind's "function of unreality." With it, we integrate our intentions. He sees human lives, from infancy onward, as proceeding in a dialectic between being "home" and "away from home." We go home, collect, and form images brought from our activity outside. (Bachelard evokes the sense of what we do there by describ-

ing the feeling of being snug in a house during a snowstorm. There is a diminished sense of the outside world and an increased quantity of intimate data within.) Then we go out again. Thus we live in alternating security and adventure. "A creature that withdraws into its shell is preparing a way out."

3. As children, we learn about space from our house. It is an instrument of "topoanalysis." It is geometric. We learn vertical/horizontal, inside/outside, secret/open, from it—as a gradual extension of infantile learning from our own and our mother's bodies. And all this cognitive and spatial learning takes on meaning in the "inner plane" very early. Bachelard points out that the "attic" and the "basement" have atmospheres, values, bodily and spiritual analogues, which gradually accrue. As we grow, "simple geometry becomes tinged."

Though his own work was not child related, Bachelard intuited and spoke many of the insights we express differently as the interweaving and mutual influence of developmental lines. He recognized what we know as developmental stresses and arrests. For example, he remarks on how sharp a dialectic "outside and inside" is, for small children: almost, he says, as sharp as "yes and no," which "decides everything." "Unless one is careful," he says, children may even use these polar opposites as a basis for images that govern *all* thoughts of positive and negative.

4. Our space *is* ourselves. "I am the space where I am." Bachelard sees daydreaming as "inner immensity." It is the link between "full and empty." This is an interesting idea for clinicians. Children negotiating separation-individuation, and adult patients with narcissistic disorders, struggle most especially against experiencing emptiness. When separated in space or thought from loved objects, they are often less successful than the snails and rabbits Bachelard describes—in their shells and holes, where a "living creature fills an empty space." The normal child, of course, has growing awareness of his power to recapture "fullness" in thought and imagery. That will be essential to his stable sense of identity. It can well be thought of as being able to "fill the inner space."

Bachelard remarks on children's great interest in "large and small." Their hopefulness about their own future powers is maintained in seeing that in nature "large comes from small." In the story, the oak is said to come from the acorn. Also, looking at small things is restful, pleasant. And "small is the center of decision." Tom Thumb can dominate much larger people. Here again Bachelard is speaking of what we express as the adaptive interweaving of cognitive and psychosexual progress, as our child patients develop toward health.

Many interesting subjects are raised in the *Poetics of Space* which can enrich our play therapy. Bachelard considers nooks and crannies seriously. He remarks on the human orientation toward what is secret. What is hidden behind locks, in small spaces, in boxes nested within each other, is most valuable. "There will always be more things in a closed than in an open box" (1969, p. 88). Piaget (1969) has explained the cognitive stages of the child's understanding of that matter. Bachelard reminds us of the deep persistence of early childhood attitudes in all of us. Those are some of our vital links with the children we treat.

5. To "change space" is psychically innovating. By leaving the "space of our usual sensibilities, we change our nature." We become different, as the caterpillar is changed in becoming a butterfly; as the convalescent is changed, when at last he is allowed to go outdoors.

6. When two persons' "daydreams"—two diverse "images"—meet, they strengthen each other. In fact, in their convergence, the images of each person lose their "gratuitousness" and gain more weight of meaning. As Bachelard sees it, then the free play of the imagination ceases to be "a form of anarchy."

He makes these last two points, 5 and 6, in regard to poetry and the effect of the poet's images upon the reader's images. They seem equally applicable to the effect of our "therapeutic space" upon the child, and of the interplay of patient's and therapist's images in that space.

CASE PRESENTATION

COURSE OF TREATMENT

Paul was brought for consultation at age 4½ because after a year and a half in nursery school he still did not mingle with his classmates. He appeared unhappy there. This was in contrast to his comfortable boyish play and talk at home with his 7-year-old brother and the brother's friends. He also chatted intelligently with his nursery school teachers and with teen-age girl baby-sitters, but he steadily avoided his age peers at home and school. He imitated his older brother constantly. Whatever Mark preferred was what Paul valued. He seemed generally accepting of his 2-year-old sister Margaret, but little involved with her. During her infancy, Paul had alarmed his parents by wanting to wear Margaret's clothes and be "pretty" himself. But they had effected a "cure" of this by buying him Superman underwear and teaching him to be "proud of his penis." His lack of 4-year-old social skills clearly made them very anxious.

Paul's was an academic family. His young professor father was intellectually outstanding, as well as socially affable, a family man, and especially keen on his boys' athletic progress, though he was not an athlete himself. His mother, a small, tense and intense woman, said her fondest wish was to mother a brood of happy children. She "retired" from intellectual pursuits after earning a Ph.D., to begin her family. She remembered her own childhood as miserable. Her father was a successful, unempathic professional man, whom she spoke of with dislike and contempt. He had had several periods of psychotic depression, during her adolescent and adult life. At these times he "collapsed" and required the total absorption and care of his wife. Their home life was bleak. Her own sister "never talked for years."

Paul's early history and development were normal. He had no serious illnesses, no intense fears, temper tantrums, etc. He did have a picky appetite, and was very small and thin, like his mother. She regretted his self-weaning at 7 months: she had enjoyed breast feeding immensely. The parents had noticed Paul hitting himself in the stomach, hard, when he made mistakes of any kind, from the age of 4. They also thought him excessively modest about his toileting and about showing his body.

My initial evaluation showed Paul to be age-appropriate or superior in all developmental areas—with special precociousness in language. His play was very serious and self-contained. He wanted only to make models, or play board games. Fantasy play was inhibited. At nursery school where I observed him, he was aloof and solitary, and engaged alone in intense fantasy play about space ships—to my surprise. He talked only to teachers. I did observe him very surreptitiously stealing away the play materials of a little girl—then pretending to be solicitous.

I recommended that Paul continue at nursery school rather than begin kindergarten; and I made a few other suggestions for more comfort at home. He did, over the next 6 to 8 months, become more outgoing and active in nursery school. At home, however, he engaged in a more and more focused "passive-aggressive battle," as his mother put it, with her. He drooped around the house, would not dress himself, picked at his food, would not play by himself or with others, and was bored. His extreme attachment to his brother had paled, but he seemed to have nothing or no one to put in his place. He would not play ball. He would not play at the beach or on vacation. He often "collapsed" when confronted with expectations. This distressed and angered both parents, His mother described the fury she felt, daily, when he "won't admit he enjoys *anything!*"

We began a course of twice-a-week individual play therapy for Paul, for 1½ years; along with counseling meetings with his parents every 2 to 3 weeks.

Paul's behavior at home, school, and in the neighborhood gradually became more zestful and age-appropriate. His appetite and self-care improved. He was willing to play ball, and to learn to swim. His range of interests and conversation became richer. "He's living in the moment for the first time," said his mother in a relaxed moment. But the relationship of mother and son remained very difficult. Even when he was lively and happy in his father's company, he continued to maintain to *her* afterward that he had been miserable. And in our parent consultations, it became more and more obvious that the mother did not wish to see the improvement in Paul that the father documented. With increasing tension and anger, the mother at last returned to the psychoanalytic treatment she had ended some years before. She reported that she was now reliving there her fury at her own parents—and realizing how similar were her feelings toward Paul.

After a year of our treatment, mother's father died suddenly. The family traveled to his funeral—and this was the occasion (unexpected to all of them) for mother and all the children to feel closer to grandmother. Paul especially demonstrated a responsible and caring and intelligent mien which very much pleased his parents. His personal growth after this time was noticeable. He was in kindergarten doing well. He made some friends, and learned various new skills. At home, he was a buddy of his father and a vigorous competitor of his brother. Only his manner remained somewhat aloof and serious and watchful, in general.

By the end of our therapy, Paul's mother still often openly disliked Paul. Especially in the termination phase, she could speak of him as "defective, sadistic, unloving." However, the two coexisted somewhat more comfortably. And Paul seemed to maintain a better opinion of himself. His play with me—which had initially been very controlling and sadistic—had become much less so. In our last weeks together, he reverted to his controlling mode. But at the actual ending of therapy, he was able to be warm, and even sad—and also to talk with me seriously *and* boyishly about the fine things he was "going to do."

THE USE OF SPACE AND TIME

Paul presented as a small, neat, quiet, watchful, well-modulated, constricted, 4-year-old boy. In evaluation and through our first four therapy sessions, he would sit quietly in one place in a small chair. He set himself one after another impossible task: making a complicated ship model, or playing chess, as his father and older brother liked to do. It was dogged and depressing, though he hurried in purposefully each time. I began to notice, however, a small increase in the aggressive force of his blows with the hammer on the wood—and the sawdust began to fly more wildly from his saw. There was sometimes a hint of pleasure in his eye. Then at the fifth session, Paul ran across the room, took up a bear hand puppet, gave me a fox puppet and his bear bit, and killed the fox. He was off on a total use of our playroom and its contents which continued at this level for many months. At each session he was the invincible and evil-minded bear. He had many slaves: animal puppets and robots. The persons I was assigned to be were always hunted and killed. With agility, Paul ran to every corner of the room to head me off. He climbed to the top shelf to reach the globe I keep there, showed me the snowy mountains in which I could *try* to hide—then shook me off into the Pacific Ocean where I drowned. His "top power gun" killed every living thing in the room, to his grim enjoyment. I asked him why the bear was so mean. "Because somebody was mean to him. Then he shot a fox, and he liked the feeling, he decided to kill more and more. He's *glad* of it!" In answer to my next question, he assured me that the bear is "*never* lonely."

It was spelled out for me in a hundred ways, in my assigned roles: what total lack of personal space can mean. My hiding places were known to him. When I thought of new strategies to escape or attack, he took them over. I could have no secrets. He kept *all* good things for himself. He even had a corner on all the "good colors." The blue rays of his space ship could enter my soldiers' minds and confuse them and "make them fight each other." He offered me small vistas of hope; for example, at the end of a session, the bear *could* be killed by being shot in the left ear. But next time he would immediately kill my fox, "because the bear has a secret shield, he hears your plans."

Paul usually sat in the waiting room glumly with his mother and his sunny sister, before these sessions. He was silent and still, with a lax, babyish face. Afterward, he emerged with a little more buoyancy, but with scant hint of the vigor of what he had been doing.

Our own relationship was a curious one. This play was clearly serious "work." For several months I could not feel that Paul had any personal investment in pleasing me, sharing with me, or even in tormenting me. I was a work partner. Throughout, he was always careful not to break things, and not to collide with me despite all the dashing about. Gradually, we began to have what I would call a workaday *familiar* relationship. Paul would ask me amiably for help in dividing up the puppets (so that he could kill mine, a moment later). He asked my aid in dressing up in a "bear cape." As an aside, he would finally agree with me that *some* of my men should survive just so there would *be* a next time. Also, there began to be moments of play in which his aggression did frighten him. I was allowed to point out to him that he would feel better if he went to the bathroom, when he was frantic; or to reassure him that next time the murdered puppet would be quite all right again. Around this time, he sometimes looked at me briefly with warm, smiling eyes. Once he came in companionably and started singing. After 3 months of treatment, he volunteered an "outside" fact of his daily life for the first time: he had been to a picnic and he told me what he had eaten. To be sure, this was in the context of play he was directing, in which my man was to be killed by eating a poisoned apple. A second instance of Paul's volunteering outside information came after 4 months. He mentioned that it was his father's birthday. He told me just how old his father was now, how old he had been a year ago, and where exactly in the house (drawing a picture) he had hidden his father's present.

During these months, Paul's parents were reporting that he was a little less negative, and less prone to "collapse" when they expected him to conform at home. But he still would never tell his mother when he had enjoyed anything.

Over the next few months, up until the summer vacation, Paul continued to play vigorously, using every part of the room each time, and almost every toy available. This did not feel chaotic or overhurried. It seemed rather that Paul needed to make meaningful contact with every material in the room—use it, incorporate it in his fantasy, under his control, and become comfortable with it. For example, he found the spare paint bottles on an upper shelf. He brought them down to be weapons of the bear, handling the bottles carefully and never spilling. The red paint was "lethal": the bear, as "Dr. M.D." now, could put just a speck of it on people and kill them.

He brought out toy horses from a corner. First, one horse was changed into another by the bear, with his "color magic": much as the horses pleaded to keep their own identities. But in ensuing sessions, we began to have contests that were zestful and fun—galloping all over the room with his bear on one horse and my wolf on the other. Drum and xylophone salutes were added, to honor the winners. Also, later, the "changing" of horses by the bear was used in other ways by Paul. Boy horses were mysteriously changed to men or mother horses—girls to mothers or boys—and back again. We discussed how they felt about all that. It is interesting that at home, Paul and his mother's relationship was especially tense and angry at this time. His mother in fact returned to her psychoanalysis then. One day in Paul's play, he used not horses but human dolls. The kids were changed into adults, and vice versa. The children were now the parents—and they refused to change back, despite the parents' pleadings. The new "children" were sent to their rooms and told to stay there!

Paul's vacation at the seashore came earlier than my vacation. By his and his parents' account, he enjoyed the swimming and the water and sand—in contrast to his droopy negativism on previous vacations. He told me in words, at greater length than ever before, what he had done. This led to thoughts about time and age: he reminisced about being at the shore "before Margaret was born." He was proud of how late he had stayed up, and described the dark night and the moon. Then we pretended swimming and diving, with the puppets, from one corner of the room to the opposite wall, for a few sessions.

As my vacation approached, however, themes were the opposite of expansive. The bear glued all my people to their seats, and forced them to drink nasty drinks, and "rearranged their minds." Or he captured and cooked my puppets and ate them. And my puppets were forced to eat their friends and to *like* eating them. I asked the bear why. "I get angry when I'm empty. But eating people makes me not empty."

Paul started kindergarten after the summer. This last year of therapy began with the bear killing or dominating others sadistically as usual. Paul looked anxious—and was sometimes rougher with the dolls and puppets than he had ever been. Then little by little, themes and problems from his life outside of therapy were brought into the bear play. I will divide these into their general themes, for clarity, though of course they came and went many times as the sessions proceeded.

The bear ran a school for a few months; he stopped doing so a few months later, about when Paul himself was reportedly well settled in school. The bear posed arithmetic problems to dolls tied at their desks: such as, "50 + 50 + Imbecile + 1000 = what." Puppets were put in rocket ships and sent to outer space, as punishment for dumbness. A puppet tried to do arithmetic with his feet, but "That's not right!" said the bear. "And you can't think out a problem, you have to know!" My fox kept being sent into orbit around the top of the room, by the schoolmaster. Some boys went up in their planes to save him, but they couldn't.

Then Paul remarked one day, "School is good." He sometimes told me about the assemblies, and sang some of the school songs for me. This led to discussions about the World Series, Hallowe'en, Passover, and so forth, with comparisons he made between various years of his life, and times of the year. Fantasy school play largely disappeared, but we could *talk* about school sometimes.

Paul's relations with his father and brother grew warmer. His increasing athletic skills, and his decreased fearfulness, allowed his bond with them to flourish in a newly "manly" way. The World Series and the Olympic Games—both watched avidly on TV by the male members of the family—entered the bear play. In the beginning this consisted of Paul's animals and dolls jumping and swimming and batting balls with incredible speed and distance: again the whole room was used. Over the days, a careful setting up of the scene, and the rules, evolved, and the action became more circumscribed. Paul made one especially interesting use of this play. I was asked several times to play a Russian athlete who *thought* he was just great, but really was clumsy and stupid. In the interests, it seems, of world peace and personal ethics, Paul's American athletes were very kind to me, and never jeered at my stupidity (though they giggled audibly at me). In fact, they sometimes let me *think* I was winning.

Meanwhile at home, Paul's relations with his mother varied from testy, mutual anger to some glimpses of humor and pleasure. Now Paul made a move. He developed a nighttime routine with his mother involving a stuffed animal named Foxy. Foxy talked baby talk, and wanted to be fed, and tucked in. However, he would be "nice and nasty." Paul explained to me, it's a fox's job to hunt, and to eat chicken eggs. "She has to lay them, and he has to eat them." Paul's mother was required to feed Foxy every night, to talk to him, and to tuck him and Paul in. She said she was delighted with all this—since it was the most intimacy Paul had allowed her for a long time, and she'd always wanted him to be a "cuddly boy." They both were aware of the controlling aspects of this play. Yet it seemed to work for both, as a rapprochement scenario tailored to *them*—and one could see a teasing closeness developing between them at times.

Paul brought Foxy to his sessions with me after awhile. Foxy ate the eggs of my chicken puppet, over and over, with great excitement. Then Paul began to arrive for his hour with a clothes basket full of *all* his stuffed animals from home. Often he announced he was tired, as he entered the outer door, and his mother had to carry the basket into the waiting room. I finally encouraged mother to revolt about this. But meanwhile, all Paul's home animals had come in and met and fought with and had adventures with all our office animals. Remember Bachelard's words: "To change space is psychically innovating."

Paul took up many developmental tasks in our play, and usually in fantasy play in which spatial relations figured large. For example, his fascination with toileting and with sexual bodily differences was first expressed in play in which we built a tinkertoy telescope at one end of the room—and the children dolls peered through it, through a bathroom window, at a lady doll going to the bathroom in a three-story apartment building at the other end of the room. The children all got arrested by a chicken. In ensuing hours, the theme became more focused. A girl doll was winning all the broad jumps at the Olympics. I said, "That's unusual, you boys usually win." He told me this girl has a penis. When I doubted that, he said loudly, "Yes! She pees standing up!"

Another space example contained some of Paul's puzzlings about aggression. A wolf, in a spaceship, zoomed from planet to planet all over our room, eating and biting and beheading creatures wherever he landed. Then some good guys came in a large spaceship, and simply *told* the wolf that he was the weakest creature in the world. He was only made of tinfoil! The wolf was crushed. Then, generously, the men allowed the wolf to get a little stronger by eating healthy foods.

I described earlier the workaday relationship between Paul and me in the first 6 months of treatment. During the following year, it developed more facets. A certain seriousness about the therapy was always our tone together. Once I asked Paul why he came here, and he said, "It helps." Also, though we played together in many moods, he always made clear his wish for a say about his privacy. He would admit me voluntarily or not at all. In play, one day, we were companionable spacemen in a rocket over Mars, eating dinner. Then we went to separate rooms in the rocket and read books.

We played board games again and cards; and Paul struggled against his impulse to cheat. At the same time, I had become important to him. He touched me or leaned against me, sometimes, quite naturally. In the later months, he prattled on about his doings, "like a regular kid," as his parents now described him. When I missed a session, or especially when we talked of ending, he turned again into the sadistic cold-hearted bear.

An especially meaningful period of the therapy centered on our using a rock-polishing machine. This seems to me a good example of Bachelard's thesis that when two people's daydreams or "images" meet, they strengthen each other. Then "the free play of the imagination ceases to be a form of anarchy."

Paul had taken to bringing to sessions, to show me, little rocks he had picked up on a path to and from school. He would pull from his pockets a few green or red or striped rocklets he thought special. He would point out their color and form. I remembered I had a small rock-polishing machine at home; and he thought he would like to polish some of these. The polishing process took several weeks: ten minutes or so at the beginning of each session. The polisher would run, in the closet, from one session to the next—then we would take out the stones, wash them, put them into finer and finer grit each time, and repolish them. Paul loved this. He would finger the various grits and powders, run his hand over the stones, or put them to his cheek or my cheek to judge the smoothness. He would divide them into groups by color, or lines, or shape; discourse (rather fantastically) on just how old he judged each to be; and so on. The beauty which emerged from the dingy rocks pleased him. The mixture of sensory and cognitive elements in the experience seemed very comfortable.

Paul talked about the age of the rocks. His general interest in time frames had become much greater this year—with a particular spurt after the death of his grandfather. Paul returned from the funeral with some sadness and anxiety: for weeks remarks that reflected his worry about where his grandfather had disappeared to. But he also had a new interest in the generations of his extended family, many of whom he had just met. We drew a diagram of aunts and uncles and cousins, and who was older. (His mother's new tolerance and recognition of her own widowed mother, which I remarked on earlier, I think had something to do with this.) He talked about the different seasons, and what one did in them. He became an expert on time, and asked for a watch. One day he began our session with, "You kept me waiting 2½ minutes!" He himself had made a plane trip. When I went for a long weekend to California, he told me it was *foolish* to go millions of miles for just three days, it costs too much!

DISCUSSION

Following Bachelard, I shall use this material as a "contained space" in which to sort through potentially useful thoughts, then venture forth again into the clinical work. The "change of space" may be psychically innovative.

Paul's therapeutic course illustrates many of Bachelard's concepts. And for me, these illuminate that therapy. Paul seemed to test the literal and emotional space of the therapy, in our first sessions; then finding it safe enough, his vigorous wish to use it for "image-making" erupted. He brought to it everything and everyone important to him. He filled our space with objects and thoughts, and grew less lonely. (He had said, as the bear, "I get angry when I'm empty.") From images and feelings in the sessions, he concocted strategies for managing in his outside world. (For example, he renewed contact with his mother at home through the bedtime ritual with Foxy, using the stuffed animals at home like the puppets in the playroom, for expression and protection and negotiation. Then he reinforced the strategy by bringing Foxy to the "safe place" of therapy.) He used the playroom for "topoanalysis": wide and narrow, far and near, inside and outside, large and small were investigated in ways he had not previously allowed himself, at home or school. Now he also permitted these dimensions to become "tinged" with meanings on the "inner plane," as Bachelard says. Our cozy enclosure in the spaceship together, reading our books in adjoining but separate rooms of the capsule, while orbiting in outer space, was an experience of comfortably chosen spatial relations and the emotional tone which accompanies them. Paul used the "changing of space" to innovate, to change his own perceptions, his "own nature," when, for example, he hit upon the idea of investigating the female body in our play by peering at a female doll through a Tinkertoy telescope, through a window in a tall building, and with a puppet chicken standing by to arrest him for so doing. He clearly used the convergence of our mutual interest in rocks, colors, and textures, during our rock polishing, to deepen his own satisfaction. It gained more weight of meaning.

Paul's increasingly sure and mature location in space and time was one benefit of his progress in therapy. He did become more comfortable in action in space, in his daily life—in playing ball, swimming, skating, traveling, walking, and running vigorously. The "spatial" difficulties he particularly tried to master, in our sessions, seemed central to his difficult relation with his mother. One could be glued to a chair forever, immobilized, forced to eat terrible things, by the evil invincible bear. Or one could be sent forever, alone, into orbit in outer space, by a capricious cruel schoolmaster, for not knowing some small thing. Both he and his mother were that schoolmaster, that bear. But the danger of mutual aggressions seemed to become more manageable for Paul, when he found some safe, well-surveyed space for himself within the therapy. Mother's return to her analysis undoubtedly did the same for her. The way opened for both, to make some movements toward and away from each other without becoming glued in paralyzing rage, or catapulted alone into space.

Also, while Paul had an age-appropriate cognitive understanding of "time" even at the start of therapy, his interest in his time location rose rapidly in later months. He wanted a watch. He commented on the duration of the time he spent waiting. The ages of his relatives intrigued him, as did the recurrence of seasons and holidays and their associated meanings and feelings. Some glimpses during treatment of Paul's relationship to his little sister seemed to indicate elements of his progress along the developmental "time line." As he sat glumly in the waiting room with his mother and lively Margaret, in the first months of treatment, his flaccid babyish mouth and his low activity seemed to erase any age advantage he held over his sister. The idea of his being older, "farther along," seemed not to have occurred to him. But late in the therapy, he discussed his activities on vacation at the beach, comparing them to what he had done there "before Margaret was born." That is "operational thinking" as Piaget (1969) defines it: the ability to keep in mind and compare two or more sequences of events. And gradually, Paul seemed to *own* more of his own history.

Each of these examples of Paul's perceptions of space and time speaks, moreover, to the rich interconnections of developmental lines. His motor competence and range increased, in daily life, as he found a safe space for its exercise in treatment. His motor competence was, in turn, used to explore Arctic snows and outer space, in our playroom. He manipulated and mastered them and their associated feelings; thence, perhaps, to "explore" toward a closer relationship in the new bedtime ritual with his mother. His psychosexual development proceeded apace through play experiments: outdoing girls in the Olympic games; spying on them through telescopes; being changed into them, and back again, by the all-powerful bear. At the same time, he was becoming aware of his precedence in *time* over his sister Margaret. And he was bonding more proudly, at home, with his father and his brother, in the context of his increasing skill at skating and playing baseball, and daring to swim.

These rich interconnections are largely beyond our understanding. Nevertheless, we do know that a healing, developmentally promoting effect will occur in many psychological sectors in a young child, if his family can be helped to allow his growth; and if he can be encouraged to progress along even one developmental line. Our availability to him as transference objects and as new objects, and our interpretations, promote this. It is also the thesis of this paper that the child has a great capacity and urge to use the therapeutic space. There he can collect and sort the intimate data central to his conflicts. We can contribute images, ideas, to match and contrast with his. In the protected space, he can play with all of these, and gain confidence in those he chooses as reliable "meanings" about his world.

BIBLIOGRAPHY

BACHELARD, G. (1969). *The Poetics of Space.* Boston: Beacon Press.
———— (1964). *The Psychoanalysis of Fire.* Boston: Beacon Press.
FREUD, A. (1965). Normality and pathology in childhood. *W.,* 6.
PIAGET, J. (1969). *The Child's Conception of Time.* New York: Ballantine Books.
WHITROW, G. J. (1979). Introduction. *Time and the Sciences.* Paris: United Nations Educational, Scientific, and Cultural Organization.

Play and Reality

MORTIMER OSTOW, M.D.

THE OXFORD ENGLISH DICTIONARY DEDICATES FIVE PAGES TO DEFI-
nitions of "play," as a substantive and as a verb. The primary
significance as a noun is given as: "Exercise, brisk or free movement or action." As a verb the emphasis is on exercise or energetic movement. My own sense of the word, based upon its usage, is
that it implies freedom from restraint, as in such expressions as:
"The phonograph record is playing," or "There is too much play
in the steering wheel." With respect to children's play, or play as
a synonym for drama, the freedom is a freedom from the constraints of reality, established, for the moment, by transition into
the world of make-believe.

Play may be free in any of a number of ways. Playful thinking
may be freed from the restrictions of logic, compliance with
reality, and thereby become fantasy. Games are transactions between two or more individuals who are freed of the many considerations that ordinarily impinge upon interactions among
them, and are limited to one or a few prescribed and permitted
procedures. The author of a drama starts with a given situation
and can make it turn out any way he wishes.

In the playing of games, however, there are indeed constraints
in the form of rules, without which there would be no game.
That is true, but the rules still offer a relative freedom from the
restraints to activity or to a two-person encounter in the real
world. Playing the game, the participants agree that they will be
constrained only by these considerations. Similarly, although
theoretically the dramatist is free to express whatever fantasy he

Attending psychiatrist at Montefiore Medical Center; President of the Psychoanalytic Research and Development Fund, and Sandrow Visiting Professor
of Pastoral Psychiatry at the Jewish Theological Seminary of America.

chooses, unless he satisfies some need in his audience, that is, unless he complies with some rules, he will not be heard.

The definition would be incomplete without taking into account another freedom—freedom from expectable consequences. Play is an activity that is enjoyed for the moment; after it is over, nothing that has happened is to carry over into the real world. The child who is playing is expected to do no damage to the furniture in his room or to his playmates. Activity that damages is no longer considered play. The child learns these rules from adult caretakers as soon as he starts active play that impinges on others. During a two-person or team game, it matters very much who wins, but after the game, it is understood that there are to be no enduring consequences. The loser who remains resentful and angry after the game and the winner who humbles his antagonist are considered "bad sports."

On reflection it becomes clear, however, that in fact few games have no enduring consequences, and much individual play takes cognizance of, and responds to, aspects of reality. A person skillful in a game may achieve renown by virtue of his skill, with consequent improvement in social status, access to partners for romance, and business opportunities. An individual engaged in solitary recreational activity, reading or watching a performance, may be influenced in political or social views, or even in his or her affectionate relations.

Although play is, in the first instance, distinguished from nonplay by virtue of its unrealistic and inconsequential nature, the spice of play is contributed by whatever reality factors are invoked. A game becomes more exciting if there is even a small reward to the victor, or a prize for the winner of a contest. A novel or a drama becomes more engrossing if the reader or viewer recognizes himself in a character and identifies with that character in his fictional experiences. The historical novel, the roman à cléf, the drama that portrays the human situation— these are all more compelling than the fantasy in which no aspect of life can be recognized. In fact one can list a number of human activities in which it is difficult to sort out the play from the serious elements, for example, social activities, sports, sexual relations, and humor.

A playful attitude, which I should like to distinguish from readiness to play, can be considered the converse of play. The fully engaged player disengages himself from reality, enjoys the disengagement, but obtains even greater pleasure by reintroducing a small amount of reality. The playful attitude on the other hand (and here I am not using playful in the sense of the readiness of play) takes full cognizance of reality but, by treating it as if it were a joke, attenuates, to some degree, its accompanying pain or stress. The tendency to play and the tendency to be playful are not necessarily correlated.

THE PSYCHODYNAMICS OF PLAY

Let us look at some clinical examples of pathological play, or rather, play used in a pathological way.

Mr. A., an intelligent professional, oscillates between two states of mind: in the one, he is depressed and scarcely able to fulfill his professional duties and family obligations because of his depression; in the other, he is usually hypomanic. But in this state, too, he is unable to engage reality, and so he busies himself in a driven way with one or another form of pleasure-seeking such as promiscuity, heterosexual or homosexual, growing plants, playing music. Again, both his professional life and his family suffer.

Here the motivation for play is provided by the patient's need to distance himself from reality's demands upon him, which he feels he cannot satisfy, and from reality's frustration of his unconscious needs. The erotic, aesthetic, and activity pleasures can be considered a kind of "secondary gain."

In a state of melancholic depression, a patient, if he is not psychotic, is tied not only to reality, but to an intransigent view of reality, to an unyielding, irresistible, constricting reality. If play means first of all retreat from reality, it cannot be invoked in a state of depression, and to a large extent neither can any of the partial play activities to which I referred above, namely, social activities, sports, sexual relations, and humor.

Mr. B., in his 30s, had changed his name and occupation several times. He came to treatment asking himself, "Who am I?" and "What will I be when I grow up?" There were many features of the classic impostor personality. He had left school before completing his education and traveled around the world, inviting adventure, and supporting himself by his cleverness. Because he was brilliant and personable, he could earn relatively large sums of money with little effort. Whenever he received payment of any size, he spent it on frivolous self-indulgences, giving little thought to how it would be replaced, and he attached little importance to establishing a steady stream of income. When he married, he and his wife spent many hours each day playing games of all kinds, traveling abroad together, and conversing. Their mutual play was interrupted only briefly to permit Mr. B. to do another job when the money ran out.

Life for Mr. B. was not serious. He was cynical about people and the world. Although he enjoyed the acclaim and success he attained by his business activities, when he found a similarly minded wife, he retreated with her into a mutual, playful isolation. Analysis revealed that behind the behavior lay a profoundly low self-esteem: he felt unequipped to deal with the world, treated his contact with it nonseriously, and retreated from it into compulsive play.

Mrs. C., in her 70s, presented a series of dreams during her depression, all of which portrayed her as playing enjoyably with small children. She had left school at age 16 without evident reason, had done very little remunerative work, and in recent years had engaged herself principally in gardening, flower arranging, and painting. She had tutored children for a while in a public school. She had very much enjoyed puzzles and humorous word play. She took little interest in the realities of life, but she had fulfilled her family obligations properly and engaged seriously in philanthropic activities.

This case demonstrates that the inner reality of depressive anguish, when it is not too severe, may prevent actual play but need not obliterate the wish to be able to play—a kind of expression of hope.

Motivation for Play

Among children we can recognize normal play as a preparation for the assumption of the responsibilities of the next phase of development. Here it serves a progressive function. As analysts we also recognize that the child may attempt to play in order to repeat and perhaps find a solution for inner problems that cause distress. The play is regressive, though the hope, usually unfulfilled, is for relief.

In the case vignettes I have cited, I would infer that the motivation for play in adults resides in two complementary qualities. First, play effects a disengagement from the world of frustration and disappointment, a world whose requirements the individual must strain to meet, at the cost of some discomfort. That disengagement permits a reduction of tension, effort, vigilance, and distress, and a partial replacement of these by a lesser degree of effort, usually in a different type of activity, in which a frustrated need achieves illusory gratification. Play that requires the exercise of the same faculties that are employed in one's work is disparaged as a "busman's holiday." Play can also provide surcease from discomfort and anguish arising internally, as in the case of Mrs. C.; or though internally generated, nevertheless projected outward, as in the case of Mr. B. Second, play encourages the enjoyment of the exercise of physical and mental faculties, a functional pleasure. Play offers relief from sustained and mildly distressing effort, or from inner anguish, or frustration; it also affords the pleasure of engaging in alternate and enjoyable activities.

Mrs. D., a mother who had worked as soon as her children were old enough to permit her to leave the house, led a seemingly normal life: a good marriage, a wholesome family, comfortable involvement in community activities, and adequate and skillful engagement in recreational play with friends as well as with her husband and children. She came for treatment after a severe anxiety attack. During a prolonged analysis, she seemingly flourished. She acquired full professional training and functioned well in her new profession. She became less angry, envious, and erratic; but she continued to be plagued by frequently recurring episodes of fairly severe hypochondriacal anxiety and by expectations of being fired by her employer and rejected by her friends.

During one analytic session, I observed that several times she left her eyeglasses lying next to her on the couch in such a way that they were not easily visible to her, or she managed to brush them off onto the floor. Each time she missed them, or heard them fall, she gasped and momentarily seemed panicky, until she reassured herself that they were not lost or broken.

It seemed to me that she was playing a game with the glasses, deliberately provoking immoderate anxiety for brief periods. I called her attention to this behavior and compared it to her apparently spontaneous episodes of hypochondriacal anxiety and her unjustified fears of criticism and rejection. These too were self-generated, I suggested, for the purpose of providing her with the thrill of the anxiety and the gratification of being able to overcome it, much as small children make themselves dizzy to the point of falling, by turning themselves around and around. She told me that she had done that often as a child, and over the next few days was able to confirm that she found herself initiating the episodes of anxiety.

One could argue that the analytic procedure, from a patient's point of view, can be compared to play, in the sense that nothing that the patient says is to have any "real" consequence for him. For the duration of the session, he lives in a make-believe world, in which he is not held responsible morally for anything he says and his fantasies and dreams are taken seriously. In fact, the transference relation is often symbolized in dreams as a game between the patient and another player.

Even within the analytic session, however, Mrs. D.'s adventures with her glasses can only be described as play. She enjoyed her sessions and felt relatively well protected in them from the harsh judgments of the outside world. But the play with the glasses deliberately induced discomfort, and in subsequent sessions we were able to see under what circumstances she undertook it. Thoughts about fatal illness or accident or about criticism and rejection could not be treated as fantasy; by attributing reality to them, she started the generation of anxiety or despair which then acquired its own momentum and escaped her voluntary control.

We may recognize in Mrs. D.'s glasses game and in her self-induced bouts of anxiety an example of reintroducing reality into play. In the glasses game, the threat of loss is immediately canceled when they are retrieved and the game is concluded, evidently with some pleasure. But in the case of the more serious threats, illness, dismissal, and rejection, the possibility cannot be eliminated for the moment, and anxiety rapidly intensifies.

What is the "reality" that is introduced? It is the prospect of realistic injury. The situation can be compared to gambling. The individual who plays cards for token stakes, or bets trivial amounts on horse races, is making his play more interesting by adding the possibility of a small gain or a small loss. The individual, on the other hand, who plays for stakes that represent his entire fortune or more, is introducing the realistic possibility of becoming either wealthy or really impoverished. Whichever the outcome, the affective response may be overwhelming.

Without the possibility of realistic gain or loss, the play may be enjoyable but scarcely exciting, and after a while it is likely to become boring. With it there is the real possibility of pain as well as pleasure, but in either case there is a true arousal, a heightened state of tension. The tension seeks prompt discharge, but after a while the individual craves to repeat it. In other words, the glasses game can be considered successful play because Mrs. D. confronts her neurotic anxiety in the game symbolism and overcomes it. When she plays more directly with the neurotic fears, teasing herself with self-induced anxiety, the introduction of the possibility of grave consequences makes the neurotic fear seem realistic, and the play terminates in failure.

METAPSYCHOLOGICAL CONSIDERATIONS

The pleasure principle tells us that we shun pain and pursue pleasure. Why then, in the midst of play which is invoked to escape the pain of daily life, do we introduce reality factors that, if they do not directly cause pain, at least threaten to do so? Freud in *Civilization and Its Discontents* (1930) provides, I think, a reasonable explanation: "What we call happiness in the strictest sense comes from the (preferably sudden) satisfaction of needs which have been dammed up to a high degree, and it is from its nature only possible as an episodic phenomenon. When any situation that is desired by the pleasure principle is prolonged, it only produces a feeling of mild contentment. We are so made that we can derive intense enjoyment only from a contrast and very little from a state of things" (p. 76).

Play seems to provide, not for the unrestrained pursuit of pleasure, but rather for the exposure to realistic or realisticlike challenges, the overcoming of which relaxes tension and replaces it with pleasure. The first three case vignettes I cited are atypical. These three patients use play purely as a defense against the pain that arises in their contact with the external or internal world. They are not interested in confronting challenge and overcoming it. People without their needs, on the other hand, use play not to avoid challenge, but rather to enjoy confronting and disposing of a challenge that is tailored to the severity of threat and discomfort, and to the particular modality of confrontation with which such people can deal. The successful confrontation provides for the gratification, real or illusory, which they crave. Play is a simulated, attenuated, and controllable reality. When the pain becomes too great, or the threat too formidable, the play can be terminated.

Now we can see the similarity between the play of children and of adults. In the case of the former, the play serves to test the child's ability to manage tasks to which he expects to be exposed in the future. The specific task poses certain difficulties and elicits fears, which the child, in response to his maturational drives, seeks to master. The play offers the opportunity to experiment with this task, to anticipate its dangers and gratifications. In the case of adults, the same mastery pleasure is obtained, but whereas children's play anticipates future, more difficult tasks, adult play attempts to master simplified versions of the external world, problems of limited complexity, and posing limited threats.

Under certain circumstances, adults too may fear assuming new tasks or roles, and use play to help them to master their fears, either realistically by practicing the new roles, or unrealistically by denying them.

Mr. E., obligated by age to surrender his powerful position in his business and his industry, played tennis daily, almost always with partners younger than he. When he won, he would comment to his partner or to whoever was available, "Not bad for an old man."

The more difficult the task undertaken, the greater the satisfaction in mastering it. Healthy players, both adult and child, will therefore choose and contrive play-tasks that will really challenge them and that will be manageable, but just barely.

What is it that labels a prospective game as attractive? The anticipation must include not only function pleasure and the possibility of successful resolution, but also the discomfort or threat that will be faced and that will have to be mastered. It follows then that the prospect of discomfort not only fails to discourage undertaking a particular form of play; but if it seems serious enough to be interesting and gratifying, and yet subject to mastery or control, that prospect may actually encourage its selection.

We are left then with the problem of Mrs. D.'s anxiety-provoking play during her analytic session, and the similar games of children. The best way to understand them may be to regard them as attempts to deal with inner as distinguished from outer reality, that is, to master unresolved neurotic problems. The child struggling with death wishes for one or both parents may play games that involve automobile or airplane crashes. If the game liberates too much anxiety, he will terminate it, and perhaps initiate a less transparent representation of his fantasies and wishes. Mrs. D. played the game of hide-and-seek with her glasses; rejection and acceptance in her relations with family, friends, and employers; and death and life with respect to herself. During latency, she was troubled by fears of death. A neighbor characterized her as "the saddest little girl" she had ever seen. She remembered very often weeping endlessly after having been scolded or sent upstairs by her mother, and imagining being rescued by a kind fairy. We have evidence that her early life was dominated by fantasies of separation from her mother by death, by murder, by running away to strangers. These influences and the fears that they generated obviously persisted and created anxiety attacks from time to time, constant concern with health and acceptance, and the games I have described during analytic sessions. The games were made interesting, engaging, and cogent by representing the threatening inner impulses as threats from the real world. As a matter of clinical interest, a considerable improvement followed my demonstrating to her that a preconscious but voluntary decision initiated the anxiety attack and, at least in its early stages, could either terminate it or let it acquire momentum and escape control. It is the glasses game that she conducted during the session which provides our example of successful play. It was by means of this play that she tried to master in small doses what she could not master in her fully developed anxiety attacks, namely, the fear of loss, separation, and death. Of course, she was also motivated by the desire to show me her problem and to invoke my assistance as the good fairy, much as child patients play for similar reasons before their analysts. As I observed above, when she attempted to confront her neurosis more directly by activating her fears of rejection and death, the anxiety escaped control and the attempt to play failed.

The gambler too externalizes neurotic problems. He makes his game exciting by tying realistic consequences to it. But the act of tempting fate until he is destroyed by it can be seen as an externalization of a need to overcome a sense of impotence by defying the restrictions imposed, first by parents, and later by reality. The devastation that usually results reveals the ultimate self-destructive intent.

The psychodynamic significance of solitary play is suggested by the following case vignette.

Mrs. F. was too busy with child rearing, business and community affairs to have much time for play. At times, however, when she felt especially put upon, she tended to withdraw into solitude, occupying herself with arranging her collection of family photographs or reading classical novels. She imagined taking a trip overseas to a warm climate where she would be able to rest idly and feast on pastries. At some time she intended to resume painting, a skill with which her mother had helped her. The dreams she reported at such times had similar images. In the dreams her mother appeared either manifestly or in latent content.

For Mrs. F., her solitary play, if it can be called that, represented a return to the earliest, exclusive intimacy with mother, a fantasy state, since mother had been neither reliably nor consistently affectionate or hospitable.

SUMMARY AND CONCLUSIONS

By playing, the child and adult seek surcease from the stress of living in reality and the frustration of basic needs, conscious and unconscious. Play involves rejection of realistic constraints and seeking relative freedom from restraint and from consequence.

The game that is played is usually secondarily endowed with realistic consequences; the more serious the consequences, the more exciting, and up to a certain point, the more pleasurable is the play.

In play the child and adult attempt to achieve gratification by undertaking to confront challenge and to master it.

The challenge that the player undertakes resembles a challenge of the real world, but it differs in being less complex and more manageable; it is titrated to try his capacity but not to defeat him.

Play in neurosis differs from nonneurotic play in that the player deals with inner as distinguished from outer reality, concealing its inner origin by externalizing it. It betrays its origin in conflict by its tendency to escape control and elicit the anxiety that the patient otherwise tries to master by symptom formation.

For those of us who are wearied and stressed by inner or outer struggles, by the need for self-control and self-denial, play offers a means of gratification and recuperation, less radical than the forms of major disengagement from the world with which we are familiar, and a gratifying and readily available alternative to other human diverting institutions such as religion, aesthetics, and science.

BIBLIOGRAPHY

FREUD, S. (1930). Civilization and its discontents. *S.E.*, 21:59–145.

A Psychoanalytic View of Play

ALBERT J. SOLNIT, M.D.

> . . . the urge to do theatre is a very natural thing. It
> stems from the urge to play that exists in all of us. As
> we grow we have to funnel this urge into other forms.
> And that's what theatre is all about.
> —BAR-YA'ACOV (1986)

ALTHOUGH WE ALL THINK WE KNOW WHAT WE MEAN WHEN WE
speak of or hear about play, in fact play is better described by its
functions than it can be through a formal definition. There is no
generally accepted, comprehensive definition of play. In a standard dictionary (see Webster's *New Collegiate Dictionary*, Merriam
Company, Springfield, Mass., 1974, p. 881), the list of definitions of the noun and verbs "play" takes up half a page, running
from "the conduct, course or action of a game" to the stage
representation of an action or story, and from "to engage in
sport or recreation to cause a radio or phonograph to emit
sounds."

HISTORICAL PERSPECTIVE

In his 1908 paper on "Creative Writers and Day-Dreaming,"
Freud stated, "Might we not say that every child at play behaves
like a creative writer, in that he creates a world of his own, or
rather re-arranges the things of his world in a new way which
pleases him? It would be wrong to think he does not take that
world seriously; on the contrary, he takes his play very seriously

Sterling professor of pediatrics and psychiatry, School of Medicine and
Child Study Center, Yale University; training and supervising analyst, Western
New England Institute for Psychoanalysis.
An earlier, shorter draft was presented in Jerusalem on March 17, 1986.

and he expends large amounts of emotion on it. The opposite of play is not what is serious but what is real. In spite of all the emotion with which he cathects his world of play, the child distinguishes it quite well from reality; and he likes to link his imagined objects and situations to the tangible and visible things of the real world.[1] This linking is all that differentiates the child's 'play' from 'phantasying'" (p. 143f.). Perhaps, we should add, using a line from Shakespeare, through indirection the child finds direction out, i.e., for the child play is a way, usually safe and advantageous, for getting to know the real world (Colonna and Friedmann, 1984).

Waelder (1932) indicated that children's play is a process of assimilation through repetition, demonstrating cogently how the process of recall can operate in the service of discharge. However, the psychoanalytic concept of the repetition compulsion does not include every repetition in the psychic realm.

Later, Hartmann (1964) wrote, "The role of analysis in explaining the play of children is analogous to the one it performs in explaining anxiety. In both, analysis tends to substitute a dynamic-genetic explanation for a teleological one" (p. 89). "The repetition factor in children's play must be understood from the same point of view. Here too recall serves the mastery of experiences" (p. 410).

In a survey of the psychoanalytic literature on play and adaptation, Plaut (1979) suggested that assumptions about instinctual drive energies are linked to psychoanalytic views of play as reported by Waelder (1932), Hartmann (1964), Erikson (1937, 1950, 1977), and Winnicott (1971). For example, Waelder (1932) stated, "From the standpoint of the theory of instincts, the mastery instinct, like all others, is a blending of love and destruction."

Reviewing the reports by Peller (1954), A. Freud (1965), Erikson (1937, 1950, 1977), Piaget (1945), and Winnicott (1971), Plaut (1979) has suggested that psychoanalysts have used the observations of children at play to illustrate or demonstrate vari-

---

1. Though he may not like or want adults, especially therapists, to make such linkages until he feels ready to hear it from outside himself, especially when the child was not aware of such a linkage or connection.

ous aspects of drive theory, of developmental characteristics, and of metapsychological constructs. Plaut goes on to suggest that play and playfulness throughout the life cycle are abiding human activities that also can be used to illuminate a major pathway of adaptation for children and adults. "As people grow up, then, they cease to play, and they seem to give up the yield of pleasure which they gained from playing" (Freud, 1908, p. 145). This apparent discrepancy is worthy of more study and reflection, i.e., how play changes, if it does, throughout life.

Developmental Perspective

In using Freud's statement (1908) as part of a platform on which to construct his interesting theory of play as a primary function and as a lifelong characteristic of human beings, Plaut overlooked a crucial developmental implication of Freud's statement about adults ceasing to play. Freud (1908) said, "But whoever understands the human mind knows that hardly anything is harder for a man than to give up a pleasure which he has once experienced. Actually, we can never give anything up; we only exchange one thing for another. What appears to be a renunciation is really the formation of a substitute or surrogate. In the same way, the growing child, when he stops playing, gives up nothing but the link with real objects; instead of *playing*, he now *phantasies*. He builds castles in the air and creates what are called day-dreams" (p. 145).

Freud elaborated by explaining how adults are self-conscious or ashamed of their fantasies and hide them from others, whereas the younger child is usually more comfortable to reveal them, especially in play with a trusted adult. One could say that the younger child plays and the adult fantasies.

Older children are in transition, preferring games and playfulness. For example, in school classrooms the teacher wants children to attend to the lesson, what is being taught and learned. Teachers generally discourage a preoccupation with or evidence of interfering fantasies while lessons are being taught. In one instance a 12-year-old boy enjoyed his daydreams after lunch but had to contend with a warmhearted teacher who discouraged daydreaming by always calling on an obviously daydreaming child to recite on the subject of history, thereby embarrassing the child who was not paying attention. In this instance, Charlie loved his moments of daydreaming as he looked out of the classroom window watching drifting clouds; tall buildings; flying, chattering, singing birds; and falling leaves. He planned to trap the teacher so she might leave him alone. He made it clear by his posture, drooping eyelids, and lack of attention to what the teacher was saying that he was otherwise engaged. He pretended not to listen—he played out a role. Predictably she called on Charlie who, after a brief second of hesitation, stood up and with gestures answered her questions accurately, completely with dates, sites on the classroom map, events in proper sequence, and with understanding. The teacher was taken aback. The class laughed nervously and Charlie was quiet and apprehensive, though appearing nonchalant. Then the tolerant teacher who liked Charlie said, "Well occasionally there is a student who can do two things at once." Charlie was relieved and thereafter was much more comfortable in his daydreaming. He had played at or pretended to be completely distracted in order to protect his opportunities for daydreaming. When Charlie grew up he became a child advocate who advised educators and parents not to overschedule children with curriculum or social and athletic activities. He wrote, "Children should have time to play and to daydream." Here one can see the question further elaborated: what happens to the child's need for time and settings in which to play and daydream as they become adults?

There is one more question about this vignette: that is, where it fits into the developmental frame of reference. Charlie was doing what latency children often do, playfully tricking the teacher by pretending to daydream. Is such a dramatization play? Is it the type of nongame play that late latency children characteristically use? In this case, pretending to daydream was an effort to prevent a future threatening reality and to gain some protection from that reality, i.e., to be treated as an exception. It is more accurate to use such mental and physical behaviors as examples of playfulness in the service of reducing the demands of reality. This may be one of the developmentally appropriate transformations of childhood play into adolescent and adult playfulness.

At the other end of the developmental continuum, how should we understand the so-called normative play of an infant who plays with his toes, or an infant who plays with mother's breast, and the play of infant and mother in peek-a-boo or in a multitude of activities where the parent teases the infant for an instant and then there is an interaction of touches, looks, and sounds that give each pleasure. Are these variations of imitation and teasing the precursors of later play? After the first year of life can there be play without some element of imitation and identification being involved? Most of these normative activities are examples of a parent (usually the mother) playing with the baby and the baby imitating or responding in a playful way to the mother and to the inanimate object that is commonly introduced and cathected by the mother. Can we think of these activities as those used by the parent to introduce the baby to play, teaching the infant how to play? Often, as the child becomes older, the imitative behavior is elaborated and practiced as caricature and satirical behaviors. Thus, play becomes a source for initially trying on, practicing, and imaginatively elaborating the capacity for wit, humor, pathos, and a whole host of affective experiences (tolerating the feelings) and their expressive communication to others.

From such a developmental perspective, are autoerotic activity and masturbation at some point forms of play? At least, they often seem to start as play as toddlers ride up and down on their father's foot. Genital masturbation in adolescence begins with the fantasy and activity in which one pretends to be courting, to engage in sexual foreplay, and to arouse oneself genitally as one imagines the love-making proceeding to sexual intercourse. Does this masturbatory activity cease to be play? Does it go beyond the boundary of what is play? As the degree or level of stimulation and gratification rises, the suspension of reality decreases; the pretense is lost in the reality of the sensuous experience. Masturbation may start as play, but as the intensity of the stimulation and gratification increase, quantitative changes build up to qualitative changes of experience.

Then the relationship of ego and id in play is changed. The observing ego loses its role and the capacity to pretend is lost, or at least sharply changed from one of primary significance to a secondary or tertiary role in the behavior and subjective experience of the individual, allowing for maturational and developmental changes in such capacities and tolerances. It may be useful further to explore those criteria of play that structurally and energically characterize the ego-id relationship in play states and in nonplay states as illustrated in the autoerotic, masturbatory activities of children and adolescents.

PLAY IN THE PSYCHOANALYTIC SITUATION

In clinical child psychoanalytic play interviews, how the child analyst responds to the imaginative, make-believe play of the child reveals characteristics of the child at play that can help us to a better conceptualization and understanding of the domain of play. Technically, the child analyst enters into the child's fantasies by how he responds and by how he does not respond. In general, the child analyst attempts to encourage the child's pleasurable elaboration of the fantasy-dramatizing-free play by going along with the child's make-believe. He joins the child and they play together. In a psychoanalytic treatment, for example, a 5-year-old is cuddling a teddy bear and offers it to the analyst as he holds and cuddles the teddy bear. The analyst would say, "Oh, the teddy bear wants to be cuddled because he feels left out of what Mama and Daddy Bear are doing." The child analyst usually would not say, "Oh, I see, after supper when you are tired, you want your mother to cuddle you and stop listening to your father because you feel left out of what they are talking about." The analyst knows that such interpretations directly from play to the child's reality often disrupt the play before it is fully elaborated, thus limiting what can be understood from the play as well as putting at risk the development-promoting aspects of the play.

Thus, play suspends reality, puts the child into an active position, and converts felt deprivation into felt relief and a sense of pleasurable gratification on a make-believe basis. As Freud would say, it is the opposite of the child's perceived reality. It is a trial action of a different sort than thinking, imagining, etc., because in childhood, play is behavior that characterizes what the child is feeling without expecting it to be perceived as behavior that is consequential, responsible, or unchangeable. Play can always be redone! We could say the same about playfulness in the adult.

PLAY AND PSYCHOPATHOLOGY

Play is conceptualized as a mental-physical activity that has normative, development-promoting functions. However, many of the most difficult questions about the concept arise from the so-called play activities of children and adults in certain psychopathological states.

For example, can one speak of the rhythmic, twirling behavior of an autistic child as play? Can one think of how or whether autistic children do or can learn to play? The defensiveness of autistic behavior suggests that it has little, if any, of the characteristics of play, especially the influence of a recognizable fantasy. Such behavior is mainly or exclusively a repetitive, rhythmic activity that is relatively mindless in terms of fantasies, illusions, or a mental and behavioral effort to explore, practice, or try on roles having elaborate defensive and adaptive capacities.

The autistic child's behavior and mental activity, as far as we understand them, are to engage in behavior and thinking that close down awareness, or reduce pain, warding off external and internal stimuli. They are much more like treading water than they are like trying to swim, regardless of which swim-stroke one has in mind. Whereas play not only involves physical activity and pretending, it also has a symbolizing capacity and usually has the characteristics of a synthesizing exercise or practicing to adapt or to resolve conflicts in an exploratory, make-believe manner.

Similarly, when we examine the deficits, absence, or deviations of play in children who are severely deprived or whose sadomasochistic behavior has found instant short-cuts to tension discharge, the play activity is not elaborated and tends to represent a narrow or small repertoire in terms of links to fantasies. Such play often fails to achieve that elaboration and structure which we find characteristic of a progressive development. In between are those children who do not initiate play but who can respond and borrow the capacity to imagine, try on, and use the fantasy provided by an active "playmate."

PSYCHOANALYTIC CRITERIA FOR PLAY

Play involves acting, i.e., physical behavior and mental activity—fantasy that includes cognitive and affective components. Its consequences are in the realm of pretending, trying on, imagining. When play "goes out of control," the pretend becomes real in terms of consequences, and then play is the same as—not the opposite of—reality. Then we can speak of the players losing control. They are no longer playing because the pretend element is exchanged for behavior that has reality-bound consequences. For example, the psychoanalyst becomes erotically aroused by the analysand and the child and analyst become stimulated and gratified in reality rather than vicariously (in the mind, i.e., in the realm of thinking more than doing). This is especially seen among children who in playing with each other regress and in so doing give up or lose hold of the make-believe quality as they begin to fight for real, seeking direct gratification in a manner that departs from the structure or context of the play.

In such instances, the suspension of reality in the service of play is lost, and now the play is replaced by activity that has real consequences. When play breaks down, it often leads to or is associated with poor reality testing. This is often seen when play becomes transformed from pretend to realistic consequences and gratifications, i.e., when the pretend boundary is lost. Similarly, the ability to recollect is dependent upon this line of development; i.e., to remember a person or event when they are not concretely present is a capacity which requires that the person can imagine (pretend) that the person or the event is available in the "mind's eye." One can run off that movie (or video tape) inside one's head. But such recollection is not play because it does not involve physical activity that dramatizes (in a make-believe way) a fantasy about a person or situation, or wish or longing that is being called to mind. It is play if the child explicitly pretends the person is there talking, reading, or interacting in a make-believe fashion.

Even before mentation is sufficiently mature and developed, there is an earlier form of play-remembering in which the child unwittingly reenacts certain aspects of memory in a playful way. Piaget (1945) referred to this as psychomotor memory or recall. For example, a 2½-year-old, Daniel, returned to a summer cabin in which he and his family had spent a month one year earlier. He was anxious not only because he was away from home; this was a second visit, yet he felt as though he were in a "strange" place and a different situation because now his mother was pregnant and many other things in the family had changed. He clutched his transitional object, a teddy bear, as he entered the cabin in the early evening, following a picnic supper on the way to the cabin. First, he went from room to room in the cabin, holding his mother's hand. There was no overt evidence that he remembered having been there. Then suddenly he pushed a chair to the kitchen sink, climbed up, and said playfully, with a smile that indicated he was "pretending," "Let's play bath in the kitchen sink." In fact, that is where he had been bathed during the vacation a year earlier, though he had never had his bath in a (kitchen) sink at any other place. His behavior started as a pretend, using his psychomotor memory since the parents could find no obvious evidence that he remembered the cabin in any other way. This play enabled him to reach back to a pleasant past experience in coping with the anxiety of the new situation and its uncertainties. When he took his bath in the kitchen sink that night, he played with the water and rubber whale. Bathing of his body was real. Play in the service of recollection led to mastery. Then he initiated a new play in which manipulating the rubber whale and giving it a story line dramatized his phallic capacities and fantasies.

In the case of 2½-year-old-Daniel, there was no doubt of his capacity to play, as defined above. For example, in one instance, while sitting in his car seat as his father drove him to nursery school, he pretended that he was driving the car for a ride in the country. In the instance above, having returned to the same vacation cabin in which he had been one year earlier, it could be inferred that play was to enable him to cope with certain apprehensions, but it was also using the unique, intuitive way of thinking and acting as a means of remembering. As Waelder (1932) has indicated, he assimilated through repetition the challenge of the present situation in terms of "remembering," i.e., of making familiar in the new situation (mother is pregnant, an absence of his usual supportive routines such as his favorite baby-sitter, and the tensions evoked by an exhausting trip to the somewhat isolated vacation setting).

In examining the meaning of play for children of different developmental capacities and tolerances, it is clear that all agencies of the mind are represented, though the mix is usually characteristic of a particular period of development. In younger children the drive derivatives are less disguised and superego elements may just begin to appear. However, the ego functions represented by the particular play—solo, parallel, interactional—can almost always be understood in terms of wishes, styles of creating illusions, and seeking pleasure, or in reducing uncomfortable tensions, ranging from specific (interpersonal) to interpsychic to intrapsychic domains.

Throughout, once the child has acquired the capacity for object constancy, the psychological presence of one or more primary love objects usually can be detected or inferred in the play. The distance from the play to the representation of the primary love objects varies according to the level at which the conflict, wish, tension-reduction, or practice of mastery is represented—conscious, preconscious, or unconscious.

Thus, play is pretend, another way of using the mind and body, in an indirect approach to seeking an adaptive, defensive, skill-acquiring, and creative expression. It is a mode of coping with conflicts, developmental demands, deprivation, loss, and yearnings through the life cycle. What makes play unique is the coordination of mental and physical activities that convey to both the actor and the observor the characteristics of suspended reality, the use of illusions and fantasies, and their dramatization. Functionally, the play is exploring, trying out, and pretending another approach than that which would be realistically consequential. Play is not intended to be a planned rehearsal, i.e., play does not count because the person is only pretending. Parenthetically, one can often say that certain individuals do not know what they want to do or what they are thinking until they play it out in one way or another.

Play enlarges the child's sense of himself, his capacities and his effectiveness in altering the reality in which he lives. In that sense play enables the child to explore safely how he can become active in shaping his world and not feel helpless or dependent on it more than he prefers or can tolerate.[2]

PLAY AND GAMES

Finally, in the use of games as a channel for play, we see the same principles, especially in the beginning of spontaneous, invented games. Later, particularly in the school-aged child (in latency) when there are rules to be followed, the aim of the game and how it allows for winning and losing also can be used to cover and either to encourage or to discourage the use of the underlying fantasies. In other words, though not inevitable, well-structured games with definite, mandatory rules (as in checkers) can be used either to ward off, disguise, or hide the fantasies, sexual and aggressive, with which the older child is coping. This would not be play but would be using a structured game as a defense against play. For example, playing checkers (often repetitive and monotonous) frequently is used by children to enable them to feel safer and more protected (less exposed) while having discrete underlying fantasies that they resist bringing into the analytic process initially. Such games are not playful. Rather, they serve to defend against the behavioral dramatization of play. It requires interpretive psychoanalytic work to enable such a restricted child to move from defensive games to development-promoting, age-appropriate play. Thus, playing a game by the rules may be derivative of play, but it is not play. Conversely, in the psychoanalytic treatment of latency children, the use of a table game (e.g., cards, checkers) often provides the child with an anchor for physical activities and an available opportunity to limit the pull to regressive behavior, which permits or encourages the child to talk and to use free associations for a short time.

2. Suggested by Alice Colonna.

Prelatency children mostly play, tolerating the regressive behavior involved.

Our inability to formulate a comprehensive definition of play and our inability to set forth clearly defining criteria of what constitutes play and what would not be play are both a reality and an opportunity. Realistically we strengthen our theory about play by acknowledging the limits of our knowledge, pointing to where we need to raise better questions (e.g., masturbation) which we can approach in our investigative studies. The opportunity is the realization that play is a unique activity, perhaps a line of development, that can be followed through the life cycle in several domains.[3] This can encourage us to move ahead in examining the many roots and meanings of play in children and adults, not only developmentally but in the domains of art, music, mathematics, and even certain kinds of so-called work or athletic activities. The concept of play invites a consensus from a wide variety of disciplines and experience about the characteristics, functions, and meanings of play. However, the experts often begin to disagree when the fine points and the boundaries of what should not be viewed as play are brought into the discussion.

For example, if an infant watches his own feet or fingers, moving them about in a playful fashion, should that be viewed as play? In order to be more rigorous, I propose the following developmental, behavioral, and psychological criteria for what constitutes play and playfulness, beyond which the term play would not apply.

PLAY AND ITS DEVELOPMENT-PROMOTING FUNCTIONS

Play involves physical and mental activity, and in a sense is always between thought, as trial action, and an action designed to solve

3. A. Freud's (1965) concept of developmental lines refers to basic id-ego interactions "and their various developmental levels, and also age-related sequences of them which, in importance, frequency, and regularity, are comparable to the maturational sequence of libidinal stages or the gradual unfolding of the ego functions. . . . In every instance they trace the child's gradual outgrowing of dependent, irrational, id- and object-determined attitudes to an increasing ego mastery of his internal and external world" (p. 62).

problems, and always with an underlying fantasy or state of pretend. It may be a preparation for as well as a part of mastery, defense, and adaptation. The maturational and developmental characteristics change as the child's and adult's capacities advance in regard to complexity of understanding and skills, probably retaining a continuity with earlier forms of such play activities or playful attitudes. The latter could be viewed as a unique style or analogous to a central organizing fantasy that is uniquely characteristic for each individual, beginning in childhood and in various modifications continuing throughout the life cycle as a component of progressive development.

However, though an infant's behavior (watching his moving fingers) may evoke a sense of playfulness in the observing adult or older child, we may find it useful to incorporate what Freud and others have said by indicating that our designation of certain physical-mental activities are development-promoting play if:

1. The attitude and expectation are that such activity is the opposite of real or at least implies a suspension of reality.
2. There is an illusion-creating and practicing quality to the activity.
3. It is a process of assimilation through repetition and often includes an approximation to recall from the past as well as implying mastery through recall and practice (see Hartmann, 1964, p. 410).
4. The inference that the child is playing can be confirmed by the way the player refers to it as metaphoric or pretend. This raises the question, can we confirm our inference about an individual's mental-physical activity before that person can use language or symbolic equivalents?

BOUNDARIES AND TECHNICAL IMPLICATIONS

It is also important to indicate the limits or boundaries of play by stating what is not play. Childhood play does not qualify as being on a par with the adult's capacity to work (see A. Freud, 1965, p. 123). Anna Freud (1965, p. 29) also indicated that play is no substitute for free association; it is not the same; it is not equivalent. Further, she reflected in this connection that, in child analysis, the child's play and his verbal expressions gradually lose the characteristics of secondary process thinking such as logic, coherence, rationality, and instead display characteristics of primary process functioning such as generalizations, displacements, repetitiveness, distortions, and exaggerations (p. 100). Thus play is a vehicle for regression in the service of the ego in the psychoanalytic situation.

Further, the child's symbolic play in the analytic session communicates not only his internal fantasies; simultaneously, it is his manner of communicating current family events such as nightly intercourse between parents, their marital quarrels and upsets, their frustrating and anxiety-raising action, their abnormalities and pathological expressions (A. Freud, 1965, p. 50). The child analyst who interprets exclusively in terms of the inner world is in danger of missing out on his patient's playful dramatization of external perceptions and memories that threaten to overwhelm him. Will interpretation that interrupts or focuses only on inner or outer events hinder the development-promoting aspects of the child's play as well as make the child self-conscious, discouraging him from playing in the psychoanalytic sessions?

CONCLUSIONS

Play is a unique capacity for combining thinking and acting (behaving). The mental component is between primary and secondary process thinking, tapping into the primary process while relaxing the censoring, orderliness-demanding, and inhibiting influence of secondary process thinking and reality testing. Play allows thinking and acting (or behaving) to flow into each other with a looser connection, developmentally and experientially, than nonplay thinking and acting usually permit; but it is a much tighter or more cohesive and coherent connection than, e.g., in sleepwalking.

Play that reflects or is coping with a previous trauma may be constrained by being influenced disproportionately by past experiences and its effects on both the thinking and the behavior of the individual. For example, past trauma may evoke more of the remembering than the exploring functions of play. Thus, in connection with certain experiences, developmental and those that life brings, play will in its thinking and behavioral components not only reflect where the child and adolescent are developmentally but may also bring up for its reviewing, familiarizing, assimilating, integrating, development-promoting functions what has happened and the anticipation of and preparation for what is about to happen.

As we speak and think of a dream state, a waking state, and a sleeping state, I suggest we explore how the concept of a play state could facilitate our study of the many meanings of play as well as its uniqueness as a mental-physical activity.

BIBLIOGRAPHY

BAR-YA'ACOV, SHAI (1986). In Jerusalem. *Jerusalem Post*, December 5; in report by Andrew Sofer.

COLONNA, A. B. & FRIEDMANN, M. (1984). Prediction of development. *Psychoanal. Study Child*, 39:509–526.

ERIKSON, E. H. (1937). Configurations in play. *Psychoanal. Q.*, 6:139–214.

_____ (1950). *Childhood and Society*. New York: Norton.

_____ (1977). *Toys and Reasons*. New York: Norton.

FREUD, A. (1965). Normality and pathology in childhood. *W.*, 6.

FREUD, S. (1908). Creative writers and day-dreaming. *S.E.*, 9:141–153.

HARTMANN, H. (1964). *Essays on Ego Psychology*. New York: Int. Univ. Press.

PELLER, L. E. (1954). Libidinal phases, ego development, and play. *Psychoanal. Study Child*, 9:178–198.

PIAGET, J. (1945). *Play, Dreams, and Imitation in Childhood*. New York: Norton, 1951, pp. 110–113.

PLAUT, E. A. (1979). Play and adaptation. *Psychoanal. Study Child*, 34:217–232.

WAELDER, R. (1932). The psychoanalytic theory of play. In *Psychoanalysis*, ed. S. A. Guttman. New York: Int. Univ. Press, 1976, pp. 84–100.

WINNICOTT, D. W. (1971). *Playing and Reality*. New York: Basic Books.

CLINICAL PAPERS

Mother, Is That You?

CALVIN A. COLARUSSO, M.D.

THE PURPOSE OF THIS PAPER IS TO PRESENT UNIQUE CLINICAL MATE-
rial, namely, the appearance, for the first time, of the biological
mother of a 12-year-old adopted boy during the course of his
analysis. In addition to a description of the patient's response, I
shall discuss technical issues raised by the mother's appearance
and its effect on intrapsychic representations and the transference.

Very few case reports in the analytic literature focus on adoption (Wieder, 1978; Brinich, 1980; Sherick, 1983). I could find
none that focuses on the sudden unexpected appearance of a
biological parent, especially during an analysis. This circumstance provided a rare opportunity to study intrapsychic effects,
particularly on the patient's object representations of parental
figures, as well as effects on the analytic process.

CASE REPORT

EVALUATION

Ron, a small, wiry 10-year-old, was referred because of fighting
in school, particularly with younger children. He lacked friends
and was the subject of ridicule by his peer group. Bed wetting
had been a continuous problem since toddlerhood. He expressed a vivid, violent fantasy life and had frequent nightmares. He was afraid of being alone, day or night.

Ron's natural parents had been unmarried teen-agers at the

Training analyst and supervisor in child and adult analysis; chairman of the
Child Analytic Training Program at the San Diego Psychoanalytic Institute.
Clinical professor of psychiatry and director of the Child Psychiatry Training
Program at the University of California, San Diego.

time of his birth. At 4 weeks of age he was adopted through an agency by a couple I shall call Ed and Jean Long. Ron was told of his adoption as soon as he was old enough to understand. Although he did not ask many questions, the subject came up frequently over the years.

Mrs. Long was the primary caretaker; developmental milestones were achieved on time or at an early age. Efforts at toilet training were inconsistent and casual. The boy was never dry at night and wet during the day until latency. Sexual curiosity and an infantile neurosis were evidenced by masturbation, nightmares, and fears, which increased in frequency toward the end of the oedipal phase. Ron was very close to his adoptive parents, particularly his mother. Latency was characterized by a dislike of school, lack of motivation, and growing isolation from other children.

During the diagnostic interviews Ron presented as a somewhat subdued, sad youngster who related well and readily told me of bad dreams in which people tried to kill and eat him, his loneliness and lack of friends, a consuming interest in Dungeons and Dragons and war games, and a deep love for his mother. When asked about his adoption, he expressed little interest; the subject was apparently unimportant to him.

Psychological testing revealed an IQ in the bright normal range, an intact ego, and the presence of intense anger which was defended against through the use of projection, passive aggressiveness, and withdrawal. Ron felt continually threatened by others, whom he saw as hostile and uncaring. His lack of self-esteem was pronounced, leading to a growing identification with odd, hostile figures living on the fringes of society. His phobias resulted from unresolved oedipal conflict.

Both parents, intelligent and cooperative, accepted the recommendation for analysis and were supportive throughout. Treatment began just before Ron's tenth birthday.

INITIAL COURSE OF THE ANALYSIS

During the first 2 years and 3 months of analysis the work centered on Ron's phobias, nightmares, and lack of friends. Gradually he revealed an intense interest in vampires, horror movies, and war games. These preoccupations and his dressing and behaving like a hostile guerilla fighter made his lack of friends readily understandable. Through a steadily developing transference in which I was often the victim of attacks by vampires, monsters, and Rambolike characters, his conflicts with aggression and peer relationships were explored and interpreted.

Considerable analytic work also centered on his having been adopted. Ron manifested many of the themes typically seen in the analysis of adopted children. After the defensive aspects of a seeming disinterest were interpreted, he began to describe fantasies about his natural parents. They were young students who gave him away because they could not afford to raise him. More conflicted were thoughts that he had caused them to give him away. As he grew more attached to me, Ron became very curious about my family. "I'll bet you have 7 kids," he said. "I think you're a good father." His wish to be my son was first revealed in dreams and later in less disguised ways in fantasy and play. By the time his biological mother appeared, Ron's symptoms, including his bed wetting, had nearly disappeared.

THE APPEARANCE OF RON'S BIOLOGICAL MOTHER

Ron's analysis was radically changed soon after his biological mother walked into his adoptive father's office and asked to see her son. When he called me at home that evening, Mr. Long's understated question was simple and dramatic: "I'll bet you never ran into this one before. Ron's biological mother showed up in my office today. She wants to see him. What do I do?"

The first decision facing me as Ron's analyst was whether or not to give advice. Should I beg off in order to protect analytic neutrality and the therapeutic alliance or try to guide the reunion in an effort to enhance its potential developmental and therapeutic effects? After thinking the matter through, I decided to intervene because I felt that mother and child were likely to meet sooner or later regardless of what the Longs or I thought. Moreover, because such interactions can enhance identity formation in adolescence and young adulthood, I favor having older adopted children meet their biological parents if they want to. I therefore advised Ron's father to meet again with the boy's biological mother, whom I shall call Sue, to assess her motivation and reliability. He discovered that she lived in the area, was married, and had a family. After several years of trying, she had traced the Longs with the help of a searcher and an organization of women who had given their children for adoption and now wished to reestablish contact.

Sue had been under great stress when Ron was born because neither the baby's father nor her family were supportive. The last time she had seen her lover was just before the birth, when he drove her to the hospital and left, never to be heard from again. She deeply regretted the decision to give up her baby, and her intention now was to get to know her son *without* disrupting the 12-year relationship he had with his adoptive parents. Mr. Long felt she was sincere, bright, and reliable. He was prepared to take the next step. I suggested that both parents meet with me prior to telling Ron about his biological mother's appearance.

Because of their individual strengths and the rapport built during the 2 years of Ron's analysis, the Longs were able to face their fears that Sue would try to displace them and/or that Ron would prefer her to them. Recognizing that neither they nor I could completely determine the future course of events, they decided to permit a meeting between Ron and Sue because it would be in Ron's best interest. Both of them were reassured by the fact that the boy would be able to bring his thoughts and feelings into the analysis. With considerable trepidation they told Ron what had happened. He met with me a day later.

January 25: "My mom and dad are more nervous than I am," he said. After finding out the night before, he had wet the bed. "I do want to meet my birth mother, I think. At worst I can find out more about myself. At best I can make a good friend." From the moment he found out about his natural mother's presence on the scene, Ron was concerned about his adoptive parents' feelings. "My mom is worried that my birth mother will want to take me away. She won't. The Longs are the only family I have."

His mind raced from subject to subject. "I have a new brother, I mean half-brother, and a stepfather, and maybe new grand-parents too. Wow!" Later his thoughts turned to his biological father. "Maybe I'll find out about him. Maybe I'll look like him." Then, motivated by guilt, he began to discuss his "real" (adoptive) father. "I walk like him. I even talk like him. I don't try to. I don't even want to, but I do." As he worked furiously to integrate the profound changes taking place in his real and intrapsychic worlds, Ron's ambivalence toward his fantasized, but now a bit more real, birth mother emerged. "She must have had a good reason to give me up . . . but she'll have to earn being a parent." He readily agreed with my suggestion that we take as much time as he needed to analyze his feelings about this big chance in his life before he met her.

Three weeks were to pass before he decided that he was ready. A sequential summary of some of the analytic work done during that period follows.

January 28: Ron was anxious about the first meeting. "If she doesn't like me, it's her fault, not mine." He was less willing to talk about his thoughts and feelings than he had been in the previous session when words and feelings had rushed out in a torrent. He wondered how tall she would be, fearing that both his biological parents were short. He was just experiencing the pubertal growth spurt and was keen on becoming as tall as his adoptive father.

Sue had told the Longs that her baby's father had dropped her off at the hospital and then left. Ron was incensed by that information but had avoided analyzing thoughts and feelings about his natural father. I interpreted the resistance, "Do you sense that you're having more trouble talking about your birth father than your birth mother?" "Yeah. I wonder where he is, the jerk. He dropped her off at the hospital and left." Then he built a house, filled it with toy soldiers, and blew it up.

"Could your birth father be one of the people inside that bombed house?"

"I'll find him some day and I'll give him hell for leaving my Mom."

"And you?"

"Yeah, me too [sadly]. He probably didn't have any choice in giving me up. It's the woman's choice, you know."

January 31: "I haven't thought about my mother since last time. . . . I wet the last two nights. I'll bet it's related to [in baby talk] 'Mommy, Mommy.'"

"You don't talk in baby talk. I think that's a wish that your birth mother had been around to take care of you when you were a baby."

Later Ron expressed the fear that his "new" mother would steal him away. "I'd be scared she might try and make me part of her family. Then I'd lose my own. She might try and steal me illegally. She'd toss me in the car and drive away." Yet he wanted to talk to her alone so he could "get to know her as a friend." The prospect of the meeting was overwhelming. "For all I know I may faint when I see her."

February 2: The fantasy that he would be stolen took several sessions to work through. This day it was elaborated more fully.

"She says to me, 'Ron, how would you like to live with me?' I say, 'No, I like my family the way it is!' Then she grabs me and pushes me into a box in the back of her car. I dive out while the car is going and do a couple of rolls to break the fall. She drives away thinking I'm in the car. Then I call my mom and she comes and gets me."

Ron was also concerned about the impression he would make on Sue and was thankful for the analytic work we had done. "I'm glad she didn't meet me before when I was a self-centered asshole. She wouldn't have liked me then."

He continued to struggle with the painful issue of why she gave him up, using rationalization and displacement to explain the unexplainable. "Mothers who can't afford their kid shouldn't feel bad because if they can't afford him he's better off. But they should keep in touch [with emphasis] and the kid should know why he was adopted. I'm not mad at her. She was pressured into it. I'm mad at her family for making her."

February 4: Ron's attempt to relate his emerging sexuality to his biological parents continued, as did his intense struggle with anger at the biological father. "Some day I'll make Sue a grandmother. Oh my God, my kid will have three grandparents."

"Why not four? What about your birth father?"

"He's dead."

"Not likely."

"If he's not dead, I'll kill him." The direct expression of the rage was too powerful and had to be displaced. "What do you call a person with leprosy in a hot tub?"

"I don't know. What?"

"Stew!" The sick jokes continued for some time.

"Why do you think your mind went to sick jokes just now?"

"I don't know."

"I think it's a way of continuing to express anger at your birth father. You still feel guilty when you do it directly."

February 10: Ron wanted to meet Sue as soon as possible. He'd decided when and how—in MacDonald's restaurant after school. That way he'd be safe until his mom picked him up. His biggest worry was hurting his mom by telling her he was ready to meet Sue.

February 12: Jean Long had called Sue, and the two mothers agreed again to meet to arrange details. "Yippee! I'm finally going to get to meet her, that is [soberly], if the two of them get along." He felt his mom was "real nervous" about this. "Up to now she's been my only mother."

"I think your mom is worried about the same things you are, that Sue will take you away from her."

"Or try. She doesn't have to worry."

February 18: Ron tried to make light of his first meeting with Sue, but his thoughts and feelings soon rushed out. "When she came to the door, I thought, 'Oh my God, is this really happening?' She looked sorta like me. The same kind of face and hair." They drove to a nearby shopping center and ate. "I found out how and why I was adopted. She was still under the anesthesia when she signed the papers and didn't know what was going on. She thought she was signing papers to take me home. It was basically an illegal adoption. My brother, I mean my half brother's name is Sam. . . . I told her how little she would have liked me 3 years ago [before analysis]."

Ron asked Sue to meet again the following weekend, this time at her house. She agreed. She told Ron that his parents were wonderful to let them meet. She knew from her group that a lot of adoptive parents refuse. "My parents are cool. They knew I wouldn't go nuts."

Ron reported, "She asked me how I feel about having two mothers. I said, 'Fine.' I'm really lucky to have such nice people for mothers."

February 22: In this session Ron dared to feel pleasure and joy over being loved by Sue, and he began to find a place for her intrapsychically as he replaced fantasy with reality. "She cares about me a lot! She loves me very much. She told me she's waited 12 years to tell me that. She tried for a long time to find me." His increased self-esteem was almost palpable. "It's amazing that we found each other. It's kind of like 'E.T., phone home.' My parents have been great. I knew they wanted to know what was going on, but they didn't make me say anything. I think I like my mothers in the order they came into my life, Jean first and Sue second."

February 26: A subtle but distinct difference was apparent after Ron's second meeting with Sue. He was full of details about her house and family, but more subdued. He seemed to need to distance himself from the material, to allow time for integration. Although she hadn't said so, he felt his mother didn't want him to see Sue all the time. He felt she was still worried, unnecessarily. "I really like Sue, and I plan to keep seeing her, but I'm not going to jump up and say, 'Mom, let's go.' I'm sort of like a dog. I'm real loyal."

Later I asked if Ron had found out anything about his birth father. With mild annoyance he said that he hadn't asked. "I don't want to know. I know I have to some time and I will. There's nothing nice to say about a guy who leaves his kid at the hospital."

March 4: A pattern began to emerge for future meetings between Ron and Sue. Ron planned to see Sue "when I want to. My mom and dad say it's okay as long as I plan ahead." Intrapsychic integration continued. Ron joked, "I think I'll keep Sue around for a while. She ranks right up there, just behind my mom and my dad, in about the same place you are."

Ron and Sue met once or twice a month for the next several months and talked occasionally on the phone. In that time he met her extended family, commenting primarily on similarities in appearance.

Eventually Ron did ask Sue about his birth father. They had been students together, but she knew few details of his life and nothing about his whereabouts since the day Ron was born. Ron's anger continued unabated, but near the end of the analysis he did express sadness about not knowing "this guy who made me. There's a hole inside me that only he can fill." We were able to analyze some of his fantasies about physical resemblance and sexual functioning.

Discussion

As pointed out by Brinich (1980), "The adopted child must include two separate sets of parents in his representational world" (p. 108). Even under the best of circumstances he "may have difficulty differentiating between the 'real' and the 'false' parents, ascertaining which is which" (Glenn, 1974, p. 414). In his attempt to resolve this dilemma the adopted child is confronted with a task more complicated than that facing his natural peers because it is "more difficult to fuse the intrapsychic relations into a workable, more realistic identification" (Simon and Senturia, 1966, p. 864).

All children deal with the issue of real and imagined or false parents through the family romance (Freud, 1909). In an attempt to compensate for real and fantasized disappointment in his parents, the natural child imagines he was adopted into an inferior family—his "real" parents are important, all-loving people who will find him some day and rescue him. But "the fantasy solution of the biological child's conflict—adoption—is the *fait accompli* underlying the adoptee's distress. The adoptee's wish, in contrast to that of the blood-kin child's, is to deny adoption, fantasize a blood tie to the adoptive parents, and thereby erase the humiliation adoption implies" (Wieder, 1978, p. 507). Further complications occur in adolescence because the adopted child finds it difficult to locate his personal history within his family and is likely to experience curiosity about his origins and early life as conflictual and dangerous (Brinich, 1980). Such comments demonstrate the enormity of the task facing the adopted child as he moves developmentally from phase to phase, working and reworking two sets of parental object representation. (In the case of divorce, three or more sets of parental figures, real and imagined, may be involved.)

Before and during the first 2 years of his analysis Ron went about the business of modifying object representations for his adoptive and fantasized biological parents much the way any adopted child would. Like Sherick's patient (1983), he first ex-

pressed a lack of interest in his adopted state, but gradually came
to speculate. What were his natural parents like? Why had they
given him up? Did he cause it? Did he have any siblings? And so
on.

The sudden appearance of Ron's natural mother shattered
the ongoing work and precipitated a major psychic reorganization of object representations which became a central aspect of
the analytic work. Unlike the typical adopted child who experiences his *curiosity* about his early life as conflictual and dangerous, this boy had detailed factual information thrust upon
him. For him, *actual knowledge*, not fantasy, was the threat.

At first Ron was unclear about his feelings about all three real
parent figures. But gradually he achieved a new, more comfortable, and lasting integration as he came to the conclusion that his
adoptive parents were his "real" parents. They had raised him,
taken care of him, loved him. They were at the center of his life
in the past and present. They would remain there in the future.
This case material also demonstrates how an older adopted child
can think abstractly enough to differentiate the functions of
progenitor and parent, roles performed in his case by different
people. Although he already had a "mother," his progenitor's
determined effort to find him, her intactness and interest, allowed him to develop a more narcissistically gratifying object
representation of her, replacing the ambivalent one that preceded it and which still existed for his biological father. Still, she
remained less important than his adoptive parents.

What made this integration possible? The analysis facilitated
the process but undoubtedly did not determine the outcome.
Ron's solid, lifelong relationship with his adoptive parents was
clearly an important factor. So was the age at which his biological
mother appeared and her desire to occupy a constant but secondary position in his life.

At age 12 Ron had developed considerable capacities for reason and judgment and thus was able to compare the impact of
each parent on his development. For instance, he recognized
that his adoptive parents were a proven commodity. They had
demonstrated over 12 years that they loved him and could take
care of him. Further, he reasoned (correctly) that they were well

educated, financially secure, and in a better position than his biological mother to further his development.

But probably the most important factor was the de-idealization of the biological mother. She was no longer the forlorn, unmarried teen-ager forced by circumstance to give him up; that predominant, persisting fantasy had been based on the scrap of information he had been given that his natural parents were young and unmarried. That fantasized mother had been much like him: young, vulnerable, a victim of circumstances beyond her control—a figure to be cherished and protected as well as hated for rejecting him. That object representation could not be sustained in the presence of a real, not too pretty, middle-aged woman who, although she had sought him out, had also, disloyally, found time to find a husband and have another child. In some way the fantasized mother was more gratifying than the real mother, for her representation could be manipulated without fear of contradiction by reality. The luxury of such intrapsychic manipulation was rudely taken away from Ron by the presence of the woman whose object representation had to be based on reality.

The power of such fantasized constructions remained obvious where Ron's biological father was concerned. The image of him as an unloving cad who abandoned both mother and infant (confirmed by the biological mother) was now intensified and unyielding to analytic consideration. There was no actual contact to modify the fantasies. The fact that his biological mother had no knowledge of his father's whereabouts further fueled Ron's increasingly hostile feelings. In addition, the boy resisted learning more about his progenitor because of a strong sense of loyalty to his adoptive father. Other determinants of this behavior included (1) the pleasure of having won the oedipal victory over the biological father—mother obviously loved him more than she loved his father; and (2) an ambivalent attitude about learning whether he looked like his natural father, an important developmental concern for a preadolescent boy. Once this was interpreted, Ron began a systematic comparison among his adoptive father, his fantasized natural father, and himself concerning all aspects of physical maturation. For example, following his first ejaculation, he began to wonder about his ability to father a child (Glenn, 1974). Would he be potent like his natural father who had obviously fathered him, or defective like his adoptive father (pure speculation on his part) who had to "pay money to get me because he couldn't make me."

CHANGES IN THE TRANSFERENCE

Even when an adopted child has little or no knowledge of his biological parents, he uses the transference as a major vehicle for the expression of feelings. The fact that an adopted child has little or no information about his biological parents does not prevent him from constructing elaborate fantasies about them in order to make sense of his adoption (Brinich, 1980). In this case, the transference became even more important after the appearance of Ron's biological mother and was significantly changed in three ways.

First to appear was a tendency to see the analyst as the powerful preoedipal mother (Brunswick, 1940) who had made his natural mother appear. These feelings were heightened by my unambivalent attitude (in contrast to those of his adoptive parents) to Ron's wish to see her. He voiced the fear/wish that I might find his natural father as well and create a situation in which his natural parents, now reunited and in love, would take him away.

This was followed by an intensification of positive oedipal feelings and fears. In discussing the oedipal dilemma in adopted children, Feder (1974) points out that "with the adopted child, the position of not being wanted is almost the whole" (p. 492). In a very real sense Ron went from being oedipal loser to oedipal victor overnight. His mother wanted him very much; she had gone to great effort to find him. Further, his oedipal rival was nowhere in sight and was despised by her. This change altered the transference by producing an upsurge of powerful competitive and hostile feelings toward me as I became the fantasized oedipal father. After considerable resistance we discovered that Ron was fearful that the father/analyst would want Sue for himself. Having made her appear, he would now take her away—for the second time in Ron's life. Once these feelings and fears were interpreted, Ron began to express intense curiosity about me and my life. Where did I live? What kind of car did I drive? How many children did I have? These questions had been asked at the beginning of the analysis, but now my refusal to answer was greeted with intense rage.

A discussion of some of the technical decisions thrust on an analyst by this unique situation is in order. My decision to facilitate a meeting between biological mother and son was based on developmental considerations, namely, the complicated struggle with identity facing the adopted child in adolescence. As Glenn (1974) pointed out, "So intense and frequent is the desire of adopted children to find their original parents, to establish their continuity with the past and their present and future identity, that an organization has been formed by adopted people to overthrow the legal barriers to receiving information about their origins" (p. 416). The key question, "Who am I?" extremely difficult for an adoptee to answer, might be more readily faced and integrated if Ron actually knew his biological mother. Further, I knew from 2 years of work with him that he was deeply curious, and I *assumed* he would want to meet her. In making this decision I had to analyze and assess my own strong curiosity to meet her and struggle with the fact that I was withholding vital, extra-analytic material from my patient while his parents decided whether to allow the contact. In addition, I was aware that some analysts, such as Wieder (1978), were opposed to contact between adoptees and their biological parents.

The question of direct contact between me and Ron's biological mother was one I was forced to consider when Mr. Long asked me to see Sue and render an opinion as to whether or not she should meet Ron. I decided against such a meeting because I did not want to usurp parental prerogative, and, more important, I did not have my patient's approval to do so. After the Longs decided to permit such a meeting, I encouraged them to tell Ron of his mother's appearance, offer him the choice of meeting her or not, inform him that I knew about her, and encourage him to analyze the matter with me if he wished.

As Ron and I worked, he stated categorically that I was *not* to meet Sue. Gradually we understood the defensive and transference reasons for his decision. Ron was overwhelmed by the prospect of meeting his mother. He wanted to control his feelings—and my access to them—as best he could. Then, as described, I came to be seen as an oedipal rival for her affections. At one point after these issues were worked through and interpreted, the patient himself suggested such a meeting. The offer was declined because I felt that I could best serve the primary analytic function of understanding Ron's *intrapsychic* response by remaining as apart from his real world as possible. The fact that I knew about his mother's appearance and had "conspired" with his father to keep the information from him while his parents decided what to do had already contaminated our relationship and produced a strong transference response. The remaining analytic work to be done could be best achieved by maintaining neutrality.

This boy manifested an amazing ability to integrate an awesome experience and achieve a new intrapsychic balance in which he found a place for his biological mother "right behind my parents." Frankly I was surprised by the result, having both feared and wished, because of my own dynamics and family romance, that he would come to prefer his biological mother to his adoptive parents. The support of his adoptive parents and the analytic relationship contributed to Ron's remarkable achievement, but they would have meant little were it not for the basic intactness of his personality despite significant neurotic problems, his excellent reality testing, clear ego boundaries and self-object differentiation, and a rapidly developing, phase-appropriate capacity to think abstractly. I doubt that the same integration would have been possible at a younger age, even with the help of analysis. The case also suggests that it may be possible for some older children to have ongoing relationships with both natural and adoptive parents that facilitate rather than impede normal developmental processes.

BIBLIOGRAPHY

Brinich, P. M. (1980). Some potential effects of adoption on self and object representations. *Psychoanal. Study Child*, 35:107–134.
Brunswick, R. M. (1940). The preoedipal phase of the libido development. *Psychoanal. Q.*, 9:293–319.

FEDER, L. (1974). Adoption trauma. *Int. J. Psychoanal.*, 55:411–493.

FREUD, S. (1909). Family romances. *S.E.*, 9:235–241.

GLENN, J. (1974). The adoption theme in Edward Albee's *Tiny Alice* and *The American Dream*. *Psychoanal. Study Child*, 29:413–429.

SHERICK, I. (1983). Adoption and disturbed narcissism. *J. Amer. Psychoanal. Assn.*, 31:487–514.

SIMON, N. M. & SENTURIA, A. G. (1966). Adoption and psychiatric illness. *Amer. J. Psychiat.*, 122:858–868.

WIEDER, H. (1978). On when and whether to disclose about adoption. *J. Amer. Psychoanal. Assn.*, 26:793–812.

Reflections on the Psychoanalytic Treatment of Patients with Bronchial Asthma

LAWRENCE DEUTSCH, M.D.

BRONCHIAL ASTHMA IS FAR MORE WIDESPREAD THAN IS APPARENT. It is not an infrequent condition in patients who are in psychotherapy or analysis for neurotic or characterological difficulties. Analysts whose patients present with physical symptoms, such as asthma, often regard these illnesses as external to the analytic situation and refer their patients for organic therapeutic intervention, dismissing the psychic meaning of the specific diseases. The internists frequently report that their asthmatic patients seem to them to be free of neurotic difficulties. This is not surprising since the intrapsychic needs of asthmatics may be handled symbolically and via fantasy by the somatic illness itself. Furthermore, during severe attacks, asthma functions in additional ways: (1) There is a narrowing cathexis of all aspects of life, as the patient focuses on the need to breathe. (2) In underlyingly phobic individuals, severe attacks necessitate and justify remaining homebound. (3) Analysts become partially decathected, and transferences are temporarily less workable. (4) The fantasies associated with the asthmatic process become further removed from consciousness. One of the aims of this paper is to demonstrate the nature of the relationship between asthma and intrapsychic conflict. This essay addresses some of the technical aspects of psychotherapy and compares the different goals of

Associate clinical professor of psychiatry, Yale Child Study Center; clinical associate professor, The Psychoanalytic Institute, New York University Medical Center.

psychotherapy and psychoanalysis in the treatment of classical psychosomatic illness. The recognition and handling of transference and transference neuroses are crucial with asthmatic patients.

Beginning in the 1970s, the term psychosomatic medicine was redefined (Lipowski et al., 1977; Weiner, 1977; Wittkower and Warnes, 1977) so that it no longer referred to the 7 classical diseases outlined by Alexander (1943). Instead, all medicine and psychiatry, including malignancies, infections, depression, and psychosis, were now under the rubric of psychosomatic medicine and defined as biopsychosocial. Authors of the texts noted above clearly state that psychoanalysis, once considered the pivotal force in both understanding and treating psychosomatic diseases, is, in their opinions, both antiquated and of little value. Pollock (1977a, 1977b), on the other hand, has reworked and updated Alexander's specificity theory to give it relevance today. My understanding of the psychosomatic process essentially parallels Pollock's in that I have noted how biological and social factors interact with a psychological readiness to produce somatic expression of psychic conflict (Deutsch 1980).

Freud (1905) stated,

> It is not easy to estimate the relative efficacy of the constitutional and accidental factors. . . . It should, however, on no account be forgotten that the relation between the two is a co-operative and not a mutually exclusive one. . . . To cover the majority of cases we can picture what has been described as a 'complemental series', in which the diminishing intensity of one factor is balanced by the increasing intensity of the other; there is, however, no reason to deny the existence of extreme cases at the two ends of the series [p. 239f.].

It is worth emphasizing that physiological factors, including allergic predisposition, as well as psychological components play definitive roles in the development of bronchial asthma. One can conceptualize an etiological spectrum from the entirely organic to the entirely psychological. However, the ends of the spectrum, in pure form, are rarely found. Yet psychological aspects are almost always essential to institute the asthmatic process. Some speak of stress as the only psychic force, but it is far more complex. Genetic factors such as the nature of the autonomous ego functions as well as very early childhood experiences help determine which individuals will express emotional conflict and react to stress via physiological (psychosomatic) pathways. Overstimulation (be it aggressive or libidinal), the primitivity and harshness of the superego, and the amount and nature of rejection experienced by the patient at the hands of the parents are some of the experiences that have a profound influence on ego and superego development. This determines the extent and nature of the psychological predisposition to an illness such as asthma. A fear of abandonment is typical in asthmatics. Thus, intense loss, real or symbolic, can usher in asthmatic attacks.

In an earlier essay (1980) I suggested that conjoint medical and psychiatric therapy is important for those suffering from these diseases, but barring physical emergency the prognosis may be improved if psychotherapists or analysts remain the primary physicians.

Bronchial asthma has been divided into two types, the extrinsic and the intrinsic. The former, which is what most of us mean by the term, applies to persons under 40 by and large who have multiple allergies, usually of the respiratory type. The latter, seen in older persons, is usually involved with nasal polyps as well as a sensitivity to salicylates. The case material that I shall present is concerned with the extrinsic type of bronchial asthma and therefore I shall limit my discussion to it.

The development and the analysis of the transference relationship in patients with psychosomatic diseases are crucial. When there is a therapeutic alliance and a positive transference, the patients may lessen the severity of well-established symptoms or give them up completely. As with all such transference "cures," the changes can be illusory in that if the transference becomes negative, life-threatening symptoms may recur. In the case of asthmatics negative transferences can lead to severe bronchospasm and dangerous sequelae.

If we carefully examine the therapeutic process, with a strongly positive transference, we see a number of alternate pathways that treatment may follow. Such a transference can obviate the patient's need to utilize the psychosomatic symptom for a greater or lesser period of time. Another utilization of the positive

transference is with asthmatic patients who develop acute symptoms shortly before or during sessions. They can be helped to
abort these symptoms if the events that precipitate the onset of
specific attacks can be identified and if the aggressive and adaptive functions of the symptomatology can be understood.

However, it is not always possible to influence the acute episode by confrontation or interpretation. Some of the asthmatic
attacks seem to require a certain length of time to dissipate or
"cycle" even with the dynamically correct psychic intervention.
This poses a problem if the physiological situation is so compro-
mising that it is life-threatening. Medical intervention is then
mandatory. This applies as well if the patient's physical symptomatology is so disabling that he cannot comprehend or use
the interpretive intervention. In some instances psychological
events are so devastating, mortifying, or enraging that interpretation produces a negative therapeutic reaction and the
positive transference to the therapist is replaced by ambivalence. The asthmatic attack then may be life-threatening
and necessitates somatic intervention. After the acute phase is
over, it is mandatory that the incident be analyzed and the medical intervention treated as a necessary, but analyzable
parameter.

When the positive transference is predominant, it can be used
to help develop insight and effect structural change, which is
more commonly the case in psychoanalysis than psychotherapy.
Under these circumstances, psychosomatic symptoms, if addressed, readily lend themselve to analysis. When these aspects
of psychopathology are worked through, they tend to become
ego alien and psychosomatic symptoms are replaced by neurotic
symptoms, most commonly phobia or depression.

From a technical point of view it is often necessary to undertake the analysis of the asthmatic symptom early in treatment,
not only because it can be life-threatening, but because it serves
as a resistance to uncovering other material. Wheezing must be
considered part of the associative process, much as mannerisms,
gestures, posture, grunting or other communications having
content and expressing affect.

There are some patients who from the very outset have a
negative transference or others in whom the therapeutic alliance

is tenuous and the transference assumes a brittle quality. The slightest miscalculation in an interpretation, or a nuance or confrontation that is accurate but ill-timed, can produce rapid symptom formation with physiological deterioration.

CLINICAL MATERIAL

The first two vignettes demonstrate different transference reactions and some of the problems arising when there is a need to have careful medical availability and help. Whatever the nature of the transference, a problematic situation arises when there is a split transference, between analyst and parent, internist, or even medication, which can be endowed with magical qualities. Specifically, the positive transference in the first case allowed the patient to work through certain conflicts so that his somatic difficulties decreased and were replaced with neurotic symptoms, in this case phobia. In addition, there is a dramatic illustration in this case of how a proved allergen, dog dander, can produce crippling symptoms when the patient is frightened or unsettled and the same allergen, in the presence of a positive transference, produced no symptoms.

CASE 1

Paul was 8 when, at the request of his pediatrician, I began to treat him for intractable asthma. He was the product of a stormy marriage. Both parents were professionals. His mother had enjoyed working, resented household chores, and was rather critical of her husband. She was very demanding of and punitive toward her four extremely bright children, all of whom had significant characterological or psychosomatic illnesses.

Paul and I hit it off from the beginning. A therapeutic alliance was established even before I met Paul by virtue of his pediatrician's recommendation of me. When the patient came into my office, it was clear that he had the greatest of difficulty in separating from his mother. He insisted that she stay in the waiting room during the entire session. When on one occasion she went on a short errand without telling him, he noticed the absent car as he looked out of the window. He was momentarily panicked, and then it all subsided as he went into an asthmatic attack and his panic centered about air hunger. I interpreted to him his anger with her and how he wished to show her what she had done to him by breaking her promise. He agreed, but this did not lead to an abatement of his wheezing. Having discussed the adaptational aspects of his attack, I turned to the extent of his aggression, but he was suffering from air hunger and all the accessory muscles of his neck and chest were under tension. He coughed up extremely thick mucous and was very cyanotic. At this point in time Paul's mother rang the bell and appeared on the scene. In a very professional manner she whipped out a syringe and gave him a shot of adrenalin. I felt that if she had not arrived at this point, I would have had to call for an ambulance. Parenthetically, she always carried a syringe with her and ampules of adrenalin for such emergencies.

In subsequent sessions I discussed this particular episode with Paul and why he in a sense allowed himself to become so sick. He said that I was the only one that his mother seemed to respect. He trusted me and he believed me that she would wait in the waiting room when I told her to do so. When she left, he felt that I had no power, or that I had not said it to her correctly or definitively, and he had a conscious feeling just before his attack that I had deserted him like everybody else. We also discussed the rage that he experienced when he felt abandoned. He had great difficulty in distinguishing between rage and panic, particularly since his anger soon gave way to panic.

I was able to point out to him that his anger always seemed to precede panic and wheezing. I suggested that he was so angry with his mother from childhood on, when she had left him with different, somewhat incompetent baby-sitters, that he welcomed any opportunity to "embarrass" her.

Some months later Paul's mother left the waiting room to get a book from her car. He had a severe asthmatic attack which nearly necessitated adrenalin. His transference was far more positive now and we talked about the episode. This was the first time that he had ever been able to reverse an attack without medication, and it was the last of the severe attacks.

Later in treatment he discussed how badly he wanted a dog. However, his allergist indicated he was extremely allergic to dog hair which was borne out by an incident when he had a severe asthmatic episode while staying at the home of a friend who had a pet Collie. His mother had to come over, give him an injection of adrenalin, and take him home.

Considering his attachment to his mother, I wondered if his attack was due to the separation and phobic anxiety being acted out in somatic fashion rather than due exclusively to a biological hypersensitivity. Then I realized that I had a dog who after hours would lie on my couch or on the floor and that Paul never became ill on coming into my office. When I shared this information with him, he wondered if he could see my dog and play with her. I checked it out with his mother, who by now was in therapy, as well as with his father. His allergist, who was consulted, called me and advised me that the boy could die from inhaling dog fur. However, both parents were extremely cooperative and allowed Paul to play with my dog, which produced no ill effects. The internist father agreed with me that Paul had no allergic response to this exposure and the parents ultimately got him a dog.

Parenthetically, underlying organic vulnerability in many instances (more likely, the majority) does not produce asthma; one needs a contribution from the psyche. Interestingly, those scratch tests that were originally positive in Paul, representing physiological vulnerability, remained positive. In all the patients I have seen who were successfully analyzed and remained free of asthma, pretreatment positive scratch tests remained positive.

One year after getting his dog Paul was able to contemplate going away to camp. His parents chose a camp that had a doctor on the premises. He went and had only one episode requiring brief medication the day after his parents had visited.

Paul was treated in three times weekly dynamic psychotherapy for approximately 2 years and then twice weekly for another 1½ years. He was asymptomatic when discharged. I met Paul's father almost 18 years after discharge. He informed me that his son was essentially asymptomatic. Paul occasionally felt tightness in his chest but took no medication. He had attended medical school in California, where he had settled. He was a pediatrician, was happily married, had two children.

This case demonstrates several interrelated issues, namely,

that a severely phobic patient can utilize bronchial asthma as a means of maintaining his attachments and that the organic allergic vulnerability can be used *or not used* in accordance with the psychological (in this case, phobic) needs of the patient. His capacity to react to dog dander when under stress and to have no physiological reaction when at peace is most instructive.

CASE 2

This history demonstrates how tenuous the relationship between doctor and patient can become. It also details the development of an addiction to steroids and other antiasthmatic medications. This addiction must be addressed for a number of reasons, not least of which is the anthropomorphization of medication and the subsequent transference splitting.

Born of grossly incompatible parents, Henry was repeatedly rejected from birth on. At 1½ years he had a herniorrhophy. At 3 he had a tonsillectomy. Both times he was not visited in the hospital by his parents who felt that he would cry less in their absence. An aunt visited once and it was she who took him home from the hospital. His father repeatedly locked him in the basement as a punishment. Henry was extremely phobic, fearful of leaving either parent's side.

Henry developed asthma at age 10 and was treated with varying medications and desensitization. Psychiatric treatment was instituted at age 14 when the following incident took place. His parents decided to force him to face his phobia and, unbeknown to him, enrolled him in camp. As Henry was coming home from school, he saw the packed camp trunk, read the label, and instantly realized he was to be forced to go to camp. He immediately developed a severe asthmatic attack and asked his mother, whom he preferred, to take him to the hospital. Instead, his father insisted on taking him. Enroute to the hospital, Henry suddenly turned blue and stopped breathing. A physician in a car behind noted the despair of the father and stopped. He fortunately had oxygen and adrenalin which he administered and then took the child to the nearest hospital. It was touch and go for the child who was bronchoscoped to remove mucous plugs and given steroids. The closeness to death prompted the internist who learned of the precipitating events to suggest psychoanalytic psychotherapy for Henry.

The treatment was difficult and the transference was extremely brittle. The hostile feelings Henry felt for both parents obviously pervaded the transference. After 1½ years of psychotherapy, Henry, still very phobic, continued to insist that he be driven by one of his parents the 10 blocks to my office.

However, I shall focus on the split transference between myself and the medications which were taken by Henry and which he had both hypercathected and anthropomorphized. Shortly after beginning therapy with me, the patient himself chose a new internist, a neighbor who was very cordial to the family. Dr. R. became extremely concerned at the extent of Henry's self medication. For example, Henry carried several medihalers which he used in a fetishistic manner. He was also overdosing himself with Elixophylline and prednisone.

As he improved in psychotherapy, his attacks of asthma became less frequent, but he refused to disclose which medications he was taking, how often he took them, and what the dosages were. His parents and the internist put enormous pressure on Henry to go into the hospital to be withdrawn from the medications, particularly the medihalers and the prednisone. The medihalers were found at that time to cause a rebound phenomenon, which in certain instances could lead to death. Henry willingly agreed to hospitalization, perhaps too willingly. In the hospital the internist idly thumbed through a book Henry was reading and found it was hollowed out; 50 prednisone tablets were secreted there. When Henry went to X-ray, his room was searched. He had hundreds of tablets hidden in every nook and cranny. He had 10 medihalers in his jacket pockets. It was necessary to change his room and to search him too in order to be certain that he was without medication. He remained free of asthma for one day and then became enraged with his loss of control and swore to die of asthma if he could not have his medications back. It was interesting that he said he wanted physically to hold a medihaler, as a talisman, but insisted on having access to prednisone at will. The theophylline drugs did not intrigue him, and he had not brought Elixophylline along. He then went into status asthmaticus and was maintained with oxygen and intravenous aminophylline. It was a precarious situation and I visited him daily. As dyspneic as he was when I visited him, he could come off the oxygen and would talk with me.

For the first time he described the full extent of his addiction to medihalers and to the prednisone. His feelings about each were quite different. The medihalers reminded him of eating ice cream cones, of thumb sucking, of magic, of comfort, and "of course you will say the breast." Prednisone was magic personified. It could stop any attack within minutes and of course had psychotropic effects. For years he had carried both with him to feel safe. Henry left the hospital taking minimal dosages of Elixophylline, but made as a condition of his leaving that he and his mother go to their summer house together for the rest of the summer. He had completed high school and decided not to go to college. Instead, he went into his father's lucrative business which was located adjoining their home. I followed Henry for another 6 months during which time he remained relatively free of symptoms. He decided that he would discontinue treatment because he had worked out a satisfactory deal with his parents who would not "desert me anymore."

It was my feeling that the transference to me was always tenuous. As he said, he felt more secure with the right pills than with the right doctor. His mother had agreed to get analytic help when Henry began therapy with me. It was really as a result of her analysis that it was possible to withdraw him from medications and for her to effect a reconciliation with him so that he could stay relatively free of asthma. Several years later I spoke with her analyst who told me that she was finishing her therapy and that Henry occasionally wheezed, intermittently took Elixophylline, and remained free of steroids and inhalers.

I have presented this vignette to describe two factors: (1) a form of habituation to steroids and inhalers which really took on the characteristics of addiction; and (2) a splitting of the transference between myself and the internist on the one hand and on the other between myself and the medications which almost seemed to be anthropomorphized. Henry's inability to form a transference neurosis severely limited the psychotherapeutic influence.

A unique opportunity to study the effect of psychoanalysis on bronchial asthma presented itself in 1965 when a set of adolescent identical twins, Steve and Ted, were hospitalized for status asthmaticus. The pediatrician felt that psychiatric intervention might be helpful at this time and referred them after discharge to the outpatient psychiatry clinic. Steve was treated on a twice weekly basis, in a low-fee clinic, for 1½ years by a well-known analyst interested in these illnesses. This treatment resulted in a marked reduction in the frequency and intensity of Steve's asthmatic attacks. In fact he never was hospitalized again for asthma, whereas prior to psychotherapy he had been hospitalized several times each year. The other twin, Ted, was referred to me for private treatment. I saw him in psychotherapy for 1½ years and then in a four-time weekly classical analysis for 4 years. Since then he has kept in touch with me over a 20-year period of time and I have had an opportunity to compare the results of his analysis with those of his brother's psychotherapy.

I should like to begin by presenting an overview of this case. Although Ted was at ease in the sessions, outspoken and rather unsophisticated, he had a negative transference to me which colored the sessions for quite some time. Manifestly, he was angry at being treated by a less senior person than was treating his brother. In addition, I had to be paid (whereas his brother paid no clinic fee). At his parents' insistence, Ted had to work to contribute to my fee. The displacement of affect from both parents to me was not yet recognized by the patient.

Early in psychotherapy we dealt with those things that precipitated asthmatic attacks. He was aware that he wheezed during situations of great anger or rage, particularly when he could not express his feelings lest there be serious reprisal; a close friend dated a girl with whom Ted thought he was going steady; his parents made demands on him that in reality were unfair and unrealistic; he was accused of cheating in class when it was someone seated next to him. His descriptive vocabulary particularly in terms of aggression related directly to asthma, as discussed by Sperling (1978). For example, Ted would speak of "being all choked up," of "not being able to catch my breath," of being "so angry I want to throttle him until his tongue comes out." A favorite punishment was to wish his enemies were "put in a guillotine or hung by the neck."

As he became aware of the relationship between frustrated aggression, both in and outside of the transference, and asthmatic attacks, he had fewer and less severe attacks. He seemed to speak freely of his sexuality, his masturbation, his fantasies, and his awkwardness with girls. An early association was: "I masturbated with the fantasy of a woman with one child who arranged for me to baby-sit while she went out. She came home drunk and I slept with her." Ted then began to tell me about the structure of his household. "My family sleeps nude—all free and easy. We always were able to see everything. My brother and I both got asthma when we were about 3 or 4."

His associations were not difficult to follow. He had reported a masturbatory fantasy of seducing an older woman, followed by comments on the fact that his family slept nude. Then he discussed his mother's feeble attempts at covering up when she emerged from bed. This only served to further excite the twins. Ted was able to see the connection in his associative train between his masturbatory fantasy and the seduction at home. He did not at this point connect frustration at the seduction with his rage. Although a connection between overstimulation and asthmatic attacks was clear to him and logical, it lacked the necessary conviction or the emotional insight necessary for structural change. What did transpire was that a flood of material emerged detailing further overstimulation. Early childhood was an intense and exciting period. He frequently got into bed with his mother or both parents if his father was at home. He vividly recalled the tactile sensations and the smells in the parental bed. He could also remember "accidentally" touching his mother's breasts and her giggle.

Ted had applied to various analytic clinics while he was in psychotherapy. He was notified that he was accepted at one where twin studies were in progress, but would have to wait 10 months for treatment. He was advised to phase out psychotherapy at least 3 months prior to beginning analysis. After he received this information, he had an asthmatic attack and had to take Tedral. Despite the medication he came to the session wheezing audibly. He felt that this was a brutal situation and that it was typical of all clinics. He had decided himself that he liked me and wanted to work with me. He planned to leave day college at the end of the semester, to switch to evening college, and to work and pay for his own analysis. He wondered if I would make time for him, arrange a fair fee, or would I insist that he attend the clinic lest I be embarrassed after having sent a summary about him.

He seemed genuinely surprised when I said that I would enjoy working with him. He felt that on some pretext I would refuse to analyze him. He had many fantasies about this. Would I insist on seeing both him and his twin? Would I prefer treating someone who could pay more? Or would I continue the psychotherapy with him so that I could have two people in the 4-hour opening that he would need.

Ted's associations now referred to his past experiences in bed with his mother during the time his father had left the family. The marriage was unstable, although no divorce ensued. He missed his father then, but there were the rewards of being with mother. "Your giving me to the clinic is like my father giving me to my mother. The clinic is like a mother, big tits I could play with, a promise of something to come, but nothing more." With this insight, a feeling of constriction in his chest vanished.

I suggested to him that he equated me not only with the depriving father but with the mother who constantly teased him with her nudity and then did not come through with the goods. I also indicated that I was cognizant of the tremendous sacrifice he would have to make to undertake full analysis.

He now began to discuss analysis—its meaning, the differences between it and therapy, and the obligations it imposed. He was excited at the prospect of getting to know more about himself faster and wryly noted that he had been born with the umbilical cord around his neck; he was delivered first and had to be resuscitated and was considered more fragile than his brother. Now for the first time he did not feel second best and was eager to make something of his life. This was one of the very few times he showed direct competition with his twin.

At this point prior to undertaking an analysis, two major

things were clear to both Ted and myself: (1) Asthmatic attacks occurred when he felt unexpressible rage—when his aggression was not neutralized. (2) Libidinal overstimulation could precipitate severe asthmatic attacks, particularly if his parents were directly or indirectly involved. After 1½ years of psychotherapy, Ted was much like his brother; the edge had been taken off, "We both can still wheeze, but we don't let it get near where it used to be when we nearly died."

Analyzing Ted was very different from doing psychotherapy with him. His lying on the couch and a certain amount of abstinence led to a revival of the dormant negative transference. I certainly was the absent father and the mother who, in ways that he came to enumerate, was quite narcissistic and depriving. Having a twin brother meant a forced sharing of everything and a lack of a clear-cut feeling of belonging. My silence reminded him of the noises he would listen for from his parents' room. In this sense he reminded me of the meaning of the Wolf-Man's dream as reported by Freud (1918). His schoolwork began to suffer as he rapidly developed a transference neurosis. It was possible to demonstrate to him the various displacements from his father to me. Not only was the negative transference fraught with danger, but the positive transference was equally disquieting in that homosexual feelings abounded. He recalled wrestling with his father in the mornings, in bed, nude, and the panic he experienced when his father held him down and pinned him.

His asthmatic attacks increased in number and severity during this period. It was necessary to arrange for medical assistance, an injection of adrenalin on two occasions. However, at no time did he develop status asthmaticus or require hospitalization. As he worked through the negative transference in terms of the projection and displacement from his parents, his brother, and his grandparents, his asthma markedly diminished. As we reworked the overdetermined meanings of bronchial asthma, he was faced with ever-increasing rage at the overstimulation during childhood. With the virtual disappearance of asthma after about 8 months of analysis he became overtly phobic. He feared travel, airplanes, driving with other drivers, and essentially kept to a routine which involved traveling in a square from his home to work, from work to treatment, then to school, and back again home. Understanding the phobia, which involved multiple fixations, occupied a great part of the analysis. He also came to recognize that bronchial asthma served as a phobic equivalent for him by, for example, limiting the distance he could travel. With the diminution of the recurrent asthma, he was able to concentrate on schoolwork, utilizing more neutralized aggression, and fared well there.

Ted took to the analytic process very readily. He spoke freely and the observing aspect of his ego was in evidence as he frequently would stop to reflect on what he had said. Most of what he had discussed in psychotherapy was repeated but in much greater detail and with affect and actively involving the transference neurosis.

By the time he had completed his second year of analysis, Ted no longer had symptoms of asthma, was doing respectably in night college, and worked at a semiskilled job by day. His twin still had chronic asthma, had not done well in school, left college, and was working full-time at a similar job to Ted's but somewhat more skilled.

The analysis at this time took on the characteristics of the analysis of a person with a phobic character disorder. Ted had multiple fixations, acting-out tendencies, areas of psychopathy, and an intense, somewhat ambivalent transference. I shall allude to but a few items of the latter phase of his analysis because this essay focuses on the issue of analytic approaches to bronchial asthma, which was no longer a symptom. However, it was important to work through the psychic meanings as a barrier to recurrence.

Fantasies dealing with asthma and phobic feelings provoked intense anxiety. Ted thought of a spot of dust wandering in his lungs. This could be blown about anywhere in the two balloonlike structures which constituted them. There was no escape for this spot of dust. He thought of "Huit Clos" (No Exit), the existential work by Sartre. He easily identified the spot of dust as himself, and this image could produce panic in him at anytime, particularly when he saw himself lost in a maze.

The two balloonlike structures seemed obvious to him; they were breasts. He spent considerable time discussing his fascination with "mommary glands" and his recognition that he fought off sexual excitement when he would watch his mother in the bath or dressing. Despite a myriad of associations along these lines, it was my feeling that this fantasy was indeed more primitive.

After associating further, he saw his lungs as a womblike structure, one in which he once was imprisoned. He now recalled that from early childhood on he had trouble swimming underwater and wondered if this phobia was related to an unconscious fear of drowning in the womb. His mother, who freely discussed all matters pertaining to procreation, had told him when he was quite young all about the water bag in which babies live. As he got into late latency, he would frighten easily at the image of the spot of dust lost in his lungs. A profound fear of drowning would cause him the same type of anguish from early latency on.

The patient had other interesting fantasies concerning his asthmatic attacks which were related to his phobias. He began by noting that he felt the same things that his twin would feel. Once when his father hit his twin and Steve cried, Ted also cried and felt as if *he* were hit. He then wondered if when he wheezed, he was in reality furious; then by a process of "taking in" the enemy, he would be subjecting him to the same discomfort he felt. This caused him to realize that the spot in his lung could also represent the "enemy," not just himself. He now associated bronchospasm, along aggressive lines, to incorporating and then killing or choking his foes, who would suffer oxygen deprivation, much as he had during asthmatic attacks.

During early adolescence he had many thoughts about life and death, the concept of infinity and the boundaries of space, all of which provoked extreme anxiety. When he developed severe asthma during one of these reveries, he felt better because with the onset of asthma he no longer thought of these disquieting fantasies.

In this phase of analysis we learned that Ted had always been phobic. During the oedipal period he was petrified of spiders. In latency, he felt fearful if he had to travel any distance. However, during preadolescence and adolescence he became counterphobic, a bully and a street fighter. He did not want to "play wrestle" with his father anymore and took up boxing in school. When asthma was no longer a prime mode of communication, the counterphobic attitudes seemed to melt away, and phobic symptoms returned.

In addition, Ted had many anal associations to wheezing. Asthma involved spitting and thereby making a mess. Toilet training was difficult and the patient recalled a great deal of anal preoccupation. He and his brother and other prelatency friends would expose their buttocks to each other and play doctor. He still felt badly when he remembered the instability of his parents' marriage and his father's hostility to the family. Yet he admired cruelty and had many sadistic fantasies. He frequently thought of spanking his girlfriend during or instead of having sex. He interpreted his street fighting as an identification with his father.

Ted kept two girlfriends, a steady and a spare, much as he felt his father had done. In analysis, Ted recalled that when he was 3 or 4 his father disappeared for brief periods of time. Parenthetically, this was when the twins first developed asthma. When the boys were 7, their father, living away, would take out his sons on weekends, frequently bringing a woman with him.

It was during the final year of analysis that Ted, free of asthma and not phobic, began to identify with me in manner, dress, and in his attempts at problem solving. He completed night college and then was accepted for graduate work for an M.B.A. He did well, apprenticed, and passed his exams for a C.P.A. He has changed jobs but twice in the past two decades and currently holds an important position as chief financial officer of a very prestigious midwestern corporation.

Ted has called me every 3 years or so to keep me abreast of his progress. He has remained free of asthma during the past 20 years. He is happily married and has 3 children.

Ted's brother still is prone to asthmatic attacks. He was married and divorced, is childless, and has not completed college, but works as an artisan and is well paid in his field. The brothers who had been inseparable now lead different lives, in different parts of the country, and with different goals and aspirations.

DISCUSSION

A computer search of asthma cross-referenced with psychology and psychoanalysis for the past decade produced over 100 cita-

tions; however, there was not a single citation in any of the
classical psychoanalytic journals. The majority of the articles
were in journals dealing with asthma, asthma research, psychosomatic medicine, or psychosomatic research. These articles can
be categorized in several groups. Some assessed the role of emotions in asthma in a "fact-finding" manner. Levitan and Winkler
(1985) compared dreams of asthmatics in psychotherapy with
those of patients with the other classical psychosomatic diseases.
Asthmatics showed significantly larger numbers of dreams in
which they were depicted as victims of aggression. Many articles
refer to MMPI and the Panic-fear Personality Scale as an index
of the rate of exacerbation or prognosis (Dirks and Kinsman,
1982). Hollaender and Florin (1983) discussed expressed emotion and airway conductance in children with bronchial asthma;
they noted that "the frequency and duration of expressed an-
ger/rage, enjoyment/joy, and surprise/startle were lower in
asthmatics." The data also indicated "a relevant relationship between facial expression of emotion and breathing function" (p.
307). Another study (Mook and Van der Ploeg, 1980) shows that
expiration improved in asthmatic subjects when they verbalized
freely. No improvement was noted when subjects were either
interrupted or forced to listen.

Other articles in the asthma research journals showed a greater awareness of the role of psychodynamic factors in the development of disease but were more likely to be data-based and thus
not involved with the specific nature of fantasies or the techniques of psychoanalytic psychotherapy. For example, Jackson
(1976) notes,

> . . . major biological arousals may occur when an individual fails
> to cope with stress. A visceral expression of distressing conflict
> typically appears when its affective expression is inadequate.
> Asthmatic attacks may be regarded in some cases as visceral
> expressions of psychosocial stress which a person is unable to
> confine effectively to the ideational sphere. The psychic aspect
> of the stress is preverbal phantasy of a primitive and concrete
> kind which give meaning to the symptoms. Denial is the main
> defensive method used by an asthmatic person with an impaired
> capacity to express affect; it can range from an inability to think
> about feelings to a splitting or discontinuity within the person-
> ality. Engaging an asthmatic person in psychotherapy can be

difficult where denial is the main defensive method, for insight is likely to be repudiated [p. 250].

Ago et al. (1979) point out that although allergic reactions occur in "individuals who have a hereditary or congenital allergic constitution, clinical symptoms often disappear due to changes of the individuals' life situations and/or their adaptive patterns" (p. 197). A controlled study of university students with asthma and another group who had been completely free of childhood asthma for more than 3 years (without specific treatment) found no significant difference in allergic predisposition between the two groups. "Findings suggest that allergic predisposition does not influence the prognosis of allergic disorders as much as do sociopsychological factors" (p. 197).

Most of the articles concerning asthma and the psyche agree that stress and conflict are central issues in the development of extrinsic bronchial asthma. A variety of therapies are described—biofeedback, behavior modification, hypnosis, family therapy, group therapy, and psychopharmacology. None claims to do more than to aid in the therapeutic process. This is in contradistinction to those cases that have been analyzed where an effective cure was sought.

An interesting single case report of the psychoanalysis of a 13-year-old girl with severe bronchial asthma is detailed by Karol (1981). In this report the role of primal scene trauma in the development of a sadomasochistic character structure is clearly delineated. Wilson (1981) corroborates Karol's findings and discusses Sperling's (1949) hypothesis that unconscious conflicts of the mother or father predispose a child to psychosomatic reactions; if the fantasies involve the lungs, bronchial asthma is most likely to occur. Mintz (1981) essentially agrees with Karol's formulations but feels that a more global view is necessary in that other types of conflicts can be at the core of asthmatic reactions.

A number of authors have written about the relationship between early trauma and the development of somatic manifestations of tension or anxiety in the infant (Spitz, 1965; Greenacre, 1967). Ritvo (1981) noted:

The disturbances in the parent-child relationship stem in large measure from the personality disorders and neurotic illnesses of the parents, particularly their anxiety, aggression, and depression which result in qualities of parenting that aggravate rather than mitigate the traumatic condition. Other disturbances in the parent-child relationship may stem from inherent vulnerabilities in the child. The somatic illnesses that appear most frequently in the infantile history of these patients and often continue into adult life are skin, gastrointestinal, and respiratory disorders.

Apart from their severe anxiety and psychoneurotic symptoms, these patients are characterized by their polymorphous-perverse sexual development [p. 340].

Ritvo described multiple psychosomatic symptoms in his patient, Mr. A., who also suffered from phobias. I do not believe that the connection between phobia (or depression) and psychosomatic diseases is incidental, but rather is an interchangeable expression of the same process.

The majority of patients with bronchial asthma who come to analysis do so in seeking relief from neurotic symptoms that are not bound by the psychosomatic process, rather than for relief of asthma. Some patients are referred by medical specialists who have become aware of the extent of the psychogenic components in the precipitation of acute asthmatic attacks. In either case, asthmatic patients almost always enter the psychotherapeutic process with multiple medications and multiple transferences. It is my belief that those doing psychotherapy or analysis with asthmatic patients should be aware of the physiological pathways involved in this illness and of the medical management based on an understanding of these, much as I believe those involved in medical management should be familiar with psychological issues, such as those I have outlined.

Conclusion

The thesis of this essay is that extrinsic bronchial asthma is a multivariant disease where biological factors may be necessary but not sufficient to cause the illness. In the patients presented, bronchial asthma did not appear unless a particular psychic constellation was operant. Whether this is true for all cases of bronchial asthma is not clear. I suspect, however, that it is true in the majority of cases of extrinsic asthma. Furthermore, I have attempted to show that analysis is an effective method of treatment. My study of a monozygotic twin is most instructive in view of the utilization of different therapeutic approaches with the brothers and the long-term follow-up.

From my experiences with asthmatic and other psychosomatic patients certain concepts have emerged:

1. When the psychic structure of the patient permits, psychoanalysis is the most effective psychological intervention. Psychoanalytically derived psychotherapy is a close second.

2. Joint management of a patient by a psychoanalyst and an internist is feasible and desirable if the transference is strong enough and positive enough to keep transference splitting to an acceptable level and the analyst is essentially in the role of primary physician. The use of medications by asthmatics in analytic therapy may be necessary at times, though not ideal. Since medication can be invested with magic or anthropomorphized, its use must be seen as a parameter and analyzed as such.

3. Overstimulation, libidinal or aggressive, predisposes to defective ego formation involving difficulties with the synthetic and reality testing functions of the ego as well as leading to pathological defenses, such as denial and ultimately to the psychosomatic symptom formation (in those vulnerable to somatic representation of psychic conflict). The twins presented in this essay suffered from traumatic primal scene experiences, much as Karol (1981) has described. Libidinal overstimulation also took the form of parental nudity and exposure of the child to parental toileting. The frequent arguments and aggressive acting out have been described. In addition, frequent hospitalizations constituted traumatic overstimulations.

4. Rejection, as experienced and described by asthmatics, most often took the form of threats of abandonment by the parents. Sperling's formulation (1978) concerning the nature of the abandonment is an important contribution. She describes the parents of psychosomatically ill children as rewarding them when they are sick and dependent, and rejecting them when they attempt to individuate.

5. My experience in analyzing a number of patients with asthma and other pyschosomatic illnesses is that when the somatic manifestation leaves, the most common neurotic symp-

tom complex is phobia, which I have found to be a good prognostic sign. Parenthetically, the psychosomatic illness itself serves as a phobic equivalent.

It is my hope that my experiences will encourage others to treat psychosomatically ill patients and to treat the psychosomatic illness as an analyzable manifestation of the patient's psychopathology. There is a great deal of satisfaction to be gained by patient and analyst in undertaking psychoanalytic treatment, a treatment that can resolve both somatic manifestations and intrapsychic conflict.

BIBLIOGRAPHY

Ago, Y. et al. (1979). Psychosomatic studies of allergic disorders. *Psychother. & Psychosom.*, 31:197–204.

Alexander, F. (1943). Fundamental concepts of psychosomatic research. *Psychosom. Med.*, 5:205–210.

Deutsch, L. (1980). Psychosomatic medicine from a psychoanalytic viewpoint. *J. Amer. Psychoanal. Assn.*, 28:653–703.

Dirks, J. F. & Kinsman, R. A. (1982). Death in asthma. *J. Asthma*, 19:177–187.

Freud, S. (1905). Three essays on the theory of sexuality. *S.E.*, 7:125–243.

———— (1918). From the history of an infantile neurosis. *S.E.*, 17:3–123.

Greenacre, P. (1967). The influence of infantile trauma on genetic patterns. In *Psychic Trauma*, ed. S. S. Furst. New York: Basic Books, pp. 108–153.

Hollaender, J. & Florin, I. (1983). Expressed emotion and airway conductance in children with bronchial asthma. *J. Psychosom. Res.*, 27:307–311.

Jackson, M. (1976). Psychopathology and psychotherapy in bronchial asthma. *Brit. J. Med. Psychol.*, 49:249–255.

Karol, C. (1981). The role of primal scene and masochism in asthma. *Int. J. Psychoanal. Psychother.*, 8:577–592.

Levitan, H. & Winkler, P. (1985). Aggressive motifs in the dreams of psychosomatic and psychoneurotic patients. *Interfaces*, 12:11–19.

Lipowski, Z. J., Lipsitt, D. R., & Whybrow, P. C., eds. (1977). *Psychosomatic Medicine*. New York: Oxford Univ. Press.

Mintz, I. L. (1981). Multideterminism in asthmatic disease. *Int. J. Psychoanal. Psychother.*, 8:593–600.

Mook, J. & Van der Ploeg, H. M. (1980). Speech activity and respiratory function in asthmatics. *Psychother. & Psychosom.*, 33:166–177.

Pollock, G. H. (1977a). The ghost that will not go away. *J. Amer. Acad. Psychoanal.*, 5:421–430.

———— (1977b). The psychosomatic specificity concept. *Annu. Psychoanal.*, 5:141–168.

RITVO, S. (1981). Anxiety, symptom formation, and ego autonomy. *Psychoanal. Study Child*, 36:339–362.

SPERLING, M. (1949). The role of the mother in psychosomatic disorders in children. *Psychosom. Med.*, 11:377–385.

————— (1978). *Psychosomatic Disorders in Childhood*, ed. O. Sperling. New York: Aronson.

SPITZ, R. A. (1965). *The First Year of Life*. New York: Int. Univ. Press.

WEINER, H. (1977). *Psychobiology and Human Disease*. New York: Elsevier.

WILSON, C. P. (1981). Parental overstimulation in asthma. *Int. J. Psychoanal. Psychother.*, 8:601–621.

WITTKOWER, E. D. & WARNES, H., eds. (1977). *Psychosomatic Medicine*. Hagerstown, Md.: Harper & Row.

A Child Analyzes a Dream

ROBERT D. GILLMAN, M.D.

THE ANALYSIS OF DREAMS IN THE PSYCHOANALYSIS OF CHILDREN IS a neglected area. Ablon and Mack (1980), in their review of children's dreams, state, "despite their richness as a source of knowledge about childhood, children's dreams have been little investigated by psychoanalysts, and there are relatively few reports of their use in the evaluation, psychotherapy, or psychoanalytic treatment of children" (p. 213). Although Harley (1962) and Fraiberg (1965) referred to dream interpretation with latency children, such case reports have remained isolated examples. Ablon and Mack conclude, "If this review has any overriding purpose, it is to encourage a return to the study of dreams, especially the dreams of children" (p. 213). This paper shares the same purpose. The following case report describes a latency-age girl who was able to work on the analysis of a dream over a period of five analytic sessions.

CASE REPORT

Jenifer was almost 8 when she came for analysis. And almost exactly one year later, 2 months before her ninth birthday, she reported the dream that we worked on together. Jenifer was brought to treatment by her parents who had numerous complaints. She was rebellious, brooding, disobedient to her mother, and tyrannical to her 4½-year-old sister. She masturbated openly, had hand-washing rituals, and sometimes used the entire roll of toilet paper before she could feel clean. She could not stand

Training and supervising analyst, Baltimore-Washington Institute for Psychoanalysis; clinical professor of psychiatry, George Washington University; President-elect, Association for Child Psychoanalysis.

the smell of certain foods, but gorged herself on her favorite foods. She had nightmares despite going-to-bed rituals that involved the exact placement of toys and furniture. She was afraid of shots and insisted that her mother or sister accompany her to the bathroom. She had tantrums when possessions were lost or broken. Because things had to be her way, she had no close friends.

Jenifer was the first-born of two children, much wanted after several years of marriage. Her father was an obsessional accountant who shared a special interest in reading myths and legends with her. She had the same lighter skin and blond hair as her father. Her mother, although college-educated, felt less bright and inferior to her husband and daughter. Jenifer's birth and infancy were not remarkable except for toileting struggles that began at 2½ and continued until training was completed at 4 years. At 3½, 3 months before her sister's birth, her father was hospitalized for a brief but serious illness. When the mother too entered the hospital, Jenifer was cared for by a worried grandmother. Around this time open masturbation and fear of shots began.

Jenifer's intense jealousy which began at her sister's birth remained unabated at the time of her referral. Her mother had read to her while nursing the sister in order to diminish the rivalry. Jenifer was now a voracious reader. She had a tantrum each day on her return from nursery school with the feeling that her mother and sister had some especially good time in her absence. Jenifer's mean attitude toward her sister, with whom she shared a room, brought her into repeated conflict with her mother.

On psychological testing she achieved a very superior IQ with outstanding verbal ability. Projective tests showed distrust, hostility, negativism, a feeling of maternal rejection, and much concern with punishment.

Jenifer was a sturdy, attractive girl. In the playroom she spent much of her time drawing women and girls—endless princess and Cinderalla pictures filled with stories of envy and rivalry. It was striking that they all had long straight hair like her mother and sister, and all had stubby arms that did not reach below the waist—almost like thalidomide victims. When she confessed her masturbation, she explained that she rubbed against a corner of the bed, that she did not use her hands at all.

Early in the analysis she showed a strong positive transference. The princess fantasies seemed to compensate for inferiority feelings. It was surprising that in the presence of such prominent obsessional defenses and symptoms, triangular rivalry themes were there from the first. She told about her rituals; she confessed her loneliness and her feelings of being ugly. There were robber fantasies with many ramifications. Sometimes the analyst was a robber. Robbers scared you at night. Pirates took you prisoner, but the pirate chief chose you above all the others. Robbery was also a projection of her wish to take from the analyst, and above all to deprive his other patients. Later she became the crippled pirate who took revenge for his damaged state.

Jenifer usually reported her dreams to her mother rather than to me, though early in the treatment she had told me a dream: "There were four bugs or spiders, each in one corner at the ceiling in this office." She did not associate to or work on this dream.

One Monday Jenifer came in eating cheese crackers, wiped her hands carefully, and said, "What should we talk about—I had a dream. My mother took away my Mary book because I had nightmares. I have to ask my father to get it back." Mary was Jenifer's heroine, a teen-age girl who led her friends in detective work, solving mysteries. She then told her dream:

> I went to see the Mona Lisa, but the museum had tables we were eating at. I looked up and saw the Mona Lisa was missing from its frame. It had torn, cut edges. I was the first to see and told the guard, and the next day told my class in school, and I felt proud I was the first to know.

I asked in various ways for associations to the dream. Jenifer added more details to the manifest content and to the day's residue. She said in the course of the session in answer to questions: "I went with my grandmother and mother to see the Mona Lisa [on loan to the local gallery]. My father and my sister went to our office—I mean his office. She was too young to go," she added contemptuously. "The Mona Lisa has brown hair, her eyes follow you, she has a smile. It was cut out like with a knife—

like an apple is cut. It spoils after it's cut. It had jagged edges like
it was cut with a knife or a saw." She said that the tables had old
catsup bottles on them. To my question about something missing, she told about losing a mitten and said that it was sad to think
about things missing. "I don't want to talk about it." To questions
about being proud she told about correcting her sister who had
been talking baby talk.

While she was talking, she got very busy drawing. Aside from
her usual supply of rich girls and poor girls, she drew (1) a two-
headed lady, and (2) a series of Zoo animals and a horse (of
significance because my office at that time was across the street
from the Zoo, and sometimes Jenifer's mother would drop her
off for her hour and take the sister to the Zoo).

Tuesday was spent mostly drawing pictures of girls of all sizes
and ages, some with blond hair. The 1-month-old was the favorite of the king and several wore crowns. The 8-year-old looked
"different" from the rest of the family. When I asked about that,
she drew a Cinderella girl in rags with a broom, adding, "She
smiles to hide her downcast feelings so she won't be pitied."

She went over to my couch looking at the picture above it
(this was a scene of Rome with buildings and an equestrian statue; Jenifer had studied it carefully, intrigued by the legend that
labeled each part of the picture). "Is this the frame behind the
frame?" she asked. I asked if it could be connected with the
Mona Lisa dream since both were about Italy. "Oh, no. It's not
the same, it wasn't in my thoughts. I forget your picture as soon
as I leave." I said that thoughts stay in the back of your head
and come out in dreams. She replied, "That's the trouble with
thoughts, they come back up and interfere." She then talked
about pictures at home in the dining room. I reminded her that
there was eating in the dream. She said that it wasn't the same
at all. Then as she said good-bye, she said cheerily, "I get popcorn today!"

On Wednesday she came in with a series of pictures of "Annette and the two-headed people." She had made up a play she
hoped the children in class would act. It was about Annette
eating an apple, falling asleep, being waked, given food, and
living happily ever after. She had been proud, but had been
scared when the teacher asked her to take a paper to the differ-

ent classes for signatures. She then drew a series of college girls ranked according to meanness and popularity. The second prettiest was mean and the least popular. She said, "Kindness is more important than being pretty. I'm mean a lot of the time and don't have friends. Being pretty doesn't matter at all." I said that sometimes people say it doesn't matter when it really does. She shrugged it off, "Not with me. My parents say it's what's inside not what's outside and I believe it." I said that a person could believe one way but inside feel the opposite. "Yes," she said, "You can't help your thoughts and feelings. Sometimes I feel so miserable I want to die. My father took my book away. I was rude."

On Thursday she offered me some of her cheese crackers, then said, "Let's play museum." She had chosen this theme several times in the past. The various furnishings of the office became statues. She herself was a 4,000-year-old statue that had drunk from the fountain of youth and had been struck by a sword so she couldn't be killed. I was a visitor who had overstayed and was locked in. She came to life from her statue state and in a sepulchral tone announced, "It is I, and the stones are turned to food." I reminded her of the food in the Mona Lisa dream. "Yes," she said, "Maybe it does remind me of your office picture. The doors are locked, so we stay here forever. There is an endless supply of food, drink, and medicine, and drawers full of toys for children." As an afterthought, she added, "In case some time some children are locked in." Then she had us sleep, and later told of her earlier life when she had many servants.

The following Monday she announced, "This is my second year here" (the anniversary of her starting analysis). She set up the museum again, bringing me food and drink. I commented, "An office with food and drink." She replied, "It's not an office, it's a museum." I reminded her, "But your sister went to your father's office" (I knew something about his office). She then told me that her sister had had Sprite in her father's office. "There was Sprite in the dream," she added. I said, "Sarah was with your father, and even though you believe you oughtn't to feel jealous and believe it would be rude, you still might feel it anyway." She countered, "But I've been there." I insisted, "You might feel it anyway." This time she agreed, "Yes, you have feelings even though you don't want to, you can't help it. Let's think more about the dream and solve it." I said, "The picture was torn out." She corrected, "Cut out. I know. It means that I was out of the fun. We've solved the dream." I remarked that she had solved that part of it, it was a good idea. She thanked me.

I then wondered if it could also be that when Sarah went with her mother last week to the Zoo and got popcorn, she felt cut out even though she thought she shouldn't feel that way. "But she never gets popcorn without some for me," she protested. "But even though you know that, you might not be able to help the feeling," I said. "Yes," she said, "We've solved the Mona Lisa dream."

She told of lying awake worried and crying because she heard some boys talking about the sun getting cold and did not realize it would not happen for a long time. She said, "It's easier to forget pleasant things. Unpleasant things keep coming back, even though you try to think of something else. Sometimes I'm rude when I don't want to be and then I'm sorry and want to apologize but don't do it for a while." We talked about how miserable she had felt when she was rude to her father and he took the book away. I asked if she might feel some danger in being rude to me.

She then turned on my air conditioner (it was winter) and my electric heater, saying, "Cold on one side, heat on the other. What about the other dream, the four bugs," she asked. "Maybe it's four friends, the three other girls I wanted to make up the play. I made the title 'Annette and the two-headed girl.'" I said, "Cold on one side, hot on the other—like two feelings at the same time, like a two-headed girl who wants to see the Mona Lisa but wants to go to her father's office, who wants to come here but wants to go to the Zoo." She replied, "That solves the four bugs. Ask me some more about the Mona Lisa dream." I asked about the old catsup bottles. "This old office," she exclaimed, "Who wants to come to this old office." I commented, "Yes, two feelings at once."

"How long do I have to keep coming here? I try to solve my problems. I told two dreams. I can't remember any from last night."

Suddenly she said, "What about the frame?" She looked up at

my picture, "I know, I was framed into coming here. That's it!" I replied, "You thought you would come a short time and now it's a year." She agreed and took a small piece of paper on which she wrote with a flourish of triumph: "We think that we have solved the Mona Lisa mystery dream."

At that moment I could think only of Freud's fantasy that there would be a marble tablet that said: "In this house on July 24, 1895, the Secret of Dreams was revealed to Dr Sigmund Freud." But Jenifer had further thoughts, "What's an analyst? It's like a psychiatrist. An analyst doesn't know all the answers— he helps you figure them out. If he needs help, he goes to another analyst."

DISCUSSION

The analysis of the Mona Lisa dream was an important step in bringing Jenifer's ambivalence into the transference and in helping her to relinquish her denial and reaction formations. She now faced the anger represented in the cut or torn-out picture and the anger in the depreciated "old catsup bottles." She was then able to reveal her feelings of being miserable, formerly hidden behind her Mona Lisa façade, just as she had expressed it in the drawing of the 8-year-old girl: "She smiles to hide her downcast feelings." The pride of the manifest dream had hidden her misery. The dream brought into the analysis her feelings of being left out, recapitulating the unresolved feelings from her first nursery school days when she was so jealous of her sister and angry with her mother. In the dream it is the mother figure who is cut out. At this time she was also representing her oedipal and sibling struggles with repetitive Cinderella drawings and drawings of girls ranked by beauty, kindness, and popularity. Her wish to be popular was represented in her identification with the Mona Lisa, the most popular picture in history. Jenifer felt like Cinderella, discarded and rejected, in need of pity.

Many aspects of the dream were, of course, not analyzed at this time. The capturing of the father-analyst in the museum play, like the earlier robber and pirate fantasies of being the chosen one, eventually led in the analysis to an intense, positive, oedipal transference neurosis. The emphasis on food and her rage at her mother which were both in the dream and characteristic of her current life were only later related to Jenifer's experiences around the birth of her sister. The manifest dream theme of something missing, cut or torn out, did not enter the work until much later. In the course of a long analysis we did work with the relationship between feeling ugly and her castrated state, and we worked with her sadistic masturbation fantasies that involved torture and beating of other children, finally achieving a successful resolution of her neurosis.

What made it possible for Jenifer to work so consistently on this dream? Under the stress of the intensifying transference she told most of her dreams to her mother, and she had begun to confess to her mother the problems that came up in her analysis, probably out of guilt and to dilute the transference. Further, she told all of her nightmares to her mother and kept them from the analysis. Analysts have long noted how children shy away from associating to nightmares because talking about them leads to reexperiencing the traumatic anxiety.

It is significant that the dream that Jenifer was able to work on so long was not a nightmare or anxiety dream. The narcissistic manifest content, "I was the first to know and told the others," was an identification with Mary, Jenifer's favorite, the self-styled detective-book heroine who led her friends to solve mysteries. This identification was intensified when her parents took away her book because of her bad dreams. And her parents' action must have influenced her choice to bring the dream into the analysis. It is no accident, then, that Jenifer wrote, "We think we have solved the Mona Lisa mystery dream." By proclaiming the dream "solved," Jenifer served notice that the work on the dream had come to an end. This illustrates the episodic nature of work with children, where work on a particular conflict may be circumscribed, and an intense transference may be short-lived.

Jenifer was a "voracious reader," and reading was a source of sublimation and pride. She was widely read in fairy tales and myths, interests she shared with her father. Her dream became one of the story plots she worked to unravel in a father transference.

Ordinarily it is considered difficult to induce latency children to explore the hidden aspects of dreams because of the nature of latency itself with its emphasis on objective reality and rejection of the kind of primary process mental functioning elicited in dream associations. Relatively few dreams are used in the analysis of latency children as compared with other age groups. Dream analysis is not infrequent in the analyses of prepubertal and older children, and in the analyses of naïve prelatency children. Becker (1978) writes, "The latency child's primary task is to develop defenses against incestuous wishes. Secondary process thinking is becoming consolidated. Free association would tend to undermine both of these and is therefore rigorously avoided" (p. 358). Unconscious material is then defended against and disguised. However, Becker adds, "There are exceptions. Certain children who possess superior intelligence and suffer from obsessional neurosis may be capable of episodes of free association" (p. 356). Jenifer was certainly one of these: she could associate to parts of a dream. Ablon and Mack (1980) reached the same conclusion: "However, bright children in the latency period with strong obsessive-compulsive defensive patterns may readily take to reporting and analyzing dreams as an enjoyable intellectual challenge" (p. 207). Neither author cites a clinical example. Perhaps it is the obsessional child's capacity for isolation that permits it to analyze dreams without mobilizing too much anxiety.

What customarily takes place with latency children's dreams is that the analyst bases his interventions not on the direct verbal associations but on his understanding of the play material during that session, the current stage of analysis including defenses and transference, parental information about the child's life, and the analyst's translation of the likely latent significance of the manifest content. Silverman (1985) stated that because of their "incompletely matured cognitive and emotional development," these children cannot "communicate through words alone but also resort to drawings and to the action sphere of play to express themselves" (p. 14f.). I made use of all of these ancillary aids in the beginning of the analysis of Jenifer's dream. She was able to go beyond this, however, and in the final session of dream analysis supplied meaningful verbal associations of her own.

Other authors have suggested certain transferences and character traits that lend themselves to the analysis of dreams. Becker (1978) describes a special kind of transference in his case report of a 12-year-old boy who worked well with dreams. Martley's hostility, rivalry, and aggression were mainly repressed and expressed in masochistic compliance. Harley (1962) concluded from her work with a latency girl for whom dreams played a significant role that the dreams were a "safety valve" for the child who suffered a high pitch of excitement, excessive stimulation, and weakening of defensive barriers at home. This same constellation of latency children whose dreams reflect the struggle against being overwhelmed in an overstimulating environment was characteristic of Fraiberg's (1965) Roger and Furman's (1962) severely disturbed child who entered latency during analysis.

Jenifer's transference was quite different from that of Becker's patient since hostility and rivalry were so close to the surface. She had a good alliance with the analyst partly in her recognition that the analyst was there to relieve her considerable pain, and partly in her experience with the analyst who, unlike her mother who limited supplies such as toilet paper, let her use as much paper as she wanted for her drawings. She called it "an endless supply," and rewarded me by providing an endless supply of food in her dramatic museum play. In the alliance I was the helper-analyst: together we solved the mystery. Jenifer's ego structure and home environment stand in sharp contrast to the overstimulated, weakly defended cases cited above. She serves as an additional model for those latency children for whom dream analysis has been significant.

Summary

Dream interpretation is a generally neglected area in the analysis of latency-age children. Analysts are more influenced by reports of children's inability to work with dreams than by sporadic reports of success. This paper reports one child's dream interpretation. It discusses the factors that make working with dreams difficult for latency children, and the factors that contributed to this child's success.

BIBLIOGRAPHY

ABLON, S. L. & MACK, J. (1980). Children's dreams reconsidered. *Psychoanal. Study Child*, 35:179–217.

BECKER, T. E. (1978). Dream analysis in child analysis. In *Child Analysis and Therapy*, ed. J. Glenn. New York: Aronson, pp. 355–374.

FRAIBERG, S. (1965). A comparison of the analytic method in two stages of a child analysis. *J. Amer. Acad. Child Psychiat.*, 4:387–400.

FURMAN, E. (1962). Some features of the dream function of a severely disturbed young child. *J. Amer. Psychoanal. Assn.*, 10:258–270.

HARLEY, M. (1962). The role of the dream in the analysis of a latency child. *J. Amer. Psychoanal. Assn.*, 10:271–288.

SILVERMAN, M. A. (1985). Progression, regression and child analytic technique. *Psychoanal. Q.*, 54:1–19.

Fathers and Their Homosexually Inclined Sons in Childhood

RICHARD A. ISAY, M.D.

IN A PREVIOUS PUBLICATION (1986B) I HAVE SUGGESTED THAT THE most important erotic object of the homosexually inclined child is his father and not his mother. The homoerotic fantasy or derivatives of this fantasy may be recollected from ages 3 or 4 by some homosexual men. In other cases, early homoerotic fantasies related to the father may not be remembered, but as an analysis or therapy progresses, they appear in the transference and are usually recollected as repression and other defenses lift. I have called this developmental stage with its early homoerotic fantasies the acquisition stage of homosexual identity formation. This paper examines further how this early erotic relationship with the father manifests itself in the analyses of patients and how the defensive distortion of this relationship affects the development of the love life of gay men.

Freud's formulations about homosexuality included both constitutional and environmental or "accidental" factors. He was convinced that homosexuality had a strong organic basis, and that the relative strength of the masculine or feminine disposition decided whether the final outcome of the oedipal conflict was identification with the father or the mother (1923, p. 33). He felt an "obligation" not to lose sight of the contributing factors and mentioned on different occasions both the child's fixation to his mother (1922, p. 230) and the absence of a strong father that may "favour the occurrence" of homosexuality (1905, p. 146). However, Freud's theory of innate bisexuality, his openness to

Clinical associate professor of psychiatry, Cornell Medical College. Faculty, Columbia University Center for Psychoanalytic Training and Research.

new clinical data, an emphasis on the cooperative relations between constitutional and accidental factors, and his libertarian
instincts all caused him to equivocate about both the nature and
origin of homosexuality. He never altered his view that early
environmental influences were insufficient to explain the acquisition of a same-sex object choice.

After Freud's death psychoanalysts, especially in America,
were intent upon resolving any ambiguity in Freud's theory of
sexual object choice and decisively settled on a medical model
with early environmental determinants as the pathogens of this
"illness." Rado (1940) first dismissed the concept of bisexuality
as being biologically unsound and of little heuristic or clinical
value. Later (1949) he elaborated a theory of homosexuality as a
reparative attempt on the part of men who were incapacitated by
their fear of women due to hostile, close-binding mothers.
Bieber et al. (1962) have stated that the presence of a "constructive, supportive, warmly-related father precludes the possibility
of a homosexual son" (p. 311). They determined on the basis of
clinical histories that the absent, detached, emotionally distant,
or hostile father is largely responsible for the development of
homosexuality, by failing to break the adhesive bind of the "pre-
homosexual" child with his overprotective, possessive, seductive
mother. Socarides (1968, 1978) emphasized the presence of an
engulfing, binding mother who, he believes, interferes with the
normal identificatory processes and masculinization of the child.

My patient population shows no consistent pattern in the reporting of engulfing or binding mothers by homosexual men
(Isay, 1986b). But gay men in treatment often report that their
fathers were distant during their childhood and that they lacked
a sense of real attachment to them. In my clinical experience, this
appears most frequently to be a retrospective, defensive distortion based upon the anxiety these men have about their early
erotic attachment to their fathers. These recollections are similar
to the defensive distortions many heterosexual men have of
their mothers because of anxiety evoked by their early erotic
attachment to them. In making inferences about the etiology of
homosexuality we have not been careful to distinguish between
the nature of the actual parenting and the retrospective perception and distortions of the nature of this parenting by our pa-

tients. In our clinical work with heterosexuals the nature of these early distortions is considered to be important. The same emphasis has not been placed on these distortions in our clinical work with homosexual men. While this paper focuses on the early erotic attachment of the gay man to his father, I do not intend to minimize the importance of the primary relationship with the early, care-giving, nurturing mother. Of course, all relationships, and especially loving and intimate ones, are influenced by the nature of this earliest relationship and by the sense of security and self-esteem imparted by the care-giving parent to the child (Isay, 1986b).

CHILDHOOD ROMANCE WITH FATHER

1. Alan was 27 when he initially entered analysis. He was quite depressed, feeling dissatisfied with his life in general and with himself as a gay man. Although he was aware of being sexually attracted to other boys and men from age 8, he remained extremely anxious about his sexuality and the absence of any gratifying relationships. Alan had extensive consultations with another analyst prior to seeing me, but had left him because he felt demeaned and threatened by the analyst's explicit assertion that he should change his homosexuality. This advice contributed to a significant increase in his depression, somatic complaints, and anxiety due to the further undermining of his already impaired self-esteem. His symptoms suggested severe, early, narcissistic injuries that were apparently exacerbated by his contacts with the consulting analyst (also see Isay, 1985). It became clear during our consultations that dissatisfaction with his sexual orientation was a result of his injured self-esteem and not the cause of it.

At the start of this analysis Alan's sexual activities exclusively involved hustlers whose attention he could control with money, and with whom intimacy was never possible. He was often in physical danger, since many of these hustlers were addicts. As time went on, he faced even greater danger of contracting AIDS from these young men, a risk about which he appeared oblivious and unconcerned.

Alan's family seemed to fit the conventional formulations about the genesis of homosexuality. His mother was reported as binding and engulfing, relying on her son's dependency and accomplishments for her own gratification. Alan's father was initially perceived as being cold, emotionally distant, and often absent because of his preoccupation with work. Alan had a younger brother to whom he was very attached, feeling he was the good parent to this much younger child.

Alan's fears of intimacy were related to his anxiety about his early sexual attachment to his father and to fears of engulfment. After he had recollected some of his early feelings toward his father, he became less resistant in his analysis. He started to give up his self-imposed distance in the transference, became increasingly aware of sadistic fantasies that were related to his mother and his brother, and started to give up his masochistic behavior. Within one year he had stopped having sex with hustlers and after about two years of discouraging attempts to meet someone and begin a relationship, he did fall in love, and he has been in a solid and stable relationship since then. The following vignettes from my work with this man illustrate how the clarification of his perception of his father affected him.

Alan's early dreams were largely of frightening mother images, and getting close to a mother meant destruction. During the first two years the transference took the form of seeming indifference to the analysis and a self-imposed distance from me. During the third year of his analysis he started to have some recollection of homoerotic feelings for other boys from about age 3 or 4, and both his dreams and the transference began to change.

> I'm on a roof with these people. They first look pale or white and then they become more distinct. They begin to move across the roof in patterns that I find exciting.

He associated to people who had been placed in concentration camps and then freed at the end of the war, to someone he knew who seemed free of his old "hangups" and now was "living in the moment," to his younger brother and how much he loved him, to his father and me as oppressors, and to meeting someone in a bar the night before whom he found attractive. "He reminded me of a thief I once knew. I was very turned on by him." After thinking about his father's having questionable business dealings, he wondered whether he had been "turned on" by his father as a child.

Over the following weeks his hours centered upon his wish to be dominated both outside the analysis by men he encountered and within the analysis by me. A short while later he dreamed:

> A horse comes between me and Jack [his boss for whom he has considerable affection]. Jack reaches up and cuts the sheets near the pillow to cover the horse up.

He associated to sleeping in the same room with his parents at times as a child. His mother slept "like a horse" and sometimes lay between him and his father. As he was speaking he had a vague sense of sexual excitement and of attraction to his father from about age 4, recollecting the warmth and sexual arousal he experienced as he slept next to him. "Fatherlike" smells and voices evoked "sexuallike" feelings and sensations. In the transference there were some erotic feelings, including the wish at times to fellate me or for me to penetrate him anally. It was also around this time that he met his lover. The closer he felt to him and to me, the sicker he felt physically and emotionally. Even though in his previous, casual, sexual contacts he could be anally penetrated or do the sucking, now the evocation of these desires in the intimate relationship with his lover and in his relationship with me, combined with the memories of his father, made him feel very anxious and "full of pus."

In the transference he felt increasingly "helpless," which reminded him of the way his mother acted in order to get his father to take care of her. It also reminded him of how his maternal grandmother behaved. He frequently referred to vague sexual feelings evoked by sleeping next to his father when he was about 4. He perceived me as being distant, and felt certain that I was not friendlier because I was anxious about his increasing sexual feelings about me. Of his father he said, "I think he knew I was in some way attracted, that I was in love with him, and then he withdrew."

Such vignettes cannot capture the complexity or subtlety of the many determinants of feelings and behavior in a long and difficult analysis. I use them to highlight Alan's deeply repressed, powerful, erotic love for his father from early childhood, and to illustrate that anxiety about this erotic interest was one important factor in defensively distancing himself from other men. Guilt over this attachment was also one determinant of his masochistic sexual attitude. The gradual clarification of this erotic love for his father greatly enhanced his capacity to get close to other men. Furthermore, as his analysis progressed, Alan grew to perceive his father's remoteness, and mine as well, as not being inherent qualities of us, but of a defensive need on his part to view me and his father as cold and uncaring. As he began to recall and to experience in the present his father's warmth and acceptance, his relationships with other men improved, ushering in his successful attempt to find a lover.

2. Bradley started his analysis with considerable anxiety about his sexuality. He had had sex with both men and women, including one relationship with a woman over an extended period of time. Nevertheless, he felt detached from his sexual experiences with women and more connected, involved, and attracted to other men. His sexual experiences with men and women lacked passion, and he felt that his enjoyment of life was hampered by what he perceived as his sexual ambivalence and inhibitions. He saw his mother as an attractive, articulate woman, but somewhat removed from him and overinterested in her own life. His father, a successful executive, was perceived as being highly intelligent, more affectionate, and more open than his mother. Bradley's father always seemed to be a much more vivid presence in his life than his mother, a contrast to the way in which many gay men describe their parents. Bradley had more of a bisexual current than many gay men I see, and there was some repression of his sexual attachment to her, perhaps contributing to his experience of her as being distant.

In the first year of analysis Bradley's sexual ambivalence continued, and he remained depressed and anxious. In the second year he began to notice that he was mainly attracted to aloof men with whom he could not form a relationship. If a friendly, attractive man liked him, he felt "turned on" and then he would begin to hate himself, feeling foolish and repulsive. He said that "in the arms of a cold man, I wouldn't feel this way." Of course, such an attitude in love and sexual matters led to no intimacy and unsatisfying sex.

While on vacation, Bradley had noticed a father and son enter the dining room, and he remembered that he had felt attracted more to the father. He became uncomfortable acknowledging that he had always wanted to be "daddy's little girl." He began to identify feeling foolish and repugnant with thinking he was "like a woman," to which he connected his feeling helpless and wanting to be taken care of. He became aware of the fact that his father liked to take care of people, "strays" whom he occasionally took into his business. Bradley had fantasies that if he were a girl both his father and I would like him better. There was no evidence in dreams, associations, or the transference that these wishes and fantasies were a regressive retreat because of castration fears. He wanted to be "daddy's little girl" not because he was threatened by harm and wanted to appease him, but in order to acquire him. And he recognized this.

It was only when he made these increasingly clear connections to old erotic longings for his father that Bradley's fears of closeness began to diminish. He became involved in a relationship with a man who, like his father, enjoyed taking care of other men. These recollections also prompted a gradually increasing capacity to enjoy sex more comfortably, and to surrender himself to "passive" sexual fantasies as well as what are traditionally viewed as more active modes of sexual expression.

3. I use one further illustration to demonstrate how the repression of erotic desire for the father in the early childhood of gay men may contribute to the inhibition and neurotic distortion of their love for other men, making it difficult to form intimate relationships. Calvin was in intensive psychotherapy for several years, entering treatment at age 25 because of moderate depression, stemming in part from his loneliness. He had little conscious anxiety about his sexuality, feeling that he had always been homosexual. He recognized that in early adolescence he had felt attracted to certain teachers. In mid-adolescence he had his first sexual encounter. He had a proclivity for "mature" men, 5 to 10 years his seniors, but these relationships never worked out. He only went to gay bars with friends and never picked up sexual partners there. Only on one or two occasions had he had sex outside of a relationship. Nevertheless, such relationships were short-lived, because he rapidly grew bored, dissatisfied,

and felt little passion. It soon became clear that, like Bradley, if he did feel the stirrings of passion for another man, he was not interested in going out with him, feeling there was something wrong or, as he said, "lower class" about it.

Calvin was always close to his mother, described as loving and intelligent. His father was perceived as remote, opinionated, and somewhat domineering. When he was 7 his parents divorced, and Calvin's mother remarried a man with whom she had a long-standing relationship. He loved his stepfather, and continued to view him as a model of intellectual strength and honesty. His articulated anger at his father was motivated by many factors, including his father's leaving, but it also was used to mask repressed, explicit, sexual longings and fantasies, displacements of which, such as crushes on boys in his class, he remembered as having been present from childhood.

One form his anger took was his spiteful refusal to feel close to or passionate about any men. During one hour he became aware of a fantasy of going to a bar to get picked up by an older man, then of some vague sexual wishes toward his stepfather and me; then he reluctantly acknowledged warm, erotically tinged feelings about his father. With great embarrassment he recollected an incident that occurred when he was 7: he was fondled by an older man. While previously he had recollected this incident with only fear and disgust, now he could recall some excitement. In the same hour he remembered his first masturbation with ejaculation: dressed in his mother's clothes, he had fantasies of an older man lying on top of him. Passive sexual wishes, which were associated in fantasy by and large with older men, filled him with self-loathing and disgust. As the repression and denial of childhood recollections of erotic feelings toward both his father and stepfather lessened, the fantasies became more vivid and more easily acknowledged. Calvin then became able to tolerate his own passion in relation to men who desired him and who were closer to his age.

Although case vignettes always fall short of demonstrating the intricacies of any history and the many determinants of any conflicted wish and behavior, I hope that they give the flavor of the childhood romance of gay men with their fathers, a romance that may be disguised, distorted, and always to some extent repressed. Like the heterosexual man's childhood fantasies toward his mother, their repression may lead to inhibited and impoverished relationships in adulthood.

Each of these men illustrates another normal developmental issue in the early sexual life of some gay men: they assume opposite-sex characteristics in order to acquire and maintain the attraction and attention of the father. There is no evidence that such identifications are associated with castration anxieties or with the wish to appease the father, a dynamic that I have found to be more frequently associated with the homosexuallike fantasy and behavior in heterosexual men than in homosexual men (1986a). Although partial identifications with both parents are inevitable in all children, I am stressing here the attempt to acquire the father's love and attention as one important motivation for identification with the mother in some gay men. I am emphasizing that in my clinical experience, the same-sex object choice appears to occur before the homosexually inclined child makes such identifications; i.e., when such partial identifications with the mother or mothering person do occur, they *follow* the manifestation of the homosexual orientation and the erotic attachment to the father. There are homosexual men who, it seems to me, have not as children identified with behavioral characteristics of the mother in order to attract the father, and there are also some homosexually inclined children who have done so but who have taken on characteristics of the mother that are not conventionally feminine. From my clinical experience with gay men, when such identifications with the opposite-sex parent do occur, they are significant in determining the nature and quality of sexual relationships, but, occurring after the sexual object choice has been established, they have little significance in determining the gender of the sexual object.

I return to the gay man's early attachment to the father to see how the child's attachment appears to affect the father's attitude toward his son. My clinical data suggest that the father who appears "detached" or "hostile" may become so as a result of his son's homosexuality. One determinant of Alan's proclivity to feeling sick and helpless was to get his father to care for him, as his father had cared for his mother. At times this led to somatic symptoms that could attract a great deal of attention but also evoked a lot of anxiety in him. He recalled that as a child his sickness seemed to overcome his father's self-preoccupation and to attract him away from his mother. Similarly, Bradley spoke of an element of helplessness in his relationship with other men. Wanting to be taken care of was like his mother but also aimed to please his father, who enjoyed taking care of other men. Bradley also had the feeling that his father might have preferred a girl, or at least he could have been distinguished in this way from his older and younger male brothers. Both of these men at some time during treatment began to recall that their fathers withdrew from them as they perceived their attraction or because they appeared different from their brothers or other boys of that age. Furthermore, when they recognized during their analyses that a shift in the father's attitude toward them had occurred sometime in their childhood, the perception of their fathers as always having been aloof or uninvolved began to change.

4. Edward also illustrates the issue of a father's withdrawal from a son perceived as being "different." He had been in analysis for 6 years beginning when he was 20; he had entered treatment because of ambivalence about his sexuality. His major problem in relationships centered about difficulties in getting close. He had frequent casual sexual activity, but he could not enjoy sex within a relationship. He always felt closer to his mother than to his father, whom he initially perceived as having been distant and whom he viewed disdainfully for a perceived lack of business acumen. Repressed erotic wishes and fantasies for his father were reflected in the transference and in his resistance to and anxiety evoked by intimacy with other men.

In the early years of his analysis he complained of his mother's withdrawal from him at the time of the birth of his younger brother when he was 3½. However, later in the analysis he became acutely aware that his father had also become remote at that time. He began to talk about his father always favoring this brother who was more conventionally masculine and not "different" like Edward. Withdrawal of the father in favor of another, usually younger, more conventionally masculine male sibling is frequently noted by gay men. When the rage and rivalry with such a sibling are understood, along with the rage at the father for favoring them, the erotic feelings toward the father become less repressed, and the father becomes a more vivid presence in the patient's childhood recollection.

These two factors, then, often account for the perception and report of gay men that their fathers were distant. First, the homosexually inclined child perceives him as being distant because of his erotic attachment to him and the consequent need to make these feelings less threatening. Second, the father may become aloof and often favor another male sibling, both because of the child's atypical, "different" behavior and because of the anxiety evoked by the father's perception of his child's erotic attachment. Thus the "distant," absent, or "hostile" father is often the *result* of his son's homosexuality and not the cause of it.

Repressed Passive Sexuality in Gay Men

Alan, the first patient, described himself as feeling "sick and full of pus" when he began to feel close to a man after years of almost exclusive sexual activity with hustlers. The closer he felt, the more disgusted he was made by his sexual feelings. The analysis of these feelings revealed his response to an erotic attachment to his father. In any relationship he felt like the woman, and he recollected how as a child he would feel sick in order to be taken care of by his father. It became increasingly clear that his attachment to his father filled him with passive sexual longings and fantasies that were deeply repressed, and made him feel "like a woman." It is of interest that Alan had always preferred being the recipient of anal sex when he was with hustlers. It was only within a relationship that the early desires for the father were reevoked and his passive desires became consciously conflicted.[1]

Bradley's difficulties with intimate relationships were specifically related to ways in which they evoked the feeling that he was

1. This is of interest in view of the APA's recent decision to remove ego-dystonic homosexuality from DSM III-R. As any treatment progresses, a gay man's homosexuality may become conflicted as he becomes increasingly aware of his early erotic attachments. The transient but intense anxiety may result in temporary symptoms such as sexual inhibition or impotence. Such symptoms may also occur in heterosexuals when there is a loosening of repression around the early erotic attachment to the mother.

"behaving like a girl" to get his father to take care of and attend
to him. The man he loved "directs and takes care" of him. He
was terribly ashamed of what he labeled as his "girlishness." He
did not like and did not participate in passive anal sex which he
perceived as feminine. Although he did perform fellatio, he did
not attribute any "feminine" significance to this activity.

It was only with great difficulty that Calvin could talk at all
about his fantasies of passive sexuality. He felt anguished and
disgusted by these desires that he also described as being "girl-
like." Most of Calvin's sexual fantasies were about being the
recipient of anal sex, and he found the "feminine" feelings associated with these fantasies to be so repugnant that he could only
occasionally permit himself that kind of sexual pleasure.

Edward was perhaps the most terrified of any of my patients
of his passive sexual fantasies. Although fantasizing about men
with larger penises who could have anal sex with him, he was
always too tight to permit it to occur. Random, anonymous sexual encounters that he described as being "compulsive" and frantic were in part motivated by his desire to avoid the passive
feelings evoked by any such intimate, warm, loving relationships. His avoidance of feeling any attachment in the transference was similarly motivated. He hated his passive, receptive
longings. He also believed that anyone who was close to him
would hate him for them as well.

Fred, whom I have not previously mentioned, could permit
himself intimacy within the context of a relationship, but he
could not permit himself to be the "passive" partner. He felt that
his "feminine" mannerisms, which were not obvious, had driven
his father away. He also hated the "feminine" side of his nature.
In order to avoid such feelings, sex with his lover had become
ritualized so that it always concluded with his being the active
partner in anal sex.

Although I have only briefly recounted the histories of five
patients, the same self-hatred associated with what is perceived
as passive and feminine in their sexuality was articulated by most
gay men during their therapy. This included even men like Alan
who appeared to enjoy being the passive sexual partner in anal
sex in casual encounters, but such pleasures were deeply con-

flicted and could not be tolerated within a loving relationship. Anxiety about evoking these fantasies contributes to the difficulties some gay men have in forming relationships, and is also one of the reasons more anonymous, less intimate sexual encounters may be more pleasurable (Isay, 1986b).

Passive sexual desires and fantasies appear to be related to the ubiquitous, repressed, erotic desires for the father. There is no evidence that passive longings of gay men are generally related to a regressive wish to reunite with a dominant mother. While reunion fantasies with the mother may be one factor in the anxiety of some gay men, I have not found it to be a major factor in my patients. One would expect that if such conflicted passive longings were associated with a regressive pull toward the mother of childhood, the anxiety would be greatest in those whose mothers were perceived as being most binding. However, this does not seem to be the case, and it occurs in men who have had a variety of mothering. For example, Calvin's relation with his mother had always been close, but not binding or engulfing, and the anxiety about his "feminine" longings was intense. Nor is there evidence in my clinical experience that these passive longings are manifestations of a regressive solution to oedipally related castration fears (Isay, 1986a).

It is in large part because of the anxiety evoked by these childhood passive fantasies that the erotic transference develops only after working with a gay man for an extended period of time. What the analyst initially experiences, as I have indicated before, are the strong defenses against these erotic desires. The development of a sexual transference is, I believe, analogous to the development of a sexual transference in a heterosexual, where first the resistance must be analyzed before an erotic transference may evolve. While there are always manifestations in the transference of sexual wishes for both parents, the parental homosexual transference is most prominent in gay men. Expressions of longings for the mother in the maternal transference of gay men are similar to manifestations of the heterosexual woman's desires for her mother of childhood. That is, they are expressed most often as longings to be close to her or taken care of by her rather than as active sexual fantasies. Such passive longings are usually clearly separable from the passive erotic fantasies related to the repressed erotic desire for the father.

Most gays may, as their sexual desires become less repressed and less conflict-ridden, acquire greater responsiveness and a more flexible repertoire of sexual fantasies and behavior. They may gain increased pleasure from passive as well as from the less conflicted, active, sexual practices. This has raised important technical issues during the AIDS epidemic. Although I attempt to clarify underlying conflicts about passive sexuality, I have advised all patients to follow the public health safe sex guidelines whenever there was an indication to do so. I have not waited for patients to have unsafe sex before assuming an educative role at a time when a potentially fatal disease might be contracted through one such sexual encounter. Since I first help patients to clarify their conflicts and then in effect suggest caution in expressing their sexuality in all its forms, this at times evokes further conflict about the fantasies and desires that are viewed as reprehensible. When this occurs, of course, these conflicts must be further analyzed. It has been surprising, however, that generally the analyst's cautionary or educational stance has been accepted as caring and thoughtful, and does not evoke further conflict around the sexual issues, nor has it evoked, in my experience, masochistic acting out during periods of negative transference.

DISCUSSION

One may look retrospectively at the early history of any gay man and point to what appear to be the early environmental determinants of his selection of another man rather than a woman as a love object. We have seen that the homosexual object choice was thought to have been motivated by the close-binding, hostile mother who undermines her son's masculinity and induces a fear of women (e.g., Rado, 1949; Socarides, 1968, 1978); or that the absent, weak, indifferent or hostile father makes it impossible for the child to disidentify with his mother, who thereby becomes the only suitable object for identification (Bieber et al., 1962; Tyson, 1982). These psychoanalytic views appear to be predicated upon the position that gender identity formation precedes the sexual object choice (Person and Ovesey, 1983), the only argument for which, it seems to me, is a theoretical assumption that sexual orientation is determined solely by the environment.

From my clinical studies I have come to believe that the sexual object choice in homosexual men precedes the development of gender identity and that part identifications with the mother, when they do occur, are subsequent to and motivated by the sexual object choice of the child. Since I have found no evidence of gender identity or gender role disturbance in my 40 homosexual patients, it would suggest that such identifications with the opposite-sex parent do not usually lead to gender disorders in adulthood. Green's (1987) prospective studies of "feminine" boys suggest that there is a linkage in some boys with gender atypical behavior between early "femininity" and adult homosexuality and bisexuality. However, one cannot conclude from his studies or that of others (e.g., Zuger, 1984) that gender nonconformity precedes the sexual object choice. Nor should one conclude from such studies that all or even most gay men are "feminine" in childhood. The exaggerated feminine behavior of some gay men or the self-labeling and the labeling of other gay men with such terms as "she" or "queen" contain varying degrees of conscious self-mockery that flaunt conventional and traditional gender labeling in a society in which sexual behavior is strictly delineated along conventional gender lines. In our society a gay man is perceived as being "feminine" simply because he desires or loves other men. It is the angry recognition and flaunting of this cultural stereotype that by and large accounts for the feminine behavior and self-labeling by gay men rather than gender role disturbance or, as Blum (1986, p. 271) suggests, the "unresolved anxiety and animosity, disdain and disgust" for women that he finds in all homosexuals.

Many gay men have average expectable mothers and fathers, even in a clinical population, and we might expect to find even more frequent "normal" parenting in nonpatient populations. Furthermore, my heterosexual patients show just as much variability in parenting as do my gay patients. The evidence we have about the children of gay and lesbian parents suggests that there is no greater frequency of homosexuality than in the children of heterosexual parents (Green, 1978; McWhirter and Mattison, 1984; Kirkpatrick et al., 1976, 1981; Miller, 1979). The follow-up of children reared by fathers who fulfill the mother's traditional role, primary nurturing fathers, suggests that these children develop traditional gender identities and sex roles (Pruett, 1985a, 1985b). These studies strongly suggest that psychodynamic explanations, based on pathogenic parenting which promotes failures in identification, are insufficient to account for the sexual object choice. As Freud wrote, "it may be questioned whether the various accidental influences would be sufficient to explain the acquisition of inversion [homosexuality] without the co-operation of something in the subject himself. As we have already shown, the existence of this last factor is not to be denied" (1905, p. 141).

Some have argued that the genetic model best explains the development of sexual orientation. Kallman (1952) studied 45 dizygotic and 40 monozygotic twins and found that the concordance rate for homosexual behavior (5 or 6 on the Kinsey scale) was only slightly higher than normal for the dizygotic twins but significantly greater in the monozygotic. Although this study has been severely criticized for its sampling and methodological error (Hoult, 1983–84), a recent study by Eckert et al. (1986) with a very small sample of twins supports the significantly greater preponderance of homosexual behavior in monozygotic than dizygotic twins. Pillard and Weinrich (1986) reported that gay men have significantly more homosexual or bisexual brothers (22%) than do heterosexual men (4%). While none of these studies rules out the importance of the early environment in the development of sexual object choice, they do suggest a genetic component in the origin of sexuality. The contradictory evidence regarding the influence of prenatal endocrine influences is reviewed by Hoult (1983–84) and Ricketts (1984).

Others have emphasized the importance of personal choice in the development of homosexuality. For example, some women may become sexually bonded with another woman in our society for purposes of power, and there are women who have become disenchanted with the women's movement, who choose to leave their partners to seek more traditional lives and roles. Such political and social motives for determining the sexual object are much less frequent, if they ever occur, in the sexual bonding of gay men, in part because the price one pays in social discrimination is higher for gay men living together than it is for women. More importantly, there is no evidence to suggest that gay men can revert to heterosexual behavior without great difficulty and symptom formation (Isay, 1985). Therefore, if choice plays a role in influencing the sexuality of some women, it may be because anatomical differences make it easier for women to perform with either sex or that more women are bisexual than men. Although I have never seen a gay man who "chooses" to be homosexual, nevertheless, it is true that most gay men prefer their sexuality to heterosexuality, since what is experienced as normal and natural is usually preferred, even if such behavior is socially disadvantageous.

Although homosexuality in men is more appropriately labeled an "orientation" than a "choice" or "preference," some homosexual men find aspects of being gay advantageous to being heterosexual. For example, while many gay men mourn the fact that they may not have children and the comfort and security offered by a traditional family structure, there are some who do not want such a traditional family structure and who enjoy the economic benefits and relative independence of not having a family. Of course, this may at times be a rationalization for not having a family, but, in fact, many gay men do perceive some social assets and advantages to accrue from being gay, and prefer aspects of their life style to a more conventional, traditional one.

Sociobiologists have proposed that homosexuality has an evolutionary basis, and that genes survive that are beneficial to one's offspring. It has been suggested that the altruism of gay men toward their relatives, including economic benefits, could contribute to the fostering of the survival of genes for homosexuality, offsetting any genetic disadvantage that occurs because homosexuals reproduce less than heterosexuals (Futuyma and Risch, 1983–84; Wilson, 1978). Currently there is no empirical support for the idea of kin selection as a way of passing on a gene for homosexuality, which would first of all depend upon a definite genetic link for homosexuality, which has yet to be discovered. It is questionable as well to what extent, if any, homosexuals do have any privileged status in our society and, if so, to what extent the benefits of such privilege are shared by relatives.

In spite of the ambiguity and empirical uncertainty of all these views of the determinants of homosexuality, it seems indisputable that homosexuality has multiple and diverse roots. As Marmor (1975) has suggested, homosexuality "appears to be determined by psychodynamic, sociocultural, biological and situational factors but also reflects the significance of subtle temporal as well as qualitative and quantitative variables" (p. 1513).

My clinical work with gay men over many years has led me to consider the importance of a genetic predisposition for homosexuality. Without such an hereditary influence, environmental factors do not appear to be able to influence the development of sexual orientation, and I would suggest that the homoerotic object choice appears to be able to manifest itself in a variety of early environments. While one could not state that the nature of early parenting has no effect on the sexual orientation of the child, I would speculate that the genetic link is the necessary condition that provides for its manifestation. In effect, I view the genetic link as the necessary, although perhaps not the sufficient, factor in making the father or father surrogate the primary object of the child's sexual attention. My return to Freud's emphasis on hereditary factors not only takes into account the suggestive data from family and twin studies, but also helps to order my observation of the variation in familial environment and the lack of gender-related disorders in most adult gay men.

I have elsewhere reviewed (1985) Kinsey et al.'s studies (1948) that point to the frequency of homosexuality in our society, and mention European studies that suggest comparably high rates of homosexuality in those societies, and Ford and Beach's studies (1951) suggesting its frequency cross-culturally. It is also worthwhile to recall the many studies using projective and standardized psychological tests that fail to distinguish personality characteristics of men who are exclusively homosexual and those who are heterosexual, suggesting that gay men are no more nor less normal than heterosexual men (Riess, 1980). My clinical work in which the sexual orientation appears to be normal and certainly feels normal to those men further suggests that homosexuality is a normal variant of human sexuality. From a clinical viewpoint this also appears to be the most helpful way to view sexual orientation. Efforts to change homosexual behavior to heterosexual are usually injurious to the self-esteem of the homosexual man, and attempts to change the core sexuality are in all likelihood futile. Since in my clinical experience, the child's early experience with his parents most clearly influences the manner in which the sexuality is expressed, i.e., with pleasure or inhibition, trustingly or guardedly, sadistically or masochistically, actively or passively, and not the gender of the sexual object, it is toward these issues that our therapeutic efforts and attention must turn, regardless of the sexual orientation of our patients.

BIBLIOGRAPHY

BELL, A. B. & WEINBERG, M. S. (1978). *Homosexualities*. New York: Simon & Schuster.
BERGLER, E. (1957). *Homosexuality*. New York: Hill & Wang.
BIEBER, I. ET AL. (1962). *Homosexuality*. New York: Basic Books.
BLUM, H. P. (1986). On identification and its vicissitudes. *Int. J. Psychoanal.*, 67:267–276.
ECKERT, E. D., BONCHARD, T. J., BOHLEN, J., & HESTON, L. L. (1986). Homosexuality in monozygotic twins reared apart. *Brit. J. Psychiat.*, 148:421–425.
FORD, C. S. & BEACH, F. A. (1951). *Patterns of Sexual Behavior*. New York: Harper.
FREUD, S. (1905). Three essays on the theory of sexuality. *S.E.*, 7:125–245.
――――― (1922). Some neurotic mechanisms in jealousy, paranoia and homosexuality. *S.E.*, 18:223–232.
――――― (1923). The ego and the id. *S.E.*, 19:3–66.
FUTUYMA, D. J. & RISCH, S. J. (1983–84). Sexual orientation, sociobiology and evolution. *J. Homosex.*, 9:157–168.
GREEN, R. (1978). Sexual identity of 37 children raised by homosexual or transexual parents. *Amer. J. Psychiat.*, 135:692–697.
――――― (1987). *The "Sissy Boy" Syndrome*. New Haven: Yale Univ. Press.
HOULT, T. J. (1983–84). Human sexuality in biological perspective. *J. Homosex.*, 9(2/3):137–155.
ISAY, R. A. (1985). On the analytic therapy of homosexual men. *Psychoanal. Study Child*, 40:235–254.
――――― (1986a). Homosexuality in homosexual and heterosexual men. In *The Psychology of Men*, ed. G. Fogel, F. Lane, & R. Liebert. New York: Basic Books, pp. 277–299.
――――― (1986b). The development of sexual identity in homosexual men. *Psychoanal. Study Child*, 41:467–489.

KALLMAN, F. J. (1952). A comparative twin study on the genetic aspects of male homosexuality. *J. Nerv. Ment. Dis.*, 115:283.

KINSEY, A. C., POMEROY, W. B., & MARTIN, C. E. (1948). *Sexual Behavior in the Human Male.* Philadelphia & London: Saunders.

KIRKPATRICK, M., ROY, R., & SMITH, K. (1976). A new look at lesbian mothers. *Hum. Behav.*, 5:60–61.

———— SMITH, K., & ROY, R. (1981). Lesbian mothers and their children. *Amer. J. Orthopsychiat.*, 51:545–551.

McWHIRTER, D. P. & MATTISON, A. M. (1984). *The Male Couple.* Englewood Cliffs, N.J.: Prentice Hall.

MARMOR, J., ed. (1965). *Sexual Inversion.* New York: Basic Books.

———— (1975). Homosexuality and sexual orientation disturbance. In *Comprehensive Textbook of Psychiatry*, ed. A. M. Freedman, H. I. Kaplan, & B. J. Sadock. Baltimore: Williams & Wilkins, 2:1510–1520.

———— (1980). *Homosexual Behavior.* New York: Basic Books.

MILLER, B. (1979). Gay fathers and their children. *Fam. Coordin.*, 28:4, 12–20.

OVESEY, L. (1965). Pseudohomosexuality and homosexuality in men. In Marmor (1965), pp. 211–233.

PERSON, E. S. & OVESEY, L. (1983). Psychoanalytic theories of gender identity. *J. Amer. Acad. Psychoanal.*, 11:203–226.

PILLARD, R. & WEINRICH, J. (1986). Evidence of familial nature of male homosexuality. *Arch. Gen. Psychiat.*, 48:808–812.

PRUETT, K. D. (1985a). Children of the father-mothers. In *Frontiers of Infant Psychiatry*, ed. J. Hall, E. Galenson, & R. Tyson. New York: Basic Books, 2:375–380.

———— (1985b). Oedipal configurations in young father-raised children. *Psychoanal. Study Child*, 40:435–456.

RADO, S. (1940). A critical examination of the theory of bisexuality. *Psychosom. Med.*, 2:459–467.

———— (1949). An adaptational view of sexual behavior. In *Psychosexual Development in Health and Disease*, ed. P. H. Hoch & J. Zubin. New York: Grune & Stratton, pp. 159–189.

RICKETTS, W. (1984). Biological research on homosexuality. *J. Homosex.*, 9:65–93.

RIESS, P. F. (1980). Psychological tests in homosexuality. In Marmor (1980), pp. 296–311.

SOCARIDES, C. W. (1968). *The Overt Homosexual.* New York: Grune & Stratton.

———— (1978). *Homosexuality.* New York: Aronson.

TRIPP, C. A. (1975). *The Homosexual Matrix.* New York: McGraw-Hill.

TYSON, P. (1982). A developmental line of gender identity, gender role and choice of love object. *J. Amer. Psychoanal. Assn.*, 30:61–86.

WILSON, E. O. (1978). *On Human Nature.* Cambridge: Harvard Univ. Press.

ZUGER, B. (1984). Early effeminate behavior in boys. *J. Nerv. Ment. Dis.*, 172:90–97.

Motivational and Structural Developments and the Emergence of Selfhood in the Analysis of a Latency Child

RAANAN KULKA, M.A.

THE CENTRAL DEVELOPMENT OF PSYCHOANALYTIC THEORY OVER the last two decades has revolved around the experience of selfhood, its development, its structural aspects, and its quality as a motivational system in the personality. The theoretical status of the self as a concept has known very complex vicissitudes, and its integration in the drive theory and the structural viewpoint of the psychoanalytic metapsychology has been rife with hardship and controversies. Although the storm of the 1970s which almost caused a rupture in the psychoanalytic movement (Kohut, 1971, 1977, 1984; Goldberg, 1978; Ornstein, 1981) has abated over the past few years and the attempt at fruitful integration is showing its first results (Wallerstein, 1981, 1983, 1985; Eagle, 1984; Goldberg, 1985; Wolf, 1985), there is still a long way to go for the complete assimilation of these new developments.

Reviewing the psychoanalytic literature dealing with that integration, one is struck by the almost total absence of theoretical contributions arising from clinical psychoanalysis of children. To my mind, this is even more surprising when we consider that the psychoanalytic encounter with a child, who is in the midst of

Member, Israel Psychoanalytic Society; Faculty, Israel Institute of Psychoanalysis.

This paper is based on a presentation given to the Israel Psychoanalytic Society in spring 1983.

his growth process, provides us with the most authentic contact with the inner links existing among energy, structure, and experience, the three focuses of individual psychological growth.

Moreover, the experiencing modes for self expression and interpersonal relatedness available to the child in analysis are multidimensional and stand in sharp contrast to those of adult analysis. Only in the former does there exist the possibility for free oscillation between motoric motility in space and the manipulating of creative raw materials and structured objects, between the use of symbolization through play and drawing and communication via direct verbal dialogue. Thus, the analysis of a child as a multifaceted interaction provides us with an ideal opportunity to investigate the links among different developmental lines.

I was privileged to meet a special child who, by his full and profound use of the analytic space, brought me face to face with extremely complex developmental processes and very rich psychodynamic events which, though they could easily become controversial junctures of different theoretical concepts and trends in psychoanalysis, were living proof of the organic integration which takes place between motivational and structural developments in the personality and the complex emergence of selfhood.

The psychoanalysis of Doron began when he was almost 10 years old and ended 2½ years later. Doron was referred for evaluation and treatment with a number of disturbing problems: (1) The invention of imaginary stories and their presentation as real. This phenomenon, which bordered on pseudologia fantastica, appeared regularly in three contexts: (a) the fabrication of stories to serve as protective excuses in threatening situations, including the frequent invention of bodily complaints, bordering on malingering, in order to avoid going to school or to be excused from exams or hated homework; (b) the invention of highly detailed, self-aggrandizing stories in which achievements were substituted for real-life failures; (c) the invention of stories concerning traumatic events he was supposed to have experienced, and which focused primarily on injury to his body. Doron was usually aware of the fictitious element of his stories, but in the stories of the third group, it often seemed that the ability to distinguish between reality and fantasy was obscured under the influence of the hypochondriacal fears and anxieties which characterized them. (2) Difficulties in social adaptation. Doron belonged to the fringe of his peer group, and was often the butt of offensive name-calling and physical harassment. (3) Outbursts of rage. Although his rages were rare and appeared only in the context of quarrels with his friends, they were extremely violent and were characterized by a lack of self-control. (4) Specific difficulties in learning. His total failure in maths and gym and a completely illegible handwriting were conspicuous. Although Doron was considered a good student, the very high intelligence found in the psychological testing indicated that he was not filling his potential. (5) Night fears and nightmares, which were not known to his parents.

THE FAMILY BACKGROUND AND THE CHILD'S HISTORY

Doron is his parents' fourth child. He has a brother and two sisters, 10, 7, and 6 years older respectively.

His father, introverted and gentle, yet sensitive and vulnerable, was a cultured man with a broad education, a carpenter by trade. His approach to life, based as it was on high moral standards and conscientiousness, protected him from fully coming to terms with his own emotional life and that of those around him.

Doron's mother, a modest and reserved woman, somewhat given to depression and tension, suffered from a lowered self image and diminished self-esteem, and was insecure as a woman and mother. Her interpersonal relationships were accompanied by constant guilt feelings which were manifest by an overprotectiveness and nagging devotion. She was a teacher and worked in a kindergarten.

Both parents were from a similar background, born and raised in poor large families where the constant battle for survival and tense interpersonal relationships constituted the main ingredients of the family atmosphere. Their overall childhood experiences also bore similar marks of emotional neglect and abandonment, creating a picture of constant loneliness and sadness. It was therefore not surprising that in spite of different life circumstances they both parted from their respective families in adolescence and went on to lead independent lives. Their marriage, after a brief acquaintance, was prompted by a shared desire to have a family of their own. Although they both claimed that the union suffered from insufficient love on both sides, they perceived their relationship as normal; they seemed to have accepted mutual disappointments and to have achieved a relationship not lacking in mutual devotion and care.

Doron was born in a period of great tension between the parents, and the mother testified that she was depressed and even contemplated suicide. In deciding to have another child, she hoped to get out of her emotional difficulties and to improve her marital relations. While the father was not privy to her motives, he too wanted another child.

Doron was born after a normal pregnancy in a quick and easy delivery. He was healthy and of average weight, but the birthmarks which covered his abdomen, his left leg, and part of his face clouded his parents' happiness and caused them worry and disappointment. He was a bottle-fed baby as his mother had no milk; he was thin, but had no eating problems. His physical and motoric development was normal, although he started walking a bit late, at 1½ years, after having received special physiotherapy. In his first year of life, Doron was prone to angina and suffered a number of attacks of spastic bronchitis. This sensitivity disappeared completely after he had his tonsils removed at the age of 5.

During his first year of life, his mother stayed at home and looked after Doron. She admitted that although she functioned well instrumentally, on the emotional level she was preoccupied with herself and her mother who fell ill and indeed died a few months later. When Doron was a year old, his mother returned to work and he was cared for by a baby-sitter until he went to nursery school at 2½. His development throughout this period was normal. An alert and inquisitive toddler who learned to talk early, he was toilet-trained permissively and without particular problems, at around the age of 3. He spent 2 years in nursery school where he adapted readily both to the separation from home and to the society of the children, and was a well-liked child.

Doron's problems first manifested themselves in kindergarten where difficulties arose in his relationship with the teacher and the other children and where rages and violent behavior also made their first appearance. A lull occurred when he entered school; he adapted well, and during the first year there were no discernible difficulties. During his second year, aggressive behavior toward other children reappeared, coupled with disruptive behavior toward the teacher, and a general deterioration in performance. In the third grade, the aggressive behavior subsided, but was replaced by the invention of stories and the strange grimaces which caused anxiety and ultimately brought him to treatment.

THE ANALYSIS

INITIAL CONTACT

Doron arrived at the playroom with his mother, parted from her unhesitatingly, and seemed very eager for the meeting. He was a very thin child of average height, simply and sloppily dressed. His gait was awkward and unstable, his hands moved restlessly, and he seemed to feel uncomfortable inside his own body. His face was pale, framed by a strange and unbecoming haircut that attempted to hide the birthmarks. Doron immediately commenced with a constant flow of words which continued throughout the entire session: "You don't have to explain to me why I'm here. I already know. I have this wicked force, a cold feeling, that I've got to be shown how to get rid of. That's what complicates my life, turns my head, and causes me all kinds of trouble. There is also a warm feeling, but the cold one is stronger. I'm not retarded. I only need to be understood and explained how to get the cold feeling, the bad force, out of me. That's what I need."

When I remarked gently that he felt like a very bad boy with all sorts of thoughts and feelings that he would like to be rid of, the initial tension with which his opening words were delivered dissipated. He began to tell me when and how the struggle among his feelings arose. Doron felt that because of his physical weakness and his failure in sports, his status among the boys was inferior; in order to be accepted by them, he submitted to their humiliat-

ing domination and described situations in which he was willing
to assume the role of victim if only to belong.

"You're willing to pay a very heavy price in order to belong to
the group, but then inside you there must be much humiliation,
pain, and anger against those children," I summed up his description in a phrase emphasizing his conflict. And then Doron
burst out: "That's it, and then the cold feeling comes out, when
they call me 'face' because my face is crooked, and 'beans' because I'm so thin, then I can't take it anymore and I hit them.
That's the bad force coming out."

As I interpreted to Doron that he felt very bad when he let
himself express his anger at the insults and hurtful things he
endured, he looked at me thoughtfully, and then in a completely
associative way brought the following story: "Once, Mummy hit
our dog, for no reason. I felt the cold feeling rising, but suddenly
something happened, and I see that I'm hitting the dog too. Why
did I do to her what I so hated Mummy doing? What, can't I stop
myself? Am I crazy? Maybe I should run away from home, stop
growing, fail in life, maybe I should die. Sometimes I think that
I'll jump from the window or the roof and that will be the end."

Into his sad silence I interjected that he seemed to be walking
around with the feeling that he deserved a terrible punishment
for the hateful feelings and the desire for revenge that he had
toward Mummy. He raised his glance to me, and, as if having
caught the implicit message that his guilt was not factual but
based on an inner feeling, answered, "Yes, that's how it seems
that I think," and after a moment's silence, he added, "Sometimes the bad force in me tells me that I should hurt myself; for
example, it tells me to lie so I'll be hurt later, or to dream bad
dreams of things which will happen to me in real life."

"You turn the thoughts of hurting others—which you feel are
the worst—toward yourself, a kind of punishment that you arrange for yourself," I responded, and for the first time Doron's
face lit up with a smile, and he said, "All I need is for someone to
talk to me and help me understand, I'm not crazy, because a
crazy person doesn't know he's not alright. I'm mentally ill because I understand that something is wrong with me, and I have
to be helped."

Doron, in a manner atypical of children, displayed the proper combination of elements required for analysis as the treatment of choice: a sense of suffering and a high awareness of problems, a strong desire to be helped and to change, a willingness to form a treatment alliance, a tendency for introspection, and an impressive ability to gain insight through interpretative interventions.

FIRST PERIOD—SIX MONTHS

Doron came to the first session very eagerly and seemed fairly relaxed and at ease. As if no time at all had elapsed since our first meeting, he began, "So, what we were talking about then, about what goes on in my body—it's still going on, but now I know what happens and I'll explain the process to you: when someone insults me, the good force says, 'Be quiet, don't pay attention,' but the bad force says, 'Don't be quiet, say what you feel, fight.' And then this whirlpool begins between the forces like in the explosion of a real atom bomb." By means of the drawing of a circle which symbolized himself, which he called "a picture describing the soul" and which he would elaborate further in future sessions, Doron presented the closed system of inner forces and the complicated struggles among them.

I received the general impression that Doron felt he was a container full of seething, aggressive and destructive, overwhelming urges, originating in "parts of a mental illness" and arousing in him mixed emotions of anxiety and guilt. His feelings of helplessness in the face of these instinctual drives and the typically anal fear of losing control over them led him to search for a series of defenses against his aggressive wishes, and these were depicted in another schematic drawing: "The bad force has to be isolated from the other forces, to be surrounded by circles of an arresting 'will power,' to be cut off from the other parts, and if it wants to get out and to make me cry or take revenge, to be imprisoned deep inside." In this indirect way Doron described his drawing as representing the defenses of isolation, splitting, and repression. He called this drawing "the treatment map" and saw in the gradual achievement of the described defenses the aim of the analysis and landmarks on the way.

Besides empathic listening and the use of verbal interventions whose task was to enable him to arrive at further self-expression, I began showing Doron how he was investing most of his energies in an attempt to keep what disturbed him inside himself and gain control over it. In response to these interpretations, Doron began drawing "another treatment map" in which for the first time a new force appeared: "parts of mental health" which would expel the bad force from him. "They will penetrate me and attach themselves to the bad force, make it blow up till it won't have any more room in the system, and then it will be expelled and I'll be rid of it."

This was the first time that the struggle took on an additional, very clear—though on a purely symbolic level—sexual–instinctual significance, where questions of mating, impregnating, pregnancy, and birth appeared as Doron's passive-feminine-homosexual wishes in the context of the transference. At this stage I of course made no attempt to go into the sexual wishes and made do with interpreting the new force as representing me and the treatment, which Doron hoped would help him.

Concomitantly with his rapid absorption into the analysis, initial signs of resistance appeared, and in one of the sessions, upon my remarking that he was not sure that he could trust the treatment or me, Doron recalled hearing the following story, "Once a man invited a visitor and gave him four bottles of whiskey to drink, and when the man got drunk he gave his host everything he had, precious stones and diamonds, and when he sobered up he saw that the man had disappeared with everything he had."

Both in Doron's fears of me, which are so clearly illustrated in the story, and in his wishes toward me, the anal sexual significance was the dominant one. On the one hand was the desire to surrender to me, to be penetrated by me, and to make an offering to me, and on the other was the anxiety around the feminine wish and its implications. I interpreted the story to Doron, telling him that he was expressing his fear that perhaps I too, like the host in the story, was tempting him with four bottles of analysis sessions not in order to give him anything but to strip him bare of the treasures of his thoughts, feelings, and fantasies, and then abandon him. Doron laughed in relief, and the resistance which had accompanied us for a number of sessions for the most part vanished. This was the beginning of a period in which he produced rich and varied material relating to various aspects of sexuality.

At first Doron tested my willingness to accept his sexuality which he felt was the most animalistic part of his personality. One way he did this was by bringing along for a number of sessions his large impressive dog who was then in heat, preoccupying himself with a detailed observation of her body and bodily functions during waking and sleeping, and relating excessively to her sexual attachments to other dogs.

In my remarks I generally touched upon his sexual curiosity and his desire to see, know, and understand what happens to the body during sexual excitation, intercourse, and afterward. The effect of the interpretative elaboration during this period was remarkable. Besides lessening his anxiety and implicitly conveying my total acceptance of him, the interpretations contributed to Doron's increasing ability to differentiate and to produce an array of questions on sexual matters. One of these sessions will serve as a good demonstration.

At the start of the hour, Doron was occupied with the classification of different kinds of snakes, comparing them on the basis of the potency of their poison and the structure of their mouths, focusing especially on the location of the teeth either prominently in the front part or hidden deep in the oral cavity. In my relating to the various aspects of his juxtaposition, I also interpreted it as representing his curiosity about the differences between male and female. Doron then told me a story, deriving from a real experience, but greatly embellished by fantasy, "Once I was riding with my cousin on a raft in the sea, and we suddenly saw a kind of black and long creature under the boat. We were frightened and hit at it with our oar; it was cut in half and died, but then its eggs came out. You couldn't tell if it was male or female because they both have eggs, and in this kind the male litters and the female also has poison."

"You're awfully confused by the difference between male and female, and you're not sure then what each of them has inside its body and how the roles are divided when they have their children. And sometimes in your imagination you think that maybe each one is actually both male and female," I tried to formulate Doron's story in an organizing way. He continued, "There is a kind of balance in nature. For example, the black widow devours the male after mating, but it litters males, and if there are too many she devours some of them."

This exchange revealed Doron's confused inner picture not only of the genitals and the differences between them, but of the essence of the bond between the sexes which he saw as a chaotic combination of sexuality and aggression, with the woman assuming the dominant role. I therefore chose to end what he had produced with a rather complex interpretation which was, however, understood and well received. "Mating and birth both seem to you connected to a very aggressive and murderous act which takes place between the sexes, and you feel the ties between the woman and her husband and between the woman and her children as a momentous struggle in which the woman is the strong one, holding sway over life and death."

The fantasy world which slowly unraveled itself was not only connected to instinctual drives and wishes but related to basic questions of Doron's self perception. Following a bout of flu which left sores in his mouth, Doron commenced on an intensive investigation of his body. First his curiosity centered on the surface of the skin, the freckles on his hands, various injuries, and the scabs that covered them in the healing process. When I remarked first on his general curiosity about his body and then upon his wish to investigate and know different things about it, he said, "A person has to know himself, what and how he is from birth and to know what's in him and what's not in him."

This was the first time that a sorrowful tone, reflecting his sense of impairment and lack, crept into his voice, and it led me to say that he was not sure of the completeness of his body and that he was afraid that he might be damaged from birth. Doron in response began coming to our sessions in shorts which exposed his birthmarks. He once asked me, "Say, do you also treat cripples?" thereby hinting at a partial willingness to touch upon the wealth of feelings connected with this painful subject. I then raised the possibility that his fears and feelings of shame and humiliation also applied to other things connected to the body, trying in my suggestion to test his ability to come into contact with the feeling of phallic inadequacy and the castration anxiety coming up in the material.

Doron, however, was not yet ready for any direct encounter

with those feelings. Yet, his behavior seemed to give an indirect answer to his chosen solution: for a number of weeks he consistently hurt and bruised himself in sports and other physical activities in which he generally failed, and came to the sessions with impressive bandages, openly enjoying his condition. This enjoyment was only minimally connected to the secondary gain; it stemmed mainly from a defensive maneuver in which the physical impairment and weakness were transformed from a source of pain and narcissistic injury into a source of pride and satisfaction.

The feminine identification—through his injuries—was not only a defensive compensation and retreat for the feeling of phallic weakness expressed in the physical failure, but emerged also from a basic conflict over masculinity and femininity. Doron was preoccupied with questions of how he would like to look, fat or thin, and in associating to this, it became clear that thinness and fatness had become symbols situated at the extreme poles of the conflict. Thinness was strength, hardness, and erectness, but "If someone is thin and he runs into something he might break," while fat, the symbol of the weak softness, was also in fact a suppleness which contained a kind of strength, "When a bus runs over a rubber ball, nothing happens to it." Finally, Doron summed up his deliberations with the declaration that he would like to be "thin but with muscles which are very flexible and soft like jelly, like a heap of dough which rises as if a balloon has been inserted into it." Thus he presented bisexuality as a solution to his conflict.

While the way Doron brought the above questions did allow for a partial interpretation of the various components of their dynamics, the remoteness of the symbols from their meaning did not allow me to translate them fully to him as a conflict between masculine and feminine wishes, just as it was impossible as yet to achieve a reduction of his wish for phallic potency versus the desire for pregnancy and giving birth.

Doron's preoccupation with aspects of sexuality continued, though he preferred to relate to them indirectly and symbolically through the inanimate world and nature, and thus to remain shielded from the anxiety, shame, and guilt that his absorption in sexual matters aroused in him.

The most important subject during this phase was his fantasies on the primal scene. The gradual emergence of the subject and its working through took place along two axes: one was connected to his imaginative perception of sexual intercourse as a destructive battle for life or death in which, while the penetrating male hurts and destroys the female, he himself is doomed to be swallowed by the female and then secreted out of her as waste. Thus, for example, he described a battle between a swallow and a reptile—a tarantula. The swallow, which rises to great heights in an impressive flight, then dives into the underground burrows of the tarantula in order to devour it, but only on condition that it finds its way in the circuitous maze of the underground dwelling. Doron drew the latter as an exact replica of an anatomical drawing of the woman's genitalia and reproductive organs. My interpretation of the symbolic meaning of the picture and of the battle between the animals as representing his thoughts about the interaction between a man and a woman during intercourse allowed for the systematic clarification of several elements in the material.

On another occasion, he described similar interactions between various minute creatures that live in puddles and which he had scrutinized in the sessions with his microscope. Here he repeatedly imagined intercourse as a process of devouring and swallowing, but this time with an emphasis on the processes of digestion and secretion representing fertilization, impregnation, and birth. My interpretations in this sphere were received by Doron with a mixture of wonder and pleasure.

The combination of oral-cannibalistic and anal elements in Doron's perception of sexual intercourse as incorporation and the destruction of the object on the one hand, and the reconstruction of the object as secretion on the other, represented the pregenital levels in his perception of the oedipal situation of the primal scene, and explained the somewhat archaic quality of his fantasies. The other axis round which Doron's interest in sexual matters revolved was the creative aspect of the process, and he often expressed the wish to experience the creative act himself. The richness of his discourse and play and the creative way he dealt with the material constituted a personality style which undoubtedly drew its vitality from these wishes.

After several sessions in which he played with making up new

Hebrew words by combining two existing words, I chose to remark that he seemed absorbed in producing new creatures. This initiated a period in which, together with a friend, he engaged in a botanical experiment to grow a splendid and special miniature cypress which would be a hybrid of all the different cypresses in the world and would contain all their traits. Doron was very moved by the experience and declared that "if I can't be good at sports, at least I'll be the professor-inventor." But he eventually became frightened at the intensity of his emotional investment in the endeavor and said sadly, "I seem to be doomed to the cypress craze for the rest of my life," thus expressing his feeling that his wishes for a fertile femininity, which had at first seemed to be a compensatory solution for his feelings of weakness as a boy and magical and exciting in itself, were a sign of insanity.

The wish to participate in creation and be part of a couple was expressed even more profoundly in the transference where it took several forms. The most prominent manifestation of this wish was the invention of a secret writing known only to us, with which we wrote a play together, a play Doron wanted to publish. The play was a dialogue between two creatures. Doron took the role of the bird, the *bulbul,* and gave me the role of the lizard, the *hardon.*[1] The symbolic connotation of the creatures was no accident; they represented Doron's instinctual wishes for a sexual attachment, this time with himself in the male role, being and having a *bulbul,* and me in the female role, the creature which crawls around in its underground burrows among the rocks. But the content of the dialogue between us expressed his feelings of loneliness and abandonment and his yearning for attachment. "You have no idea, dear *hardon,* how lonely I am there up on the tree in the nest," the *bulbul* begins, and the play ends with the sentence, "Thank you my friend the *hardon* for our talk. It's been years since I talked to anyone here. Everyone is dug into their burrows."

I interpreted to Doron that he wished to create a deep and exclusive bond with me, and related it back to his bad feelings as

---

1. *Bulbul*: name of a bird, also childish term for penis, and colloquial for "confused," "nuts." *Hardon*: type of lizard, also phonetically reminiscent of the word *hara* = shit.

a single child before the parental couple. In return, Doron told me for the first time, with tears in his eyes, about the nightmares with which he was visited when he lay in bed at night with his eyes closed, just before dropping off to sleep. In these nightmares, he saw series of faces coming toward him, getting larger and larger till they passed him. "I must understand what those faces mean," Doron said, and tried to re-create the authentic situation by drawing pictures of them with his eyes closed. In the drawings, alongside faces with long noses, outstretched tongues, and scary teeth, there appeared joined pairs of distorted figures which Doron said reminded him of a heap of limbs or a mixture of materials for yeast dough. When I interpreted his drawings and nightmares as representing his frightening fantasies of the sexual activities of his father and mother in their room, he relaxed, looked at the drawings of the faces again, and sank into deep thought. When I asked him to tell me what was going through his mind, there emerged a memory, from the age of 5, of a trip to a strange city with his parents, and getting lost.

Going to bed and the nightmares, then, constituted for Doron a juncture for both exciting and frightening instinctual fantasies and for feelings of bitter loneliness, separation, and being lost. When I summed up the matter in a number of variations—thus dealing with the accumulative traumatic experience—he stopped drawing his nightmares and gave vent to his fears and sorrow concerning the impending break in the treatment during the imminent summer vacation. Doron felt the separation from me as a re-creation of the nightly situation in which he was sent to be alone again, and my interpretations in this direction were of great help to him. He left me, saying, "I feel that I understand something, but I'm not sure that I know what." And it seemed that there could be no more fitting words to describe my own feelings that in many areas he had reached a degree of insight which had remained partially unconscious.

SECOND PERIOD—SIX MONTHS

The partial insight Doron gained into the connection between his nightmare symptom and the primal scene experience constituted the first turning point of the analysis. The period which followed the summer vacation was distinguished by three changes which had occurred both in the child and in the analytic work.

The nature of the material brought by Doron changed significantly. A great increase in material relating to the reality of his life and his relationships with his significant figures was noticeable. Another change was the direct reference to other groups of symptoms which beset him, such as his difficulties in interpersonal relationships and his rages, or his fabrications, and his total failure at sports. The third factor which characterized this period was related to the thoroughness of the analytic work which became a sort of methodical sifting through of the varied material to unravel the multidimensionality of each of the main axes of the psychodynamic picture and to decode the complex interactions between them and the symptomatic picture.

The analysis of the psychodynamic picture given below reveals the dual nature of the material produced. On the one hand, it was related to the psychosexual development and the structural emergence of the personality, and as such represented intrasystemic and intersystemic conflicts; on the other hand, it distinctly belonged to the development of the self and represented conflicts revolving round the sexual identity, body image, and the emergence of a complete representation of the self.

The first differentiation to crystallize from Doron's oscillation between the sexes was the perception that the boy was the stronger sex, but his strength was basically destructive and evil, while the girl was weaker, but her passivity was the basis of her goodness. The difficulty in choosing between being strong and bad and weak and good drove Doron to seek a solution once again in the nondecision of bisexuality, and his preoccupation with the term "transvestite"—which the children used as a curse—allowed us to work through his wish to be half and half, and thus enjoy both worlds without having to choose between them.

At this point, a marked change became apparent in Doron's behavior. He was more active, free, and bold, and the "masculine" element became more striking. At the same time a fascinating transformation occurred in the defenses which had characterized him thus far, and mechanisms of identification with the aggressor, reaction formation, and affect reversals—which had been so compatible with his bisexual stance by allowing him to feel simultaneously in the position of the weak, humiliated girl and the aggressive hurting boy—dissipated and new response patterns appeared instead. Doron stopped turning the pain and humiliation he experienced at the hands of the children into a source of satisfaction and pleasure, ceased joining in and identifying with the feminine nicknames they called him, and put up a determined and at times violent fight against anyone who dared hurt him.

I interpreted to Doron that this change was the explicit external expression of his desire and determination to be a boy, stressing that, in his mind, instinctual and impulsive behavior was the ultimate proof that he had relinquished his feminine wishes and had embarked on a new path.

This interpretative work brought about a significant lull in his behavior and heralded what could be called "the flowering of the narcissistic phallicism period" which constituted the next stage in his psychosexual and self developments.

Doron at this point gathered round him a number of children and became the appointed leader of a secret adventure society which carried out his grandiose plans for trips, detective and spying activities, and for stealing into various places. While this activity was typically phallic and it was not difficult to trace its instinctual origins—both sexual and aggressive—in essence it stemmed from basic narcissistic needs for admiration and appreciation by those around him.

The understanding of the narcissistic axis in Doron's psychodynamics left its mark on my interventions during this time. Reflections gained a symbolic value of recognition and were used more frequently, while the interpretative part of my work focused on the differentiation of his wishes for admiration and on the clarification of their meaning as part of a process of building his self-esteem.

Concurrent with the expression of authentic narcissistic needs, manifest in his external behavior among his friends, Doron's imagination was engaged in a multifaceted activity to meet these narcissistic needs. In his fantasies he was a grandiose figure who displayed his omnipotent powers and earned the admiration of all around him. A few examples are his practical plans to grow an elephant in his yard, to train a donkey for a rare circus show, or organize the biggest bonfire ever seen, a plan which was accompanied by months of obsessive gathering of wood. The clarification of this imaginary world revealed Doron's defensive layer of narcissistic wishes which in fact served to compensate for a deep sense of inadequacy and worthlessness and a basic insecurity about being wanted and accepted as he was.

My interpretations along these lines illuminated Doron's fibbing symptom which appeared to have developed as a double-edged defense against the plethora of feelings with which he struggled in his loneliness and isolation among the childen over the years. One aspect of the symptom was expressed in an intensive preoccupation with inner fantasies, constituting a substitutional withdrawal from interpersonal relationships and a comforting compensation for disappointments and hurts in this sphere. "I understand today that my fantasies were my best friends because they were always there. You know, it's not easy for me to give them up," he said in tears, following a certain social disappointment, struggling between a regression to the familiar defense and a full confrontation with his pain and an adequate coping with the reality of his social relationships.

The other side of the symptom, the imaginary tales that Doron spread around him, served mainly to create a grandiose complementary shield for his impaired sense of self. "What did I have to offer the children? Football? I couldn't play. Fighting? I was afraid to. So I made up stories," he said in an exciting moment of insight.

The process of Doron's giving up his world of fantasy and tale-telling was not a smooth one. Although the phenomena and their symptomatic expressions disappeared completely or were considerably weakened, and the acuteness of the guilt feelings, shame, and anxiety which had accompanied them dissipated, the role of the imagination in the cognitive-affective functioning of his personality remained highly significant.

The working through of the defensive function of the phallic-narcissistic axis allowed Doron to reencounter his fears concerning his body and here he displayed a wide variety of feelings of humiliation, shame, and rage in relation to the various defects he found in it. His stained face now occupied the central place in his consciousness and bore the symbolic brunt of his general feeling of impaired masculinity and of his specific fantasies about defects in his genitals. My interpretations of the symbolic relationship between different parts of the body led to an impressive insight into the actual mechanism of displacement upward, an insight which paved the way for the later complete understanding of his "face" nightmares.

Doron's feelings of masculine inferiority were now grounded in an externalized conflict with his parents whom he blamed for preferring him as a girl and for opposing his unequivocal desire for a potent masculinity. By drawing incessant comparisons between himself and children of other parents, Doron revealed that in his fantasy he regarded his frailty as passed down from his parents, either as a hereditary trait, a result of their own ineffectualness, or through education by their insistence on restraint and self control, which was regarded by Doron as a demand to render up his masculinity.

The transformation in Doron from a child torn by an internal conflict into a child fighting for the realization of explicit and well-defined wishes was not only manifest in his relationship with his parents, which had become direct, open, and more assertive, but also surfaced in other spheres. His status in his peer group improved, the scope of his interpersonal relationships broadened, and, for the first time, he made friends with girls. He began participating regularly in gym classes, daring even to join in the children's informal sports activities and to succeed where his failure had hitherto been total and symptomatic.

Doron was aware of the changes in him and derived much satisfaction and pride from them. Visible "body" changes took place before my eyes, expressed in the straighter stature, in the way he held his hands, and in his walk, all of which now conveyed a sense of stability, confidence, and strength.

In this prolonged evolution to the phallic-oedipal stage, there was a short regressive phase in which Doron made himself fail out of guilt for daring to be strong. After each realistic success in a "masculine" competition, he was compelled to pay by failing in the next one. This mechanism was given even keener expression as, after every instance of the successful display of physical strength, he injured himself accidentally during play. This self-defeat and the punishing of his body by directing the aggression toward himself stemmed from his inner equation of physical prowess with evil aggression. Only through the interpretative working through which allowed for an emotional differentiation between the two concepts did Doron begin to enjoy both the inner feeling of his powers and the external exhibition of his ability. As a consequence, the self-injury ceased and the occasions of self-defeat diminished.

Doron's development toward the adequate oedipal constellation was fully expressed also in the fantasy material he produced. For example, he had a series of dreams on a subject recurring in many variations. In these dreams he stole into an exciting complex structure where entry was forbidden and dangerous. Activity wishes to penetrate and conquer, side by side with fears of retaliatory harm, were at first worked through on a general level, slowly progressing to the interpretation of the specific oedipal components. In one of the dreams, Doron was punished with paralysis by a figure holding a giant saw and denying him entrance into a secret room. My interpretations related the figure to his father, the carpenter, and this led to memories from the age of 3 to 5 in which Doron would get into his father's closet in the parents' bedroom without permission, and would be punished by his father's anger. These memories allowed me to progress to another stage and to present his dreams as stemming from his desire to conquer the exclusive property of his father who was then perceived as dangerous and threatening. A few days later, in association to a similar dream, Doron produced a memory from the age of 4, of a TV film which had impressed him: in the film a princess and a small child stole the key to the King's treasure chest and, after a series of exciting adventures in an underground maze, reached the entrance to the cave of the treasure, only to be attacked as they were about to realize their dream by a terrible fire-spewing dragon whose wrath they miraculously escaped. The analysis of the memory and its relation to his own dreams enabled Doron to accept my interpretations of his wish to covet the treasures—the daughter and the wife—of the King-father and take them for himself.

The primal scene continued to preoccupy Doron, but the symbolic raw materials for his fantasies were now derived from the world of science fiction and life on other planets. Though this scene was removed to different worlds, it brought Doron closer to the sexuality of people. Here too the oedipal factors were prominent: his previous wish to be a passive partner observing the events taking place between the parental couple was replaced by active wishes to penetrate the female genitalia, which became dominant in his fantasies. I will bring an example:

A scout's meeting in which the mysterious disappearance of ships and planes in the Bermuda Triangle was discussed fired Doron's imagination. He was fascinated by the semiscientific notion that a "black hole" in space or a "triangular opening" in the center of the globe could suck in anyone who was tempted to penetrate the area. He amused himself with imaginary plans to penetrate the place, to expose its secrets, and thus to earn everlasting fame. When I suggested that the mysterious triangle and the black hole carried a personal implication and asked him for associations, he drew a series of small black triangles standing on an angle, and beneath them added the row of faces he envisaged in his nightmares. In my interpretations I suggested to him that the triangles, like the faces, represented a part of the human body which was both interesting and tempting but in his imagination also frightening and devouring. Referring to the mechanism of displacement upward which we had learned to recognize earlier in the treatment, I told him that the lower parts of the body seemed to occupy his imagination. In response, Doron drew a series of legs topped by the upside-down black triangles, thus allowing me to complete the evolving circle of interpretations by concluding that he had lately been preoccupied with the woman's genital and that his wish to penetrate it served both to acquaint him with it and to overcome his imaginary fears of the woman as devouring the penetrating man's penis, to conquer it, and to prove to the world and to himself that he was the perfect man.

Doron's reaction was very emotional as he asked, "Do you mean to say that instead of thinking about sex and everything connected to it, I've been preoccupied with faces and science and nature, with the Bermuda Triangle and all that? Now I see what was happening here."

In the next sessions Doron continued to develop the insight he had gained with a series of three drawings. In the first, a circle was surrounded by densely drawn arrows, pointing inward and as if closing in on it from all sides. "You see, that's how I lived, like under a Communist regime which doesn't allow anybody self expression," he explained, and went on to the second drawing. In this sketch a central circle comprised an axis to a rosette of intersecting ellipses, each representing one of the subjects dealt with in the treatment so far, and given appropriate names, such as "the dog," "scraps," "fossils," "birds and insects," "detective adventures," "the cypress craze, elephant, and bonfire," "caves," "Bermuda Triangle." "All those were a camouflage, kind of underground ways for self expression, now I see that," he said and sketched a third drawing in which there was only the central circle, through which arrows like newly sprouted stalks jutted out in all directions via an opening in its circumference.

From our growing portfolio of drawings Doron took out the first three drawings in the treatment, "the picture of the soul" and the two "treatment maps." Comparing them with the new ones, he summed up his observations: "When I look at the first drawings, I see how far I've come, I see that my problem is almost solved." Pointing to the last drawing, he said, "That's where I am today. I have to become more solid, like a rock. Although it's composed of different materials and many parts, it is one solid rock."

The impressive insight gained by Doron in his gestalt concept of the parallel processes which had taken place in the treatment and in himself was indeed in my view a highly significant point in the treatment's progress.

THIRD PERIOD—SIX MONTHS

The leap forward which had marked the closing of the second phase also signaled the beginning of a change in Doron's behavior at school and in his relationship with his homeroom teacher, a change whose working through constituted the central part of the third period of the analysis.

Doron entered into an intense ongoing struggle with his teacher, whom he saw as a domineering restrictive figure, insensitive to the children's, and especially the boys', individual needs, and arrogant to the point of enraging him. In Doron's confrontation with his teacher, the needs of the self to forge an identity, to grow and be free, integrated with instinctual drives whose free expression he now perceived as an integral part of his selfhood.

The teacher's insistence on both obedience and scholastic achievement, felt by Doron as evidence that she did not want him as a boy and would not accept his instinctuality, was to Doron a symbolic expression of her intention to suppress his masculine wishes and to castrate his manhood. The clarification of Doron's struggle with his teacher allowed me a reference to the only symptom which we had not yet discussed: his partial failure at his studies; and he indeed came to recognize that his achievements, which fell far below his capabilities, were the result of an inner choice related to his wish to display manliness and to the symbolic concept of scholastic failure as its ultimate proof.

From a purely instinctual viewpoint, the interaction Doron provoked between himself and his teacher expressed clear wishes for an intimacy of a mutually aggressive quality. Through his acting out, he wished to reconstruct the situation of the primal scene that existed in his consciousness as an interaction in which sexual pleasure and satisfaction are fused with a sadomasochistic relationship. The working through of these meanings was gradually made possible through the clarification of various situations and was exhausted when Doron understood that the faces he made and the sounds he uttered to his teacher during lessons were not only means of disturbing her but a kind of active reconstruction of the sexual happenings between his parents; the central role played by faces and sounds in his fantasies about the primal scene had been recognized and worked through in earlier phases of the analysis.

I saw Doron's acute acting-out behavior as arising, paradoxically, from the achievements of the second period of the analysis. The dissipation of the fantasy world in which he had been absorbed and the pulling of the rug from under the pseudologia fantastica symptom left the child bereft of his familiar sources of satisfying his instinctual wishes and needs of the self and made him seek their gratification through overt behavior in the framework of realistic object relationships.

Doron's intensive entrenchment in doing and behaving greatly impeded the therapeutic working alliance as it took him out of the observational attitude which had hitherto characterized him. Despite the fact that the analytic-interpretative work continued, and Doron even broadened his consciousness of the internal meanings of his behavior, he did not use the insight he achieved as a lever to change the actual events.

The understanding of the essential significance of the acting-out behavior as a defensive pattern manifesting Doron's distress in relinquishing his comforting fantasy world influenced the direction of my interpretation, and gradually bore positive results. Cracks appeared in this particular defense, and his turbulent behavior at school abated considerably, and the major transferential development of that period began.

At the beginning of one of the sessions, Doron declared that he sought freedom not only in his fantasies but also in the treatment. With a sense that he was sharing with me one of his most cherished secrets, he told me of a series of daydreams in which two famous sports teams compete against each other and in which Doron, in the role of the superstar, brings about his team's victory. The elucidation of the daydreams in which the main core comprised the instinctual wishes for a competitive struggle with an oedipal rival and the desire to vanquish him and take his place caused a dramatic change in Doron's mode of working in the analysis.

Up to this point, during the sessions, we both generally sat in our chairs by the table. Doron regularly accompanied the verbal exchange with drawings on the issues under consideration, constituting a sort of graphic transcription of the verbal layer of the interaction, but also frequently complementing it with elements still unconscious to him. From here on, however, Doron abandoned his drawings in favor of playing competitive games with me, through which he hoped to express and realize his aggressive oedipal wishes in the transference, and in which I represented the figures of the boys in his group, his older brother, and his father.

The games repertoire at first included target shooting contests with weapons found in the treatment room, and later widened to include football, basketball, and handball matches with rules adapted by Doron to fit the room's dimensions and realistic restrictions. The development of the game reflected Doron's progress in three main areas: the deepening of the direct interaction in his relationship with the transference object; the expansion of his ability to express instinctual wishes in the context of object relationship; the formation of a positive body image as a narcissistic source of satisfaction and self-esteem. And in my interventions, which also revolved round these three axes, I could refer to a whole series of elements—instinctual wishes, fantasy contents, feelings, and behavioral activities, which came to a combined expression under the cover of the game.

As in the two previous periods of the analysis, this stage too ended with a further cycle of clarification of the primal scene situation and in the uncovering of its central role in Doron's psychopathology.

We were approaching the summer vacation during which Doron was to go on a tour of the Far East with his parents. This trip greatly excited him but also aroused many worries and fears. Although he was not ready to relate to the trip directly, he found an original way of showing what he was feeling. Doron brought a tape-recording of a radio program, "We Are Not Alone," for us to listen to together. The program included testimonials by people who had encountered extraterrestrial creatures on a visit to earth. The central story was that of a husband and wife who, on their way back from a holiday, met "human" creatures who landed in a flying saucer in front of their eyes. These creatures overcame them with telepathic powers, gave them a physical examination, and finally disappeared back into space after erasing the experience from the couple's consciousness. The only remaining signs of the experience were red patches which appeared on the man's groin, caused by the penetration of one of the examination implements, and an inexplicable, overpowering tension. The man, having gone for an examination and treatment, disclosed the story of his "encounter of a third kind" under protracted hypnosis.

Doron's identification with the couple, especially the man, was total and he said excitedly, "Perhaps I also lost an hour like that, a night hour perhaps, in which I was also witness to an encounter of a third kind which I saw or heard and which I forgot from fear; maybe I also need hypnosis to get what it was out of me."

When I translated for Doron the symbolic meaning of the encounter as the intercourse between his mother and father which he imagined and felt that he might have witnessed at one time, he rolled up his left trouser leg, exposed his birthmarks, and said, "And here are my patches."

This "discovery" was followed by the exposure of fantasies in which Doron, in his prenatal life from inside his mother's womb, "witnessed" his parents' intercourse; the birthmarks on his leg and abdomen were stains of his mother's blood, wounded by his father's penetration, marks that Doron felt he bore both as a testimony to the father's aggression and as a mark of shame for the dirty sexual acts of both his parents.

At the same time another group of fantasies were illuminated. In these Doron interpreted his birthmarks together with his impaired face and "all the crazy things I have in my head" as injuries sustained as a foetus by his father's penetrating penis.

Despite the great importance of the exposure and working through of these fantasies, it seemed to me that the actual emotional significance of the radio story—in which the dramatic events took place during the protagonists' summer vacation—touched upon Doron's wishes, fantasies, and anxieties concerning the imminent summer trip with his parents. When I made the connection, Doron's level of anxiety rose and he said, "You're right, I do have many thoughts about the trip—what we'll do, where we'll go, and where we'll sleep, but I don't want to talk about it now; we'll think about it when I return. Maybe I should have been more free and talked about all sorts of sexual thoughts but I'm afraid to lose the stopper." While the instinctual excitation in anticipation of the trip with the parents was essentially phallic-oedipal, it also evoked the anal conflict of letting go versus restraint, and intensified the anxiety in the face of losing control of his drives.

In light of Doron's insight into his resistance and its general reasons, and as we were only a week before his trip and the interruption of the analysis, I decided to respect his wish to avoid discussing the holiday, but I did suggest that we try and examine the sources of the fantasies and fears that were preoccupying him about the vacation. Doron responded to this with great alacrity and produced memories from previous vacations, all dealing with a single situation—the moments when he lay in bed before falling asleep and the thoughts he had about the activities of his wakeful parents. These included memories of laughter and whispers coming from their room, of light and shadow playing on the ceiling of his room, reflecting the happenings in his parents' room, and a memory of his father peeping in at him through the window of the sleeping car and his face appearing very frightening.

The analysis of these memories allowed Doron once again to appreciate the immense significance of the primal scene for him and how the incomprehensible sounds, obscure sights, and frightening faces became the realistic raw materials from which the situation was woven in his inner awareness and in his emotional experience.

While the memories Doron produced were scattered over several years, beginning at age 3, the most affectively acute ones were connected to the summer between the second and third grade, which saw the emergence of his most difficult problems and the symptoms of nightmares, tension, grimaces, and storytelling. It does not seem impossible that the crystallization of internal psychodynamic problems into a manifest symptomatic disorder took place against the background of a real traumatic experience that summer, in which Doron was exposed to his parents' sexual intercourse. This etiological hypothesis was supported by the internal structure of the analysis and its cycles of progression: each of its three climaxes of insight revolved around the primal scene and took place just before the break in the treatment for a long vacation which acted as a kind of catalyst for the reliving and reconstruction of the original traumatic experience.

FOURTH PERIOD—"YEAR OF TERMINATION"

The year commenced with my renewed meeting with Doron and my sense that he had suddenly grown up—I was facing a calm and organized boy who declared that his goal for the last year of elementary school was "to stop all the funny business, to be a good student and do well in school," an aspiration whose successful fulfillment he also regarded as the treatment's final objective. In this challenge, Doron faced anxieties from various sources, each in its turn intensifying his tendencies for regression versus his developing growth wishes.

At the beginning of this period, Doron chalked up two achievements to his credit, impressive in themselves and very significant for him: he was elected by his classmates to head the class committee and the gym teacher chose him for the school's running team. This real progress temporarily sharpened his conflict, which was given keener expression in his deliberation whether to buy an adult's bicycle, which was at the same time more vulnerable to punctures, or to remain with his disappointing children's model, whose tires were more sturdy. When I interpreted to Doron that he was torn between the desire to grow up and the wish to stay small which was related to his fear of failing in his route of growing from a boy into a man, he looked up at me pensively and said, "You know, I really must consider when to end my therapy," thus shifting the dilemma to the transference and applying it to the issue of terminating the analysis.

Doron decided to test the possibility of ending the analysis by making a chronological survey of the drawings which had accompanied the treatment from its outset, and by analyzing the progress of the analysis and his personal development throughout. For the next three months we were involved in a highly moving process of a repeated and exhaustive working through of all the subjects dealt with in the analysis, this time with Doron on a much higher level of awareness, allowing him to relinquish the symbolic material and accept a direct interpretative reference to the original problems without being overwhelmed by anxiety, guilt, and shame, and without having to activate a recurring repression and other defenses.

Doron's main sense during this process of comparing his current situation and what was reflected by the reconstruction of the analysis was of the fundamental and internalized change which had taken place in him at every level. Handing me the portfolio of drawings to keep, a symbolic act of beginning his separation from the analysis, he summarized, "Now I see how

I've changed. Once I thought I would explode from everything going on inside me; today I know I am strong; once I had lots of barriers between my feelings, thoughts, and deeds; today hardly any; once I had fantasies and stories in the daytime and scary dreams at night; today I have real things—studies, friends, running, and football."

After the survey of the changes in his condition, Doron returned to an intensive period of competitive game-playing with me, which constituted a kind of practical test of the physical and mental changes he had undergone, and their verification in the context of the transference. Two issues stood at the center of the analytic work surrounding the games.

The first was rooted in the anal dilemma between the wish for release and liberation and the anxiety of losing control, a conflict which had of course an instinctual dimension but also had far-reaching implications in the formation of Doron's body image and self. In his games, which became more spontaneous and daring, Doron revealed that he felt himself to be free and relaxed and at the same time having a consolidated sense of mastery and an inner confidence in his regulation mechanisms.

The second subject was related to the phallic wishes. The competitive aspect of the games allowed Doron to confirm his increasing potency, whether the game constituted a confrontation between oedipal rivals and the victory over me signified the vanquishing of the father; or whether the game assumed the symbolic meaning of sexual interaction where he was the man subduing me—the woman with "special goals between the legs."

Concurrently with the events in the analysis, this period saw an accelerated improvement in his scholastic achievements. It was only with the strengthening of his body and self image and an adequate crystallization of masculine sexual identity that Doron could give up his failure at school, which had served him as a symbol of manliness, and thus overcome the last of his symptoms.

At this stage Doron returned to the issue of termination with two problems: when would he be able to make the final decision about the terminating date, and how long was required for the process of separation from the moment of decision until the actual termination? At the end of the first semester at school, when Doron proudly presented me with the amazing strides he had made in his studies, he said, "That's it, now I'm sure I'm ready for Junior High, now I've attained my last goal in the treatment and I can decide when to finish it." However, the anxiety revolving around termination increased along with his growing confidence and Doron asked me not to leave him alone with his decision. When I imparted to him that I indeed shared his feelings that he was ready to terminate the analysis, he decided himself to end it in 5 months' time—at the end of his last year of elementary school. My interpretation that he wished to terminate on a symbolic day on which he felt his childhood ending and the process of growing up beginning was received with overt pleasure and great satisfaction.

The fixing of a terminating date brought about a "dilution" of the analytic process both in terms of the subjects produced and in terms of Doron's willingness to work on them. The increase in defenses and the restriction of expression of internal material together with growing demonstrations of freedom and assertiveness were adequate manifestations of a gradual separation from analysis and were also appropriate for normal development in latency and preadolescence. At the same time they comprised an element of resistance to continuing exposure and analytic work. This mixture dictated the course of the work at this stage and the nature of my attitude: I walked a fine line between displaying my complete acceptance of Doron's attitude to the analysis while making an additional effort to work through its components of resistance in order to get at new material.

On the other hand, it was precisely the imminent end which inspired Doron to reach a deeper understanding of the onset of his problems and their eruption as crystallized symptoms; he recapitulated a whole series of traumatic experiences in which he became aware of his nonacceptability by his parents and peer group. These experiences focused on two periods, one in kindergarten, when he was 5, a time when his symptoms made their first, moderate, and temporary appearance, and the second, at the beginning of third grade, when his disturbance appeared in its full-blown form. The reworking of these traumas allowed

Doron to reach a more complete and subtle differentiation of the emotional complex which accompanied the formation of the symptomatology and the onset of his disturbance.

Outside the treatment, positive developments continued. His improvement in school and sports was maintained. In his relationships with friends and parents, he showed an increased ability to express himself in a direct manner—an ability which deepened both his interpersonal relationships and the sense of a strong and integrative selfhood.

Despite all the changes in his condition and feelings, and despite all the objective improvements which reflected and verified the changes, Doron still had a nagging doubt as to whether he was different and defective. At this stage, I chose to interpret these feelings in the light of the imminent termination, relating them to his fears that not all his defects had been corrected, and to his worry that he could not yet rely on himself to continue and develop on his own without the help of the analysis.

Doron did not find it easy to relate to the termination, a difficulty reinforced by his general reluctance to come into full contact with contradictory and complex feelings and by his limited tolerance of situations of conflict. Alongside his wish to end the analysis and obtain the complete freedom waiting for him was his fear that the sought-for freedom would extract a heavy price of loneliness and that the liberation from the burden of external restrictions would lay the responsibility for controlling instinctual wishes and channeling them into new ways of fulfillment heavily on his shoulders. The parting from me, with its complex of emotions, was no less difficult. The desire for separation was accompanied by guilt feelings for leaving me behind—whether as a defeated oedipal rival from whom leavetaking was the ultimate expression of conquest, or as a nurturing mother figure from whom separation constituted a betrayal of her devotion and love.

My intensive reference to these emotions brought about not only an adequate working through of the actual separation from the analysis and the analyst as a real significant object, but also allowed us, through the combination of transference and genetic interpretations, to touch upon the essential problematic areas in Doron's psychic development. For his whole life, Doron had taken great pains not to be himself, sensing that if he did not do so, he would hurt and betray the people most important to him and thus lose them completely, whether by rejection, as a punishment, or as the logical outcome of making a free choice of development. Through a series of partial overidentifications which constituted a kind of defensive front Doron had obscured his own identity and avoided experiencing his true self fully.

Doron's struggle for a separate identity, in which the spontaneous instinctual expression would be harmoniously integrated, free of guilt, but interwoven with values, morality, and conscience, thus received a further and thorough working through in relation to the issue of separation from the analysis and parting from the analyst. This struggle, which to my mind encapsulated the inner essence of the entire analysis, reached its final resolution. A few of Doron's expressions, as they emerged in the last sessions, showed that he shared this conviction: "It's not only the treatment which will soon be over. A whole period is ending and I'm already thinking about the future, what I'll be when I grow up. I don't really know yet and actually you can't really know now, and I don't have to decide today. I do know one thing. I'll do what interests *me*, what *I* want. Once I was *yeled tov yerushalaim*;[2] then I thought that I wanted to be only bad. Now I know, that's what I've learned here, that people are not just one thing, and even when they are several things, they are a whole, that's also what I solved here for myself; I don't want to be all dried up like my parents, or like my sisters who are only interested in studying, but now I don't want to be a *chuh-chuh*[3] either, who doesn't care about anything, I have my character and soul and that's that, that's what I shall be."

The fascinating process in which Doron's determination to terminate the analysis matured was for me a kind of stepping stone of its success. It comprised an impressive testimony to the scope of the internal changes that the analysis had wrought, of the depths to which they were organically internalized in the

2. Literally "good boy Jerusalem," an appellation, somewhat mocking, given to unduly obedient, innocent, and docile children.
3. Usually derogatory name applied to vulgar aggressive youngsters.

personality, of their stability in time, and their influence on his current functioning and continued normal development. Doron's decision to terminate found me, then, fully in agreement with his readiness to do so, and with a surging satisfaction concerning his achievements.

During these months, I pinpointed in myself the sense of satisfaction and pride mixed with feelings of growing separation, feelings that are so common in a parent of a child on the threshold of adolescence. I believe that the ability to feel these emotions enabled me to be empathic and understanding, and to help Doron in the identical process he himself was undergoing on the other side of the relationship in all its transferential and realistic components.

DISCUSSION

Mahler (1975) states that while infantile neurosis does make its appearance in the oedipal phase, it is formed by the rapprochement crisis: its full understanding requires a combined view of interstructural and intrastructural conflicts connected to the concurrent development of the instinctual drives, the ego, and the superego, and developmental conflicts relating to processes of separation and individuation in the framework of object relations which determine the development of the self. This view recapitulates the essence of Doron's disturbance, the genetic sources of its development, the course of the analysis, and Doron's development throughout it.

Doron was born into a problematic emotional atmosphere in which the parents were estranged and the mother's motivation for having a child bore strong narcissistic elements. Absorbed in her mourning for her mother, her emotional presence, during the first year of his life, was not optimal and was further impaired when, after a year, she left him to go back to work, thereby also transferring a large part of his instrumental care to someone else. ·

From the reconstruction of the child's second year, made in the course of the collateral treatment with the parents, it transpired that the permissive practical approach to toilet training was accompanied by explicit emotional messages transforming restraint and control into the highest values. This attitude also marked the parents' approach to Doron's aggressive and sexual instinctuality which they were extremely reluctant to accept as an adequate expression of the child's development in his second and third year of life. These "failures of empathy" (Kohut, 1971; Ornstein, 1981), while they did not prevent Doron's continued general development, did determine the later fixation points to which he retreated.

The manifest expression of Doron's disorder began only in the midst of the oedipal phase, at the age of 5 to 6, to emerge gradually within the next 3 years as symptoms which erupted as a crystallized and acute crisis at the age of 8 to 9, probably in the wake of an actual exposure to parental intercourse. In itself a traumatic experience (Fenichel, 1939; Arlow, 1980), this assumed its special intensity as an organizing experience to a whole series of previous conflicts—narcissistic-developmental and instinctual-structural (Esman, 1973; Blum, 1979).

Doron's regression took place along two axes: in terms of instinctual development, both libido and aggression assumed anal qualities and both drives were organized around a typically anal conflict, very acute in nature, of wishes for uncontrolled release and liberation versus attempts at complete restraint and control. Doron's defenses at the time—isolation, affect reversals, reaction formation, identification with the aggressor—are also very characteristic of the anal phase and expressed a certain regression in which the child had the utmost difficulty in using the disposal defenses to cope with the anxiety and guilt that the conflicts heaped upon him.

In terms of the narcissistic development and the emergence of self, a similarly regressive picture emerged of an extremely negative narcissistic equilibrium and endangered cohesiveness of the self. The narcissistic damage stemmed mainly from an unsuccessful assimilation of instinctuality as an integral part of self representations, a failure which is thought to be connected to nonempathic object relations in the second and third years and which disturbs the normal individuation process (Mahler et al., 1975; Parens, 1980). The prominence of conflicts related to sexual identity and to issues of autonomy and growth versus regressive wishes suggested regression in the first 3 years (Mahler et al., 1975). These conflicts constituted the main threat to the integration of the self. On both levels, then, the regression was to an identical phase—to the anal fixation in terms of instinctual development and to the rapprochement crisis in terms of self development.

This was the condition in which Doron reached analysis. The course of the analysis can be described in short as a process of taking Doron back to the oedipal phase through the solution of developmental conflicts on the one hand, and via the working through of structural conflicts on the other.

In a fascinating paper praising analytic neutrality in children's analyses, Chused (1982) sees its main role in creating conditions which allow the reliving of pregenital object relations and the working through of distortions in the development of the ego and the self which occurred in the rapprochement phase. This approach is related to the assessment that since the child is in the midst of development, he experiences his relationship with the analyst as a realistic experience with a new object. Thus, the analyst's empathy and understanding both allow for the transferential emergence of object relations and facilitate their renewed development (A. Freud, 1965; Neubauer, 1971).

In the first phase of the analysis, Doron used my analytic stance to turn me into a "mirror object" through whose empathy he encountered for the first time his feelings of guilt, shame, and anxiety concerning his sexual and aggressive urges. Through the affective experience of my acceptance, he developed the ability to assimilate his instinctuality as an integral part of himself.

This served as a foundation for the production of an abundance of fantasy material, through which his archaic and confused perceptions concerning the object, the self, and the relationship between the two were exposed and clarified. Although the content of the imaginary material was organized mainly around the experience of the primal scene and touched upon genital oedipal questions such as mating, impregnation, and birth, its quality was more archaic. It showed manifest oral-cannibalistic and anal sadomasochistic layers. The primary figures were not well differentiated; and the relationship between them was seen as a chaotic blending of sexuality and aggression, a life and death struggle rather than an act of love and attachment. Fantasies about intercourse as a destructive incorporation of the male by the female, and of pregnancy and birth as its new creation by digestion and secretion, completed this inner world view, whose implications for the crystallization of the self and body image and for the forging of a sexual identity were far-reaching. This picture became clear through the child's primary identifications, which constituted a central issue in the first phase of the analysis: in Doron's feminine identifications, one could see a defensive regression from oedipal identifications arising from a sense of phallic inadequacy or from guilt feelings associated with the aggression in masculinity; but beneath those later layers, the feminine identification stemmed from wishes for closeness with the preoedipal mother and was at one and the same time a defense against the fear of being devoured by the oral omnipotent mother.

The turn to bisexuality—probably linked to later processes of identification—was, in this phase of the treatment, much closer to developmental conflicts than to instinctual development; it protected Doron both from the painful narcissistic confrontation with the recognition that neither his mother nor himself were omnipotent and world-encompassing (Sperling, 1964), and from the process of psychological separation from the mother, one route of which was for Doron as a boy to acknowledge the differentiation between his and his mother's sexual identity (Mahler et al., 1975). This acknowledgment at first involved a severe narcissistic wound related to the relinquishment of wishes of pregnancy and birth perceived as constitutive elements in the mother's envied omnipotence (Van der Leeuw, 1958).

The differential exposure and the analytic working through of the preoedipal materials brought about an internal organization, a reinforcement of the sense of self and the strengthening of the ego, and paved the way for the two-stage psychosexual development which occurred in the second period of the analysis. The quality of the conflicts changed, and the combined dilemmas of femininity-masculinity and control versus release were now linked mainly to the intersystemic interaction between instinctual drives and between ego defenses and value choices made by the superego. The bisexuality too now functioned merely as a defense against having to make choices in instinctual conflicts, and lost its acuteness as a developmental identity conflict.

Doron's inner choices brought him to the phallic narcissistic stage where the masculine sexual identity and the instinctuality related to it were now experienced as an immense source of positive narcissistic satisfaction (Joffe and Sandler, 1965; Dare and Holder, 1981; Kohut, 1984).

The transition into the phallic-oedipal phase in the analysis took place in the wake of Doron's internalization of the differentiation between destructive and evil aggression, and aggresion as a constructive driving force for individual and active growth. This differentiation generally takes place in the second year of life as part of the instinctual development accompanying the process of separation and individuation from the mother (Mahler et al., 1975; Parens, 1980) and allows for the growth of the initiating and active self (Ornstein, 1981; Kohut, 1977, 1984). This distinction was not achieved by Doron in his preoedipal development. Its absence as an internalized representation was, in my view, the main reason that, though he had reached the oedipal phase in his development, he could not remain there and had to regress to the crisis which precipitated the analysis.

The attainment of this differentiation in the analysis to a great extent dulled Doron's guilt feelings arising from aggressive oedipal wishes, canceled the self defeat and injury mechanisms which had served him as a punishment, and allowed him to establish his masculine sexual identity and reexperience the total oedipal constellation.

Doron's psychosexual development, the positive change in the inner narcissistic balance, and the strengthening of the ego, which was expressed in the change of the defense and the decrease in their intensity, brought about impressive changes in his clinical condition: besides the disappearance of most of the symptoms and an accelerated improvement in several areas of functioning, Doron developed satisfying realistic object relations within his peer group and showed positive changes in the patterns of his relationship with his parents.

The almost total positive transference and my automatic acceptance by the child which had characterized the first two periods of the analysis stemmed from narcissistic needs for reflection and admiration (Kohut, 1971, 1977; Ornstein, 1981). Doron used me as a selfobject through which, by reflection, he could encounter, recognize, and organize his archaic fantasy world and the anxieties related to it. In addition, the empathy and understanding which he interpreted as symbolic expressions of admiration (Dare and Holder, 1981) enabled him to accept his instinctuality as an integral part of his selfhood and as an inner source of positive narcissism.

In the late second period, as part of the beginning of Doron's shift from narcissistic relations with a selfobject to genuine object relations with the analyst, the transference relationship changed. There is no doubt that the most impressive gain of this period—the giving up of his fabrications which had served him in their symptomatic form as gradiose complements to a damaged self and as a substitute for object relations—was possible only once this change in the relationship was accomplished.

The combination of developmental and structural conflicts (Lichtenberg, 1975; Dorpat, 1976) continued to comprise the essence of the dynamics of the third period of the analysis, but now they were expressed in the framework of object relations with the analyst as a separate figure, in part developing into a transference neurosis in its most reductive meaning of reconstructing internalized conflicts with the parental figures in the analysand-analyst relationship (A. Freud, 1965; Lilleskov, 1971).

At this stage Doron conceived of me as the domineering restrictive and worrying mother figure, with whom he fought for free expression, for independence and autonomous growth; or as a father who aspired to see his son as his extension and as realizing his own wishes, against whom Doron struggled for his right for individual aspirations and needs. At the same time, Doron relived the complete oedipal situation through the transference, and here I alternated in his mind between a mother whom he wished to impress with grandiose phallicism and toward whom he directed sexual wishes, and a father with whom he struggled for primacy, whose punishment he feared, and with whom he wished to identify. Only through the resolution of developmental conflicts, then, could Doron return to the normal oedipal development, exhaust it, and turn it into a phase on the way to adolescence.

The revelation of his real and separate self (Winnicott, 1965; Miller, 1979; Mahler et al., 1975), the reinforcement of the constancy of internalized object representations, and the change of the inner perception of object relations from a chaotic and destructive instinctual relationship having narcissistic qualities to an emotional and satisfying relationship between separate and differentiated beings, all these transformed Doron's autonomous growth from a destructive betrayal of the preoedipal mother and from a fatal aggressive act against the oedipal father into a benign process of rewarding development existing in harmony with both internalized and real object relations.

The last period of the analysis and the separation processes served as a wide backdrop for the working through of these developments and transformed the termination phase into an essential stage of the analysis, encompassing both the child's difficulties in a nutshell and the course of his psychic development throughout the analysis.

Concomitant with the development in the sphere of Doron's object relations and the creation of a transference neurosis toward me, in the last two periods of the analysis there also occurred an essential change in me. I discovered how I reacted internally with anger both to his growth wishes and to his actual separate development, and to his contradictory need for temporary and slight regressions for refueling. This personal insight greatly deepened my understanding of how the developmental conflicts during the rapprochement phase of separation-individuation processes, combined with nonoptimal object relations, distorted the normal course of his psychological growth in the oedipal phase.

The end of the analysis and the parting from the analyst became a process which blended organically with adolescence processes adequate to his age. I ended the analysis with the feeling that Doron was entering adolescence not only free of the symptoms which had afflicted him, but first and foremost endowed with the psychic energy, liberated through the combined and mutual resolution of developmental and structural conflicts, needed for his future growth.

BIBLIOGRAPHY

ARLOW, J. A. (1980). The revenge motive in the primal scene. *J. Amer. Psycho-anal. Assn.,* 28:519–542.

BLUM, H. P. (1979). On the concept and consequences of the primal scene. *Psychoanal. Q.,* 48:27–47.

CHUSED, J. F. (1982). The role of analytic neutrality in the use of the child analyst as a new object. *J. Amer. Psychoanal. Assn.,* 30:3–28.

DARE, C. & HOLDER, A. (1981). Developmental aspects of the interaction between narcissism, self-esteem and objects relations. *Int. J. Psychoanal.,* 62:323–337.

DORPAT, L. T. (1976). Structural conflict and object relations conflict. *J. Amer. Psychoanal. Assn.,* 24:855–874.

EAGLE, M. (1984). *Recent Developments in Psychoanalysis.* New York: McGraw-Hill.

ESMAN, A. H. (1973). The primal scene. *Psychoanal. Study Child,* 28:49–81.

FENICHEL, O. (1939). The economics of pseudologia phantastica. *The Collected Papers,* 2:129–141. New York: Norton, 1954.

FREUD, A. (1962). Assessment of childhood disturbances. *Psychoanal. Study Child,* 17:149–158.

———— (1965). Normality and pathology in childhood. *W.,* 6.

———— (1971). The infantile neurosis. *W.,* 7:189–203.

GOLDBERG, A., ed. (1978). *The Psychology of the Self.* New York: Int. Univ. Press.

———— (1985). Translation between psychoanalytic theories. *Annu. Psychoanal.,* 12–13:121–135.

JOFFE, W. G. & SANDLER, J. (1965). Disorders of narcissism. Unpublished MS.

KOHUT, H. (1971). *The Analysis of the Self.* New York: Int. Univ. Press.

———— (1977). *The Restoration of the Self.* New York: Int. Univ. Press.

———— (1984). *How Does Analysis Cure?* Chicago: Univ. Chicago Press.

LICHTENBERG, D. J. (1975). The development of the sense of self. *J. Amer. Psychoanal. Assn.,* 23:453–484.

LILLESKOV, R. (1971). Transference and transference neurosis in child analysis. In *The Unconscious Today,* ed. M. Kanzer. New York: Int. Univ. Press, pp. 400–408.

MAHLER, M. S. (1975). On the current status of the infantile neurosis. *J. Amer. Psychoanal. Assn.,* 23:327–333.

———— FRED, P., & BERGMAN, A. (1975). *The Psychological Birth of the Human Infant.* New York: Basic Books.

MILLER, A. (1979). The drama of the gifted child and the psycho-analyst's narcissistic disturbance. *Int. J. Psychoanal.,* 60:47–58.

Neubauer, P. B. (1971). Transference in childhood. In *The Unconscious Today*, ed. M. Kanzer. New York: Int. Univ. Press, pp. 452–455.

Ornstein, P. H. (1981). The bipolar self in psychoanalytic treatment process. *J. Amer. Psychoanal. Assn.*, 29:353–375.

Parens, H. (1980). An exploration of the relations of instinctual drives and the symbiosis/separation-individuation process. *J. Amer. Psychoanal. Assn.*, 28:89–114.

Sperling, M. (1964). The analysis of a boy with transvestite tendencies. *Psychoanal. Study Child*, 19:470–493.

Van der Leeuw, D. J. (1958). The preoedipal phase of the male. *Psychoanal. Study Child*, 13:352–374.

Wallerstein, R. S. (1981). The bipolar self. *J. Amer. Psychoanal. Assn.*, 29:377–394.

———— (1983). Self psychology and "classical" psychoanalytic psychology. In *The Future of Psychoanalysis*, ed. A. Goldberg. New York: Int. Univ. Press, pp. 19–63.

———— (1985). How does self psychology differ in practice? *Int. J. Psychoanal.*, 66:391–404.

Winnicott, D. W. (1965). *The Maturational Processes and the Facilitating Environment*. New York: Int. Univ. Press.

Wolf, E. S. (1985). Self psychology and the neuroses. *Annu. Psychoanal.*, 12–13:57–68.

Disturbances in Object Representation

PETER B. NEUBAUER, M.D.

I HAVE CHOSEN TO DISCUSS THE TOPIC OF DISTURBANCES IN OBJECT representation for two reasons:

1. I was surprised to discover this disorder in my patients and I wondered why I had not discovered it earlier in the analysis of some patients. Presenting my clinical material is an invitation to stimulate a discussion about this topic in order to find whether others have had similar clinical experiences.

2. The data which I shall present stem from the analysis of adults. Since the history of this disorder indicates that it started early in childhood, one has to pose the question: How can we obtain information of this form of disturbed object representation during childhood?

I do not need to review the significance of object relations in psychoanalysis or the recent attention to object and self representations. The data from the study of the first years of life which led to a clearer outline of the development of the dyadic and triadic interrelationship between infant and objects are well known. Many explanations have been given of those factors which contribute to the evolvement of an inner representational world. For our topic it may be useful to remind us that *the object representational world and the inner psychic life are not synonymous, and that our understanding of the establishment of a representational*

Clinical professor of psychiatry at the Psychoanalytic Institute, New York University; Chairman Emeritus at the Columbia University Psychoanalytic Center.

Presented as the Marianne Kris Memorial Lecture of the Association for Child Psychoanalysis on March 23, 1986, Seattle, Washington.

world in the first three years of life is primarily based on inferences. We have much information on object relationships,
but the child's inner experience of the object or its representation is difficult and in the preverbal stage impossible to obtain.
As usual, we are able to learn from pathology about the normality of developmental sequences. Therefore, I shall begin by
presenting three clinical vignettes of patients with abnormalities
of visual representation with the understanding that I do not do
justice to the usual complexity and multiple determinants of
experiences and psychic structure formation, for I have to limit
myself to those data which serve the topic.

<h2 style="text-align:center">VIGNETTE 1</h2>

A middle-aged, highly articulate woman entered analysis because of difficulties with her husband and children and her
writing block. Her intense engagement in the care of her children, who were then 5 and 8 years of age, led to discords with her
husband who wanted her to pay full attention to his needs. Indeed, she addressed herself to every task with great energy and
with a channelization which excluded recognition of other daily
events. From the beginning, she expected the analysis to rescue
her from the many demands made on her. It is therefore not
surprising that she immediately formed an intense relationship
to me which included aspects of transference of her relationship
to both her mother and her father. She constantly sought contact
with me. Insatiable in her demands, she was unable to find security or gratification in it. There were many dreams, some with
anal conflicts expressing fears of loss of parts of herself; these
were related to a history of constipation and forced enemas.
There were many other dreams which had an eerie de Chirico-
like empty space, buildings and streets, without people. She associated this feeling to a painting in the living room of her parents'
home in which she saw a long arm reaching out for her. She
realized later that it was a painting of a swan on a lovely lake. This
was connected to her myopic condition since early childhood.
Unless faces were very close to her, they disappeared; indeed,
she experienced empty spaces around her, which she reex-
perienced in her dreams.

Before I went on vacation, she expressed a wish to take an object from my office, intending to return it when the sessions resumed. I thought this to be an expression of her need for a transitional object, a reenactment in the analysis of her search for reliable object relations, which she seemed to confirm by her explanation that she wished something that she could hold, touch, and carry with her in order to feel my "presence." This then finally led to the question whether she was able to experience my presence in my absence, and whether she could remember me, that is, whether she could visualize me when I was absent. She answered immediately that she had great difficulty doing so, that she thought of me frequently, but that she was unable to remember the way I looked, even shortly after she had left my office. She could remember my voice or invoke it; she could remember the smell of the room and the sound of my steps. She had always known about the problem, but she had never made any reference to it, either taking for granted that I would know it, or because she lived with this difficulty of forming visual images of people all her life. This included her parents, husband, children, and friends.

In addition to this failure of evocative memory to form visual representation, the patient also had a disorder of recognition memory. In social situations, or when she gave a lecture, she was not able to recognize her friends, even when they were close enough, and she had to remind herself before meeting them who might be present in order to prepare herself to recognize them.

During the treatment she discovered her talent as a photographer and then employed photography to document her literary work. Furthermore, when she visited with friends and family, she took photographs which were quite cherished by them. It became clear that this activity served her need for permanency of the objects, for whenever she wanted to remember, they were available to her. Similarly, she considered the written word as being forever retrievable and thus being permanently a part of history. She began to write a diary of the sessions in order, as she said, "to imbed them into stone."

It is not surprising that she had many fears of a world which for her was too unstable; headlines which referred to war or other disasters disturbed her so profoundly that she rather avoided reading the news; and she refused to go to movies or plays which depicted destruction. She confessed that when she had intense fears, it was difficult for her to differentiate between fantasies and reality.

She had found a quote from Agatha Christie's autobiography which she brought to the session with much pleasure:

> When I look back over my life, it seems to me that the things that have been most vivid, and which remain most clearly in my mind, are the *places* I have been to. A sudden thrill of pleasure comes to mind—a tree, a hill, a white house tucked away somewhere, by a canal, the shape of a distant hill. Sometimes I have to think a moment to remember *where* and *when*. Then the picture comes clearly, and I know.
>
> People, I have never had a good memory for. My own friends are dear to me, but people that I merely meet and like pass out of my mind again almost at once. Far from being able to say, "I never forget a face," I might more truly say, "I never remember a face." But places remain firmly in my mind. Often, returning somewhere after five or six years, I remember quite well the roads to take, even if I have only been there once before.
>
> I don't know why my memory for places should be good and for people so faint. Perhaps it comes from being farsighted, so that people have a rather sketchy appearance, because they are near at hand.

While I cannot examine Agatha Christie's life history, I would say that her visual disorder and the resulting inability to visualize faces appear to be isolated phenomena and do not seem to be correlated with or part of other disturbances in object interactions as they occurred in my patient. I have examined in detail the role of myopia in the disturbances in object representation. While it obviously contributes to them, it is not by itself a primary cause. There are many children who suffer from myopic conditions from earliest infancy, but they do not develop the above symptomatology.

The patient collected a family history which revealed that many other members of her family suffered from a similar difficulty. Her aunts and cousins also could never remember people's faces and had difficulty recognizing them. I have no information whether they too shared the myopic condition. Furthermore, the patient had a 15-year-old cousin who was unable to have an image of people. When I asked her how she knew this, she answered that her cousin's drawings and paintings revealed it very clearly. As a child and until her present age, she was unable to draw a figure; when asked to do so, she made scribbles and designs.

When my patient explored her object relationship, rather than the object representation, she revealed much of the usual complexity of interactions, her ambivalence, her attachments, her criticisms, and her early childhood separation anxiety. For this reason, as I have described, I at first did not conclude or anticipate that she was suffering from a visual object representation disorder.

Her need to capture and recapture the objects to make them constant and her inability to internalize objects became more apparent. They were an expression of an inability which continuously made her search for the object. Quite frequently, she would phone me in order to hear my voice; early in treatment, before she had admitted her need for contact, she would do so and justify it by referring to ever new crisis situations in her life.

VIGNETTE 2

The second vignette explores a different genetic and dynamic condition leading to a disorder in visual representation. This young man sought analytic treatment after he had left his previous woman analyst with whom he had been for almost two years. He had discontinued therapy because she could not rescue him from feelings of depression and isolation, and he left her before she went on a prolonged vacation.

This response to separation reminds us of the young child's ability to leave mother, while being unable to be left by her. His history revealed that his mother suffered from severe depression, which necessitated frequent hospitalization, the first time when he was only 3 years old. She committed suicide in a mental institution when he was 16. The father had divorced the mother and remarried when the patient was 6 years old. He had always felt that his father was not available to him; he demanded appropriate behavior and academic performance, but was unable to give him comfort.

Indeed, the patient became an unusually successful performer in his profession, but he could not find any comfort in it. All the recognition which he received did not relieve him of his sense of loneliness. During many sessions, he was silent, waiting for me to connect with him and to relieve him of his sadness. In this condition he was unable to speak about himself and appeared to be reenacting his mother's depression. When I was able to understand his feelings and express to him what he might be thinking, he instantly smiled and the sad mood was broken. Without reading his feelings, I was not present. I referred to his mother's silent presence, her absences, and then asked him whether he could now remember his mother and evoke her image. He proceeded, as did the other patient, with an immediate and unusually long statement:

> When I was with the previous analyst, I could not visualize her after the sessions, nor can I succeed in remembering my girl friend, who lives in Europe. The closer the physical contact is with people, the more I have difficulty visualizing them. When there is no relationship, I feel secure in evoking the image. With you, I have the same problem, but not to the same degree. With a woman I have more fears. She may do what mother did; to be either away; or she is not available when physically present; or she overwhelms me with her attachment and her affection. A man will keep more distance. The only true image of my mother is either her extreme silence or her screaming. I cannot recall an image in the middle, balanced. I can't recall an easy comfortable time, and still the separations from my mother and from my girl friend give me a bad time. When my girl friend arrives, for a few days, I cannot connect with her, feel close to her. We have discussed this many times. It is like with my dreams. I do not want to think about them, as if the images were a burden. When my girl friend leaves, I do not really want to think about her. When I was a child, and my mother left me, I had no contact with her, no idea where she was, no letters. When she returned, I could, after a while, retain the connection. When I went to school, I did not have an image of either mother or father. I felt separated and alone, bewildered and unhappy. I carried this longing all my life, the longing to make the connection.

I still remember when I was 3 years old how much I wanted to connect with my mother because she was so distant and silent. I wanted her to pay attention to me. I was waiting *for her* to connect with me. I carried the feeling for many years after that; when I was 9 or 10 years old, I gave up. Then I transferred my wish to be close to my stepsister; and then I was not passively waiting, I actively pursued her, and later on, when I was older, I was also active with women. There is something about my present girl friend that makes it more difficult. When I assert myself, she does not like it; it is so frustrating. It reminds me of my mother when she frightened me and intimidated me, when she was hysterical or silent. Later on, when I was older, I tried to comfort her when she was crying, but she did not stop, yet I felt I had the responsibility. It was my fault and I behaved as a grown-up who had to console her and take care of her.

In his early adolescence he turned to his father for closeness. He tried to please not only him, but his teachers as well. He was waiting to receive attention as a reward; he could never make a direct demand, for if love was to be given when asked for, then it was no longer valued.

The analytic data revealed a close link between the representational disorder and other emotional difficulties. It was apparent that he repeated his early experience with his mother in the transference. When he was silent, he expected me to find words to reach him, not by interpreting his inhibitions, anger, passivity, but by evoking in him a feeling of my contact with him, interest in him, as if he were longing for a verbal embrace. He had warned me early in treatment that he left his previous analyst because she employed a technique of waiting for his associations and expressions of his feeling and fantasies. In order to do this he needed object contact first. As he said, his reaction to her was aggravated because she was a woman.

Vignette 3

This patient, a young woman, suffered from fears and obsessive-compulsive symptoms. Her early childhood revealed a strong symbiotic need for mother, who tried to detach her daughter from dependence on her and this forced my patient to increase her demand for mother's attention. She developed somatic symptoms, longing for comfort from mother which led to severe sibling rivalry, jealousy, and envy. At the beginning of the analysis she found reasons to call her mother many times a day, in spite of her mother's unwillingness to respond.

She was occupied with the unreliability of conditions, not only of her world at home, but of the world at large. Her own ambivalence made it difficult to arrive at clear positions about her husband, children, and work. There were fears that she had not locked the door, turned off the gas, or was unable correctly to manage the elevator's "up" and "down" movement. She had to return four or five times to check whether she had indeed turned off the stove. At one time she added to her continuous complaint that the symptoms persisted; it helped her when she went through the following thought process: While she was turning off the stove, she performed other tasks, such as looking at the clock, or putting something away, or cleaning a surface. She then hoped that she would be able to know that she had indeed turned off the stove. By association, by using the memories as a bridge, she could remember that she had attended to the stove. Her inability to remember "on" or "off" and "up" or "down" led me to consider whether she could remember human objects; alerted by my previous experience, I questioned her ability to remember her parents and friends. Again, she was quite ready to speak about this and to confirm that she had always had difficulties remembering mother when she was at school and, as the other patient, she too had similar problems visualizing me and members of her family. Long ago, she learned to help herself by thinking of what people wore, what they had said, and the sound of their voices. She mobilized these other compensatory sensory-perceptual modalities to create a memory of object representation.

As stated before, under conditions of danger or panic, her capacity to remember would be more impaired. Furthermore, her fears affected her ability to decide clearly what was reality and what was fear, what was verifiable and what was illusion. These difficulties were expressed in global terms, seen as part of the conditions of life; indeed, she submerged herself fully in the study of philosophy, existential psychology, and she became expert in literary criticism. In her academic work she found a nonambivalent world beyond her usual idealizations to escape from her polarizations of love and hate. Her relationship to me (I avoid referring to this as transference) was one of extreme idealization, for she could not accept any evidence that my knowledge was limited. Such an acceptance would have created a sense of fear and defeat. My absence during vacations was viewed as a "total" absence. This seemed to reflect her "on" and "off" dilemma, her love or hate, her sense of existence or nonexistence.

DISCUSSION

These three short vignettes focused on the incapacity to evoke visual object representations. I have eliminated many clinical correlations, but I hope one can still consider the following propositions:

1. The difficulty in, or absence of, evocative memory seems to occur in a variety of diverse clinical conditions.

2. It is not easy to determine the cause of this difficulty. When the absence of evocative memory is a primary condition, does it then interfere with evolvement of identification, the achievement of individuation and separateness, and the evolvement of the beginning of object constancy? When, on the other hand, it is the result of inappropriate early relationships, this too can lead to the disturbance of evocative memory. While there is always an interplay between dispositional and environmental factors, the first patient seems to have a primary disorder of the perceptual-sensory modality, a fault of the ego apparatus, while the other patients seem to have formed the symptom as a result of early conflicts.

3. The failure to achieve evocative and recognition memory seems to reflect upon characteristics of the object relatedness and with it on the analytic process. Compensatory mechanisms are called into action, and representational features can be put together by memories of touch, smell, and auditory channels. It seems that a consolidation of the object and self representations by internalization could not be achieved. All these patients manifested an intense hunger for an object relationship with the

analyst; and in the transference, we see features of the faulty primary object relationship.

4. The male patient who had the depressed mother leads me to connect the disorder of evocative memory to depressive states, particularly where there is an early object relationship characterized by the physical and emotional absence of the mother, by her engulfing affection and alternating total silence.

The third patient who could not remember whether she had turned off the gas on the stove alerted me to the possibility that, under certain circumstances, obsessive-compulsive features can be related to the absence of evocative memory in addition to the usual conflicts.

5. None of the patients spontaneously referred to this symptom, but they were able and relieved to reveal it when they were specifically asked about their capacity to evoke memories of objects.

This alerts us to the fact that we may miss finding this disorder when we wait for associations. I have not been able to see the evocative memory disorder in child patients. Nor have I pursued the course of the symptoms during developmental sequences. I have not addressed myself to the course of the analysis and the influence of this disorder on the limitation of psychoanalytic treatment.

Some colleagues have explained this inability visually to represent objects as being caused by negative hallucinations. Freud (1905) used this term in some of his earlier papers in discussing the hypnotic condition: "Hypnotic obedience can be employed in making a number of highly remarkable experiments, which afford a deep insight into the workings of the mind and produce in the observer an ineradicable conviction of the unsuspected power of the mind over the body. Just as a hypnotized subject can be obliged to see what is not there, so he can be forbidden to see what *is* there and is seeking to impress itself on his senses— some particular person, for instance. (This is known as a 'negative hallucination'.)" (p. 297). I have some questions about negative hallucination as an explanation for visual deficits and will discuss them later.

In 1901, Freud discussed the "remarkable coincidence" of meeting someone of whom he was at that very moment thinking;

"the paradoxical fact that my unconscious is able to perceive an object which my eyes can recognize only later seems partly to be explained by what Bleuler [1910] terms 'complexive preparedness [*Complexbereitschaft*]'" (p. 265). In 1907, Freud spoke about Hanold, who according to Zoe's accusation had the gift of "negative hallucination," who possessed the art of not seeing and not recognizing people who were actually present. Freud considered the negative hallucination to be a "flight from the physical presence of the girl he loved" (p. 67). Earlier (1901, p. 109), Freud referred to negative hallucination when he read parts of the same page about Hellenistic art in the age of Alexander and each time passed over the relevant sentence.

These examples clearly demonstrate that Freud at that time in the development of his work thought of negative hallucination as an example of repression based either on hypnotic or neurotic conflicts. It seems to me that this concept does not explain the clinical data which I have presented, for they are not an expression of "I do not see what I don't want to see"; rather they indicate an inability to visualize what could not be internalized.

The following questions are central to the issue of representation:

1. Can the visual object representation stay isolated and can the other sensory modalities compensate for it?

2. Is visual perception necessary for the "knowing" about the object, that is, for the object-self differentiation and internalization?

3. Is the visual disorder linked to others in specific ways which lead to a larger ego disorder?

4. Do these children develop at critical periods the social smile, even though they are not able to observe and to interact with their mother's affective facial expressions?

5. How do children with visual representation disorders negotiate the important stranger reactions? If memory fails to remember mother, how does the infant differentiate the known from the strange? We assume here that the stranger reaction should occur by the distant reception and not by touch, smell, and voice. Whenever there is this condition, are all unknown others perceived as if they were primary objects? Or are primary objects at first also perceived as strangers? Since it is important to

learn to tolerate frustration, to make new adaptations to new objects, and to form new and varied relationships, is there an interference in these developmental tasks? It may be useful to compare the development of these children with that of the unsighted child.

The evocative and recognition faculty is closely related to the function of memory, which is necessary to deposit experience so that a representational world can be created. Memory is part of the ego, but we assume that memory traces are active during the pre-ego period. After all, perception is present at birth, and the biological part of the ego, the ego equipment, needs to be in action to prepare the evolvement of the ego and its secondary processes. The pre-ego perception is linked to primary narcissistic cathexis, the latter to object cathexis. Later, secondary processes link memory to remembering. Freud (1914) outlined sequences of remembering, repeating, and reenacting. When the infant is unable to exercise the distant preceptual organ, visual perception, he then cannot appropriately "read" mother's face or her smile, nor can he differentiate between the stranger and the primary object—at least visually. Thus we assume that there will be consequences in the self-object differentiation and object relationships.

Memory is an essential element for the achievement of object constancy, the acceptance of the absence of the object by the reliance on the internalized object. Loewald (1976) refers to it in this way: "Memory seems to be inextricably interwoven with experiences of separation, loss, object withdrawal, or cessation of satisfying external interactions" (p. 160). He proposes that memory (by primordial separation) is the result of separation and, later in development, object loss can occur only when the object can be remembered. And "Memory is the child of both satisfaction and frustration" (p. 161). Freud's (1923) formulation helps to explain patients' continuous longing for the object: "It may be that . . . this identification [introjection] is the sole condition under which the id can give up its objects . . . the process, especially in the early phases of development, is a very frequent one, and it makes it possible to suppose that the character of the ego is a precipitate of abandoned object-cathexes" (p. 29).

In all these patients, whether the visual disorder was primary or secondary, that is, related to experiences, there was still the search for the symbiotic link with the object in order to complete a step in development which demands object reliability and object incorporation. This incomplete object-self differentiation did exist side by side with later developmental conflicts. The patients experienced the therapist on one level as a primary object, with magic features. They longed for an intense and continuous contact. Every word was given significance. They seemed to show an immediate strong tie to the analyst. One can assume that the motivating force for closeness, the libidinal tie, maintains its earliest strength.

In the absence of evocative memory and, in some patients, of recognition capacity, there is an inability to differentiate object and self. How then does the patient build a representation of the self? Can there be an inner visualization of the body image? It seems that my patients were able to achieve this, but they had difficulties building a self representation, an idea of the self, an identity which integrates the various ego modalities.

Linnell poses the question: "Is there an evocative memory of the self which is required as a means to achieve self-cohesion or integration?" Or, when we follow Loewald's (1970) suggestion that one needs to focus on the representation of aspects of relationships rather than on the representational world, of the representational objects or past objects, then we have to assess the impact of the visual representational disorder on these relationships. Instead of relinquishing object and self representation, we have to link object representation with the nature of object relationships.

One will have to question whether these patients suffer from an ego disorder or a borderline condition. Such a diagnosis can be made more specific when we examine it in the context of the representational fault. This leads us to the influence of this disorder on psychoanalytic technique and reminds us of Anna Freud's (1970) prediction: "In our times, the analysts' therapeutic ambition goes beyond the realm of conflict and the improvement of inadequate conflict solutions. It now embraces the basic faults, failures, defects, and deprivations, i.e., the whole range of adverse external and internal factors, and it aims at the correction of their consequences. Personally, I cannot help feeling that there are significant differences between the two therapeutic tasks and that every discussion of technique will need to take account of these" (p. 202f.).

Robert Tyson and Phyllis Tyson (1986) discuss a similar point: "Often the child will try to use the analyst to fulfill a developmental need, for example, when a parent is depressed, absent, or suffering a prolonged illness. The analyst, by responsively and accurately interpreting the child's wishes and fantasies about him, provides a 'holding environment' (Winnicott, 1960) in which the child, while not physically held or gratified, is helped to find alternative means of gratification and control. Thus progressive structure-building and reorganization are facilitated, and development beyond the point of arrest becomes possible (Ritvo, 1978)" (p. 301).

We have referred to the primary disorder in visual object representation and to those disorders which are based on experiential failures. It is difficult to differentiate the consequences of these conditions on further development. The biological substrate of the ego equipment disorder makes studies of neurobiology relevant. I shall refer to two findings. In *Neuronal Man,* Changeux (1986) explores the development of nerve conditions that guide perceptions and memories. He postulates that an unstimulated neuron system leads to random, multiple connections. Furthermore, these random links stay labile over a period of time. This implies that stimulation by experience eliminates the random connections and consolidates into a coherent network only those which are task-specific. In the absence of appropriate stimulations, this differentiation does not occur and links are severed by the dearth of connection, which cannot be repaired. I should also like to refer to a specific organic brain disorder—prosopagnosia. The dictionary defines it as "inability to recognize faces and particularly a failure to react to the combination of those specific properties or features of an object that endow it with uniqueness. This may be congenital or acquired, but it rarely occurs as an isolated defect." In this condition the patients fail to recognize the face they ought to have known. These patients have lesions in both brain areas that link the visual system to regions involved in memory and emotions.

Thus, the facial templates which are formed by the eyes cannot be recalled.

The patients I have presented do not suffer from visual agnosia or prosopagnosia, but they have some symptoms which appear to be close to some aspects of this condition and one may therefore be inclined to pursue the neurophysiological substrates of both deficit disorders. Oliver Sacks in *The Man Who Mistook His Wife for a Hat* describes a case of visual agnosia and notes that it is especially the animate which is so absurdly perceived that "there is always a reaction on the part of the affected organism or individual, to restore, to replace, to compensate for, and to preserve its identity" (p. 21).

Hartmann (1939) addressed this issue in this way: "This distinction between a biological and a psychological *point of view* raises another important question: Can psychoanalysis, with its psychological . . . concepts, trace physiological processes of development? We reject the customary form of this question: What is biological and what is psychological in the developmental process? We ask instead: What part of it is congenital, and what maturational, and what environmentally determined? What physiological and what psychological changes take place in it? Our psychological method encompasses more than just the processes of mental development. Precisely because the psychological is part of the biological, under certain conditions our method sheds light on physiological developments, particularly on those pertaining to instinctual drives. We can trace the course of these developments, using psychological phenomena as their indicator or symptom" (p. 34f.).

I think we can be comfortable with some of these neurological findings for they correspond to our psychological propositions: the associative memory, the random activities which become more differentiated, and the definition of the disorder as a process disorder. The biologist also considers a multiplicity of specific interacting mechanisms. It is noteworthy not to exclude this dimension from our discussion.

As Hartmann (1939) states, "The biological usefulness of the inner world in adaptation, in differentiation, and in synthesis becomes obvious even in a brief glance at the biological significance of thought processes. Perception, memory, imagery, thinking, and action are the relevant factors in this connection" (p. 58). In a further extension Hartmann explains that "autonomous ego development is one of the prerequisites of all reality relations . . . [and] for many other functions. Our arguments necessitated a detailed discussion of the ego apparatuses. In this connection, I stress again that no satisfactory definition of the concepts of ego strength and ego weakness is feasible without taking into account the nature and the maturational stage of the ego apparatuses which underlie intelligence, will, and action" (p. 107).

All my patients with failure of visual object representation showed two features which have relevance to child analysis. They were aware that this inability was part of their lives as long as they could remember. It is surprising, at least to me, that they were always aware of it. It should be possible therefore to detect it in childhood and certainly during child analysis.[1] As the child reveals his object relations, reenacts the role of the primary objects in play, we can observe the child's inner world, but it seems we do not explore the representational world. *It is the recognition of the difference between these worlds which offers the opportunity to locate more accurately the disorders,* by paying equal attention to both. Still, it may not be possible to elicit this information from young children, for they may not be able to articulate it. This leads to another aspect. As I have mentioned before, none of my patients spontaneously revealed the absence of visual representation, of the evocative memory. *When I asked* about it, they *were ready to reveal it.* This alone raises many unanswered questions about our patients, about *our* attitude toward addressing ourselves to their representational world, their cognitive readiness, their revelatory capacity about associations and secrets of childhood.

BIBLIOGRAPHY

CHANGEUX, J. (1986). *Neuronal Man.* New York: Pantheon.
CHRISTIE, A. (1977). *An Autobiography.* New York: Ballantine Books.

1. In a discussion of this paper Melvin A. Scharfman and Martin A. Silverman reported object representation difficulties in their child analytic cases. Scharfman's paper was published in 1976.

FREUD, A. (1970). The infantile neurosis. *W.*, 7:189–203.

FREUD, S. (1901). The psychopathology of everyday life. *S.E.*, 6.

———— (1905). Psychical (or mental) treatment. *S.E.*, 7:281–302.

———— (1907). Delusions and dreams in Jensen's *Gradiva*. *S.E.*, 9:7–95.

———— (1914). Remembering, repeating and working through. *S.E.*, 12:145–156.

———— (1923). The ego and the id. *S.E.*, 12:3–66.

HARTMANN, H. (1939). *Ego Psychology and the Problem of Adaptation*. New York: Int. Univ. Press, 1958.

LINNELL, A. (n.d.). Object and self representation as developmental model. Unpublished paper.

LOEWALD, H. W. (1970). Psychoanalytic theory and the psychoanalytic process. *Psychoanal. Study Child*, 25:45–68.

———— (1976). Perspective on memory. In *Papers on Psychoanalysis*. New Haven & London: Yale Univ. Press, 1980, pp. 148–173.

RITVO, S. (1979). The psychoanalytic process in childhood. *Psychoanal. Study Child*, 33:295–305.

SACKS, O. (1985). *The Man Who Mistook His Wife for a Hat*. New York: Summit Books.

SCHARFMAN, M. A. (1976). Perverse development in a young boy. *J. Amer. Psychoanal. Assn.*, 24:525–546.

TYSON, R. L. & TYSON, P. (1986). The concept of transference in child psychoanalysis. *J. Amer. Acad. Child Psychiat.*, 25:1–34.

WINNICOTT, D. W. (1960). The theory of the parent-infant relationship. In *The Maturational Processes and the Facilitating Environment*. New York: Int. Univ. Press, 1965, pp. 37–55.

The Essence of Masochism

KERRY KELLY NOVICK AND
JACK NOVICK, Ph.D.

DESPITE PUTATIVE SHIFTS IN THE TYPES OF PATHOLOGY PRESENTED
to the modern psychoanalyst, our caseloads are in fact very similar to Freud's, since he too grappled with masochistic phenomena of varying intensity and pervasiveness in his daily work.
The male cases cited in his paper on beating fantasies (1919)
"included a fairly large number of persons who would have to be
described as true masochists" (p. 196) and there are references
to suicide in all of Freud's published cases except Little Hans
(Litman, 1970; Novick, 1984). The difficulties in conceptualization and technical handling of masochism led Freud to repeated
revisions of his formulations and ultimately to fundamental
changes in psychoanalytic metapsychology.

Since Freud a vast literature has accumulated around the theoretical and clinical problems of masochism. Good summaries of
the classical view are provided by Fenichel (1945), Loewenstein
(1957), Bieber (1966), and Ferber (1975). Maleson (1984) says
that masochism has acquired a "confusing array of meanings,"
with "little consistency or precision in its current usage" (p. 325).

Kerry Kelly Novick is on the faculty of the Michigan Psychoanalytic Institute;
Jack Novick is a child and adolescent supervising analyst on the faculty of the
Michigan Psychoanalytic Institute, and an adjunct associate professor at Way-
ne State University Medical School.

Earlier versions of this paper were presented at the Arbor Clinic in May
1984, to the Michigan Association for Psychoanalysis in October 1984, and to a
scientific meeting of the Michigan Psychoanalytic Society in May 1986.

Our thanks to Paul Brinich, Laurie Levinson, Steven Marans, Irene Marcus,
Ava Bry Penman, and Katharine Rees for their helpful testing of our theoretical formulations against clinical data. Special thanks to Paul Brinich for his
detailed review of the text.

For Freud, all masochism was ultimately based on erotogenic masochism. The linkage of erotogenic and moral masochism takes place via the beating fantasy; morality for the masochist represents an unconscious, resexualized wish to be beaten by the father. In this way "the Oedipus complex is revived and the way is opened for a regression from morality to the Oedipus complex" (1924, p. 169). Thus Freud reemphasized his earlier tenet that the beating fantasy is the "essence of masochism" (1919, p. 189).

If Freud's statement is valid, a detailed study of beating fantasies should help us to understand more fully the complex phenomena of masochism. In "The Economic Problem of Masochism" (1924) Freud sketched the genetic point of view; Loewenstein (1957) used a developmental perspective; and we too will apply this perspective to a study of beating fantasies to elucidate a developmental line of masochism.

A major finding of our 1972 study of beating fantasies in children was that there were two types of beating fantasies, a normal transitory one and a "fixed fantasy." The transitory fantasy was more often found in girls, was usually spontaneously modified, or easily gave way to interpretation, whereas the fixed fantasy became the permanent focus of the child's psychosexual life and was often impervious to years of interpretive work. In this paper we use the development of the fixed beating fantasy as a model to explicate aspects of the developmental line of masochism.

We use previously unpublished data from the cases of 11 children with beating fantasies as a framework. Further material from infant and toddler observation and from the psychoanalyses of children, adolescents, and adults is included. We delineate the epigenesis of masochism as an *adaptation* to a disturbed environment, a *defense* against aggression, and a *mode of instinctual gratification*. Further, we show that masochism is not only overdetermined but serves other ego functions.

INFANCY

The literature on masochism includes many controversies; one major issue devolves on the genesis of masochism in the preoedipal or oedipal stages. In our 1972 study we described material from child analyses and observations which showed that organized beating fantasies were formed only postoedipally, while the determinants could be traced to earlier phases. In the sample of 111 indexed cases at the Anna Freud Centre we found that "the beating wish, sadistic intercourse theory, and phallic beating games could be seen in some form in all the young children" (p. 239). The transitory beating fantasy seen in some girls arose postoedipally and represented, as Freud had described, both regressed oedipal strivings and punishment for them. In each instance, the dynamics followed the classical formulation of oedipal conflicts leading to regression to anal-phase fixations around aggression and the beating wish.

In contrast, the preoedipal determinants of masochistic behavior in those children with fixed beating fantasies derived from disturbances in the earliest months of their lives. Mark, who entered analysis at 8½ years of age, was later found to have a fixed beating fantasy. He was the second of two children. His mother described her "obsessive concern" during pregnancy with the older child's potential jealousy. Her concern intensified after Mark's birth to the point where she felt compelled to interrupt any ministrations to Mark, including feeding, whenever she thought of her first child. She described Mark's first year as extremely unhappy, the feeding as totally unsatisfactory, and Mark as a fussy, crying baby. Like other mothers in the sample, she described herself as depressed and preoccupied, unable to take any pleasure in her baby. Such descriptions of a mutual lack of pleasure on the part of both mother and baby were universal in the fixed beating fantasy sample and have recurred in all our subsequent cases of masochistic pathology where social history data have been available.

This finding contrasts strikingly with the histories of the children who were found to have a transitory beating fantasy. In that group, despite reports of various pathological interactions early in the child's life, there were nevertheless sources of available pleasure for both partners in the mother-child dyad. Emma's mother, for instance, said that she started her 3-week-old infant on solids and she continued a pattern of premature demands throughout infancy; Emma's precocious positive responses, however, provided intense gratification for her mother, which was returned to the child as loving praise and pleasure. Derivatives of this mutually pleasurable interaction may have formed a component in the transference relationship of pleasant working together which Emma was able to enjoy in her analysis at age 4.

While we should be extremely cautious in attributing later manifestations directly to experiences of early infancy, it is important to note the unanimous report of the therapists of the children with fixed beating fantasies that the treatments were arduous, joyless, and ungratifying for a long time.

Disturbances in the pleasure economy between mother and infant appeared in the histories of all the children with fixed beating fantasies, and were re-created in more specific forms in the transference relationship during analysis. Clinical material from child analyses suggests the links forged in very early life between the experience of lack of pleasure or unpleasure and the age-appropriate developmental needs of the infant. But in the transference relationships of adult patients the multitude of transformations which take place in the course of development to adulthood make discernment of the deviations of early infancy very complicated.

Mrs. S., a tall, attractive divorcee, sought analysis to deal with issues of unresolved mourning for her father. Although outwardly very successful, she was finding it increasingly difficult to reconcile the demands of her profession with the needs of her three children and her own social life. Early in the analysis, Mrs. S. described a beating fantasy which she used in order to achieve orgasm. In the fantasy she imagined her father telling her that she was bad, putting her across his knee, and spanking her. She only became conscious of the fantasy just before orgasm, and then habitually forgot it again. The fantasy surfaced in treatment in the context of sexualized pleasure in the joint analytic work, which was accompanied by pains in her lower back. After the interpretation that the pains seemed to be the condition under which she could experience pleasure, Mrs. S. remembered her beating fantasy and realized that she had "always" had it.

Subsequent material centered on her overstimulating relationship with her father and her unresolved oedipal conflicts and neurotic compromises. After these were worked through in the transference, successful mourning could be accomplished. After two years of work, her presenting symptoms had abated, she was functioning apparently well in all areas, and Mrs. S. wanted to finish her treatment. Despite the many positive changes, the analyst disagreed, because the beating fantasy was still central to Mrs. S.'s sexual life. She had strenuously resisted all attempts to relate any analytic material to her relationship with her mother, particularly in the transference.

During the course of her analysis, Mrs. S. had visibly gained weight and the analyst interpreted this as self-feeding to defend against her wishes and fears over reexperiencing the maternal relationship in the transference. Mrs. S. responded with stories about her childhood hitherto unreported because she considered them "irrelevant." She had been told by her mother that she had been a "poor feeder" from birth, had difficulty sucking, and had not gained weight for the first four months of her life. This history of her own failure-to-thrive had later been repeated when Mrs. S. became a mother and found the relationship with her own infant daughter unsatisfying and tense, with the outcome that Mrs. S.'s daughter was diagnosed failure-to-thrive at four months. Work on this previously omitted material revitalized the analysis, and the vicissitudes of her early painful relationship to her mother emerged in the transference to be understood as the first layer in the formation of masochistic relationships.

Reconstruction of the early mother-child relationship from analytic data can always benefit from corroborative evidence, so we will examine here some material from infant observation which pertains to pleasure and pain in infancy. From very early in life, the infant can differentiate among others via a wide range of perceptual modalities. Included in these capacities is the ability to differentiate between self and nonself at the body boundary of the skin. This takes place at the point where the skins of mother and child touch and are felt as separate, contiguous entities. Under normal circumstances, stimulation of infants occurs through multiple channels; but in a disturbed mother-child relationship, a reduction in possible channels occurs. One that may remain is skin contact, since this is not dependent on psychological or emotional synchrony, as are, for instance, eye contact, talking, or smiling.

We have been following the development of two infants who became hair-pullers. It appears that the development of this pain-seeking symptom represents an adaptation to a disturbed mother-child relationship. Both children were born to single adolescent mothers; both children were diagnosed failure-to-thrive at 4 months, when the mothers each went through a period of depression and withdrawal from the babies. While the etiology of failure-to-thrive is complicated and varied, some clear factors emerge from detailed observations, films, and interviews.[1] In films of feeding before 4 months, Nicole attempted to engage her mother in social interactions between bites. After each bite, Nicole's mother literally scraped the smile off Nicole's face with the spoon, until the sixth bite was followed by a frown. This is a good example of what Tronick and Gianino (1986) have called the failure to repair a mismatch between mother and baby. In our observations we could see the next step, in which the mother externalized her feelings of failure onto the baby: the mother then made clear that she found Nicole an unpleasant girl. Soon thereafter the mother's depression coincided with Nicole's failure-to-thrive.

Through the intervention of staff at the institution where they lived, useful feeding was reestablished and Nicole gained weight. But the effect of the sustained experience of dissynchrony persisted. Tronick and Gianino have found that infants of depressed mothers decrease their engagement with people and things and deploy more coping behaviors aimed at maintaining self-regulation. The child moves away from signaling the mother to self-comfort, such as rocking, withdrawal, or aversion. Nicole began to pull her hair, tweaking and twiddling it until it broke, just at the back top quarter of her head, the

1. These cases are selected from an ongoing study of adolescent mothers and their babies. We are grateful to the other members of the study group, Drs. Kay and Linn Campbell, Connie Silver, A.M.L.S., and Don Silver, M.D.; the views presented here are our own and do not necessarily represent those of the group.

spot where her head rested in the crook of mother's arm, the one remaining point of contact with mother. For many months the spot was nearly bald; at 2½ years Nicole's hair was noticeably shorter and ragged at the same place. Despite excellent progress in both mother and child, this symptom persisted, appearing at moments when, for example, the nursery teacher failed to answer Nicole's question.

The hair-pulling in Nicole and the other infant is an example of pain-seeking as an adaptation to a pathological situation. Pain-seeking behavior represents an attempt to substitute for the withdrawal of cathexis by the mother. In Nicole the need for the object overrides the need for pleasure. For the children with beating fantasies or for the hair-pullers, safety resides in an object that induces pain rather than pleasure. These are mothers who, for a variety of reasons, cannot pay attention to their children's needs.

In our sample of children with beating fantasies we found a preponderance of mothers who were unable to absorb (Orgel, 1974) or contain the infant's helplessness, neediness, and rage, but blamed the child and externalized their own infantile affective states. Tronick and Gianino make the point that successful joint repair of mismatches by mother and child is experienced by the child as "effectance," and this may be what Winnicott (1953) and others have called the child's normal phase of omnipotence. Winnicott suggested that a child needs a long-enough stage of normal omnipotence before it can be relinquished. It is possible that extended periods of discomfort and dissatisfaction experienced in infancy by all the children with beating fantasies may have disrupted their normal stage of omnipotence prematurely. These children may have become aware too soon of their dependence on their mothers and felt deeply their inability to exert any control over the social realm. They turn to pathological solutions as an adaptation to this dilemma, as did the 11-month-old described by Loewenstein (1957) to illustrate his "protomasochistic" maneuver of "seduction of the aggressor."

The type of intervention with both mothers and infants described by Brinich (1984) and by Peter Blos, Jr. (1985) in his discussion of intergenerational pathology could correct this pattern; however, in our sample, it appeared that the mothers themselves experienced such difficulty in relation to activity, dependency needs, and feelings of helplessness that they attempted to resolve them by externalization of these hated, devalued parts of themselves onto their children. Abel's mother was cold and irritable, withdrawn emotionally from her crying baby whom she saw as a pathetically helpless child. Eric's mother denied her own feelings of castration and passivity by externalizing these aspects of her self representation onto all her male objects: thus her husband and her infant Eric were seen as damaged, hopeless, useless people.

Rather than a relationship based on the sensitive mutual repair of inevitable moments of mismatch, the infants who later developed masochistic pathology grew up in a milieu of painful externalizations. We could speculate that externalization of blame, failure, and devalued aspects of the self onto the child served as a major and early mode of relationship and may have become the "primary fault" (Balint, 1968) leading to the evolution of masochistic structures. We suggest that the first layer of masochism must be sought in early infancy, in the child's adaptation to a situation where safety resides only in a painful relationship with the mother. Glenn (1984) too found the roots of his patient's masochism in the relationship to a "parent associated with pain" (p. 72). Valenstein's description of "individuals whose attachment to pain signifies an original attachment to painfully perceived objects" (1973, p. 389) applies also to the patients in the 1972 sample and to those we have seen subsequently. Their beating fantasies encapsulated and perpetuated the painful relationship to the object, not only historically, but also in their clinging to unhappiness through all stages of treatment.

Mark, whose early history was referred to above, was typical of the group of children with fixed beating fantasies in our 1972 sample. His beating fantasy appeared against a background of severe pathology. He was referred for frequent tantrums, periods of overwhelming anxiety, multiple fears, and being bullied at school. Once he overcame his initial anxiety, he presented a picture of chaotic drive development with little or no phase dominance. Impulses from all libidinal levels coexisted: his anxieties were often oral in form, with fears of being poisoned or eaten; he said, "in intercourse the lady eats the man." Anal sexuality was manifest in excited preoccupation with feces, bottoms, and nose-picking. Mark, like the other children in the sample, was of superior intelligence and functioned adequately in school. In treatment, however, it soon became clear that his reality perception was distorted in relation to self and object representations. Mark, a slender boy in treatment with a plump woman, complained of being fat. His feelings about himself fluctuated between grandiose delusions of omnipotence and a sense of abject worthlessness.

As with the other children in the 1972 sample, the first two years of Mark's treatment were marked by immediate discharge of wishes into action. His analyst said, "His behavior was wild and uncontrolled and there were long periods when I could make no contact with him. He would, for example, charge into the room with a pellet gun, shout, 'Alright, I'm going to kill you!' and fire the pellets at me. One moment he would be lying on the table, licking his snot, telling me he has no friends and the next moment he would shout at me, 'You fat pig, you'll die for this!'" As words could increasingly be linked to feelings and the range of affects broadened to include pleasure, Mark said, "When I'm feeling good, I feel all alone; when I'm feeling bad, I'm with my mother."

The need for pain seems to be at the core of the personalities of these patients; it arises early in life, whether from environmental causes or constitutional factors, as some have proposed (Olinick, 1964), persists throughout development, and can be seen to be at work even in the end phase of analysis. Mary was referred for analysis following a serious suicide attempt in adolescence. In her sixth year of treatment, she had graduated from university with highest honors and had a full scholarship for graduate studies where she was doing outstanding work. At the end of her first year of analysis the analyst described her as totally dependent on her mother, spending weekends and every evening in her room, sitting silently at meals and, other than studying, her only activity was rearranging furniture in her room, or spending hours trying to decide which side of the desk to put her pencils on. She was physically inhibited and looked like a prepubertal boy. At the time, the major concern was that she would become psychotic or kill herself.

After 6 years of analysis, she looked very feminine and attractive, had many friends, and had a long-standing relationship with a very suitable young man. They had arranged to share an apartment and were planning marriage. She had confronted her parents numerous times and had forced a change in the relationship which they enjoyed. Things were going well on all fronts, the end of analysis was in sight, and only one problem remained. The overt manifestation of the problem was Mary's continued difficulty in maintaining pleasurable feelings, especially with the analyst. As the suicide risk had receded, it had become apparent that Mary's primary pathology was not depression but an underlying severe masochistic disorder which subsumed both her depression and suicidal behavior. It became clear that her suicide attempt was an enactment of a fixed beating fantasy. As the determinants of Mary's underlying masochism were worked through, she could experience and maintain pleasure for longer periods of time outside of her therapy. She could feel pride and joy in her skills and competence, and take pleasure in her attractiveness and sexual activities. The conflicts around pleasure became centered almost entirely in the analysis. She would feel happy, proud of some achievement, until she walked in the door and then would feel gloomy and bad. Mary explained her need to feel unhappy with the analyst as follows:

> When I'm happy, I feel I'm not with you.
> To be unhappy is to be like you, to be with you, to sit quietly and depressed with the whole world right here in this room.
> I tell you about something funny that happened in class and then I think, oh, you should have been there, and I realize you weren't there and I feel sad and lonely.
> I sometimes think of my suicide as the best time. Everyone was with me, and loved me and felt sorry for me.

Throughout this paper, we will be examining the transformations through development of the child's involvement with pain, but what we are describing at the earliest level is a learned association. The clinical material of our masochistic patients supports Stern's (1985) view, based on infant observation, that " it is the actual shape of interpersonal reality, specified by the interpersonal invariants that really exist, that helps determine the developmental course. Coping operations occur as reality-based adaptations" (p. 255). As Mary said, "Feeling bad is something I know, it's safe, it's the smell of home."

Tronick and Gianino demonstrated the stability of the child's early coping styles, and Escalona (1968) has shown that it is *maladaptive* infant behavior which tends to persist. Thus the association of mother and unpleasure leads to the early adoption of an autoplastic, rather than alloplastic, mode of dealing with internal and external stimuli, which sets a pattern of discharge via the self which will affect all later developmental phases.

TODDLERHOOD

From the perspective of masochistic pathology, the toddler stage is crucial in determining the quality of aggressive impulses and in fixing the pattern of dealing with them. The normal developmental tasks, activities, and wishes of toddlerhood provide an opportunity to establish constructive defenses; a sound sense of self accompanied by feelings of effectance, joy, and safety; a loving relationship to constant objects; and an exponential expansion of ego control of motility and cognition. All of these are dependent on adequate drive fusion. In discussions of masochism, the concepts of fusion, libidinization, and binding are often used interchangeably, even by Freud. We feel it is important to differentiate them, as fusion denotes transformation of both drives by a mixture in which aggression is neutralized to some degree by libido, with resultant energy available for other purposes, such as defense formation or sublimation. Libidinization occurs in the formation of masochistic pathology, when aggressive impulses or painful experiences become sexualized; no transformation of either drive occurs. Binding is the structural inhibition of direct discharge. A striking feature of all the children with fixed beating fantasies was the extent of primitive aggressive behavior, apparently unfused by libido. In the first year of his analysis, Mark threw the toys all over the room, down the stairs, or out of the window. He would write on the wall, try to force open the files and lockers, and generally try to destroy the room. His uncontrolled behavior provoked the therapist to restrain him, which led to bitter accusations of attack. His mental world seemed dominated by fantasies of attack and counterattack, as he filled his sessions with complaints of being picked on by teachers, peers, his brother, and his parents.

Mary presented with alternating states of blank silence and overwhelming experiences of omnipotent rage. Her fantasies were characterized by primary process organization and her dreams were dominated by images of uncontrolled, explosive destruction. For example, the central image in one dream was of stabbing a man over and over until he was reduced to a mound of indistinguishable flesh and blood. In a later dream, a room full of babies was shotgunned to the point of indiscriminate mess. Later in her analysis, when Mary became able to associate to these dreams, a repeated latent theme was anal explosiveness which would destroy her mother, who in reality had spent an inordinate amount of time scrubbing the bathrooms.

As Furman (1985) emphasized, the mother as auxiliary ego protects the child from excessive libidinal and aggressive stimulation. Our data confirm the findings of others (Rubinfine, 1965; Orgel, 1974; Brinich, 1984) that mothers of masochists seem less than normally able to contain their children's aggression and thus promote fusion. The result for the children is unfused, primitive, omnipotent aggression. Rather than containing and modifying the children's impulses and anxieties with the help of their own libidinal investment, each mother in the beating fantasy sample intensified the child's aggression by bodily intrusiveness, constraint of normal moves toward independence and autonomy, and interference with pleasure in messing and exploration.

Further, the mothers' own conflicts over instinctual impulses were dealt with by externalization onto the children. With Mary's mother this was a lifelong process, which continued even throughout Mary's treatment. For instance, Mary's mother insisted that family members and guests always enter through the back door and remove their shoes to protect the pale carpeting from any dirt they might bring in. She cleaned constantly, reproaching others for their dirtiness and mess. Once Mary "forgot" to remove her shoes and was overwhelmed with feelings of shame which were linked via associations to having soiled her pants as a young child. During the intake interview following Mary's suicide attempt, her mother's sole complaint was that Mary had accompanied a group of girls four years earlier as they threw eggs at an abandoned house. Despite the passage of time and the intervening near-death of her child, Mary's "vandalism," as she termed it, was the focus of her attention. In analysis, Mary recounted her continuing feeling of badness over the incident and her persistent fear that the police would still come after her.

Mrs. S.'s mother had a history of flamboyant sexual relationships with men who were unacceptable to her own family. Mrs. S. reported that, as a child, she masturbated openly. Though she had no recollection of her mother's reaction at the time, she described her mother's current practice of laughing accounts to friends of Mrs. S.'s "extreme uncontrollable childhood sexuality." From early adolescence, Mrs. S. was promiscuous, imperiling herself with sexual exploits which she recounted to her mother. In analysis, it became clear that Mrs. S.'s sexual behavior in childhood and adulthood represented an internalization of her mother's lack of control of impulses; the result was that Mrs. S. hated herself and contemplated suicide. Mary and Mrs. S., like the children with fixed beating fantasies, already had a proclivity developed in infancy toward autoplastic solutions to stress. It is in the toddler phase that the earlier use of the self to restore homeostasis joins with the mother's externalizations to create the mechanism of turning aggression against the self.

We found that all of the children in our sample dealt with their aggression by denying any sign of hostility between themselves and their mothers and struggled to maintain an idealized image of mother as loving and perfect. This included denial of the mother's castration, which Bak (1968) considered an important factor in perversions. Refusal to face imperfections in the mother was linked to omnipotence of thought, as mother's failings were attributed to the boy's own aggression. Mark felt that his penis was not his own; if his mother did not have one, it must be because he had stolen it from her. He felt his own defecation was a dangerous aggressive act (a result of his own wishes and his mother's attitude), and insisted that his mother could not do anything so terrible as defecate—he must be the only one in the world, and the worst person of all, to do so.

We see the defensive aspect of the underlying masochism expressed in the beating fantasy as following upon and reinforcing the child's prior submission to a threatening environment. What was initially an acceptance of the mother's externalizations (messy, dependent, aggressive) in the service of retaining the object becomes an active internalization used by the child to maintain the image of a loving, protective, perfect mother, safe from the destructive rage of his anal sadism. From the point of view of defense, the masochism can be seen as an attempt to defend against destructive wishes from each level of development, directed against the mother, utilizing the mechanisms of denial, displacement, internalization, and, via the internalization, turning of aggression against the body.

The operation of all these defenses can be seen in the form of the later beating fantasy. All the beating fantasies contained, implicitly in that they involved punishment or explicitly, the statement, "I am a naughty boy." Mark imagined that his strict paternal aunt entered the room; he took off his clothes, said, "I am a naughty boy," and then she spanked him. Despite the evidence from the boys' material which demonstrated that their mothers were experienced as threatening objects and the fact that the mothers were often the punishers in real life, the beater in the fantasies was usually the father or a father representative. Here we see a displacement of aggression from the more frightening, but more important, primary object to the father.

In reporting the beating fantasy the children usually stopped at the point where they had been beaten as if that were the end. Further work, especially by means of the transference relationship, revealed that there was more to the fantasy, and this remainder contained the main preoedipal libidinal and narcissistic goals of the fantasy—hence the reluctance of the children to disclose it. In this extension, someone important, often a woman, felt very sorry for the beaten child and comforted him; in many versions the child was then regarded as a very important and special person. One child fantasied that the beating would be followed by both parents apologizing and the mother putting soothing lotion on his bottom. In another child's fantasy, after he had been cruelly beaten by schoolboys, the headmaster told the assembled students, "He is the outstanding boy who has been treated badly. We have never had any other boy who has gone through so much." Analyses of adolescents who have attempted suicide show that this fantasied response by the object is crucial to the goals of the suicide (Novick, 1984). Mary imagined that, after her suicide, she would hover around to see how sorry everyone was, how they would feel guilty, and turn their full attention to her to gratify all her wishes. The defensive efforts to rid the mother-child relationship of omnipotent aggression by means of displacement and turning aggression against the self are the child's contribution to the joint attempt to create a "purified pleasure dyad" (Novick, 1980).

The mothers of children with beating fantasies were psychologically intrusive, via their externalizations. Through hypercathexis of their children's bodies well into prepuberty or adolescence, for active gratification of their own needs, they were also physically intrusive. Anna Freud (1960) commented on the increased impact of parental disturbance when the pathology is not contained in thought but moves into the realm of activity. For example, one mother constantly checked the child's anus and feces for signs of worms. Mark's mother wiped his bottom until he was 11 years old; she stopped only after three years of analytic work with Mark enabled him to resist her intrusion into the bathroom. In her analysis, Mary occasionally displayed a cognitive uncertainty which contrasted markedly with her high intelligence. Work on these states allowed for recovery of a memory of a voice asking, "Are you sure?" This phrase became a pointer to her symptomatic uncertainty at many levels, but specific associations led to the reconstruction of her mother's handling of her toilet training. Mary experienced a confirming shock of recognition when she saw her mother constantly asking her toddler grandchild if she had to go to the bathroom. When the child said "No," Mary's mother said, "Are you sure?" and then peeked into the grandchild's diaper while remarking to Mary, "You have to make sure."

In normal development, the self representation emerges out of and contains the body representation. This integration starts with the experience of pleasure in one's body at the hands of a loving object. The children with beating fantasies were unable to achieve integration of body and self. They experienced their bodies as owned and controlled by their mothers, and so pre-oedipal omnipotent aggression toward mother was defended against and expressed by attacks on the body. Mrs. S. was always ashamed of her breasts and had such antipathy to this part of her body that she was unable to breast-feed her children. When this was explored in analysis, there seemed no reality basis for her negative feelings, as her breast development was normal in all respects. Later in analysis, it emerged through dreams and associations that Mrs. S. did not feel that her breasts belonged to her. Her lack of pride in her own body and her inability to feed her own children were her way of expressing her rage and disappointment at her own mother's inability to breast-feed her. Autoaggressive behavior in infants as reported by Cain (1961) and the study of suicide cases confirm this finding (Novick, 1984).

A further effect of the intrusive pattern of interaction is the hypercathexis in the child of the receptive mode. This touches upon a major conceptual puzzle—the relation of masochism and passivity. Maleson (1984) notes that many analysts continue to equate the two, as Freud did originally. It might be helpful to distinguish between passivity and receptivity. We see passivity as an ego quality linked in its pathological extreme manifestations to the experience of an inattentive caretaker. An adolescent boy who had suffered from infancy from parental inability to sustain attention to his needs and feelings showed no signs of masochistic pathology, yet demonstrated extreme passivity in all areas of his life. Masochists are highly receptive and are ready to take in any stimuli from the outside world, ranging from subtle shifts in mother's moods to what one homosexual patient described as his wish for a "fist-fuck." Masochists are very active in their pursuit of pain and failure, in part to maintain the receptive relationship with an intrusive object. For example, Mary at 19 years endured taunts because she wore her hair cut so short that she looked like a schoolboy; she revealed after years of analysis that she went to her mother for her haircuts.

We have discussed the ways in which the toddler's aggression is intensified by failure in the mother-child relationship to promote fusion and integration. Further, the normal impulses toward separation and independent functioning which arise in the anal phase are experienced as aggression by both mother and child. The struggle for autonomy first takes place in the realm of bodily activity; the mothers of the children in our group opposed independence and reacted to normal assertion as attack. These children lost the battle for autonomy and felt that their mothers needed them only as helpless anal objects. Mother and child had become locked in an intense relationship which was experienced by the child as one in which each partner needed the other for survival and gratification. The child not only feared loss of the mother, but his guilt resided mainly in his normal wishes to separate from her and function independently. As Mark said, "Whenever I do something good without my mother, I think she is going to die." The beating in the fantasy formed later could then also be seen as a punishment for wishes to separate from the mother. In the fantasy the naughtiness for which they were beaten was usually left vague, but we have often found that the fantasy followed age-appropriate behavior, independent wishes, or achievements.

Mark, at 14, was about to leave on a school trip and worried that his mother would be sad and upset, which she became. He hoped that he would be able to flirt with the girls, and at first he managed to talk to a girl he liked. Before the trip was actually under way, however, Mark created a fantasy that the school superintendent would cane him for flirting, and he spent the rest of the time preoccupied with this fantasy to the detriment of any of the social activities. Although this appears very similar to punishment for an oedipal wish, the subsequent material clearly indicated that Mark's flirting represented a breaking of the object tie to his mother, and it was for this disloyalty that he was being punished.

Similarly, other age-appropriate activities throughout development were experienced as aggressive attacks on the mother and could be performed only under conditions which counteracted any normal moves toward independence and separate functioning. For example, in adolescence several of the boys, including Mark, could not masturbate with their hands but rubbed their genitals against the sheets leaving the mess for their mothers to see and clean up. Instead of gratification in a private act which excluded mother, genital impulses were discharged in a form re-creating an anal mode of relating to their mothers. The dependent receptivity which is central to masochism and the beating fantasy can then be seen as a defense against the aggression attributed to activity, separation, and independent functioning.

Thus the child's pain-seeking adaptation to a pathological early relationship continues in the anal phase as the prime mode of attracting and retaining the object. The aggressive impulses of the anal phase are dealt with by the defense of turning the aggression against the self, which prevents destruction of the object and allows for discharge of aggression toward the internalized hated mother. In our view, the adaptive and defensive motives for the masochism which underlies the beating fantasy are preoedipal; the masochistic behavior of the child is not yet a sexual pleasure in itself but a means by which he attempts to survive and gratify other passive libidinal wishes. The clinical presentation of all the children in the 1972 sample was preoedipal. They entered treatment displaying a persistence of anal-phase ways of functioning, with excited preoccupation with seeing, smelling, and wiping bottoms, thoughts of defecating on people and smearing. One boy of 9 years still played with and hid feces, and several of them masturbated anally. The egos of these children had little ability to control discharge of the anal drive impulses; the defense systems were severely impaired, with predominant, often exclusive use of primitive defenses, such as denial and the variety of externalizations, including drive projection. Battling relationships were the norm at home, school, and in treatment. It is evident that these children carry into the phallic-oedipal phase the preexisting pathology; for this reason they will experience it very differently from the normal child. The phallic-oedipal period is crucial for the sexualization of masochism.

Phallic-Oedipal Stage

The nature of the child's theory concerning parental intercourse has a profound effect on the development of masochism and the later beating fantasy. Sadistic intercourse theories are universal, but in normal children they coexist with other theories, whereas for the children we are discussing the notion that in intercourse the parents beat or hurt each other is the safest theory available to them. Just as being beaten represents the safest form of relating to the object in the beating fantasy, so the sadistic intercourse theory is preferred to more frightening ideas, such as chaotic, uncontrollable happenings (Niederland, 1958), mutual mutilation, castration, etc. This view is in line with Niederland's suggestion that the sadistic intercourse theory and the beating fantasy serve to structure unorganized, terrifying primal scene experiences and ideas. For these patients the primal scene is not a reconstructed hypothesis or a metaphor for the universal exclusion from parental activities but an ongoing reality, as parents of patients with masochistic pathology seem unable to protect them from repeated exposure to overwhelming experiences. Indeed, they often seem to inflict them on the patients. On the eve of a 13-year-old's entry into analysis, the parents happened to leave the bedroom door open; the boy walked in to see his parents in the act of intercourse, mother on top of father; the following day, preceding his first session, the patient broke his arm playing ball. Analysis revealed that this was but the latest in a series of events in which his mother had exposed him to traumatic situations which were invariably followed by self-injurious behavior. Furman (1984) has noted the role of parental pathology in the exposure to traumatic situations of suicidal patients.

The phallic excitement of this phase and the wish to participate in sadistic parental intercourse turn what had been a means to an end into an end in itself. To submit, to suffer, to be beaten, to be humiliated now come to represent the feminine receptive position in parental intercourse. The wish to be in this position becomes the instinctual motive for the masochism, the spur and the accompaniment to phallic masturbation. A crucial transformation occurs during this phase, when the painful experiences in the preoedipal parent-child interaction become libidinized and represent for the child participation in parental intercourse.

To the powerful motives for masochism of the earlier phases is added the circumvention of the normal oedipal exclusion, humiliation, and rage. Often the parents collude at each level in the development of the pathological relationship. Their involvement in the lack of resolution of the oedipus complex contributes to the maintenance of what we have called the "delusion of omnipotence." This ego defect is an important factor in the characteristically high level of anxiety in masochistic patients.

In the children with beating fantasies, drive material from all levels of libidinal development was available in consciousness. The children were convinced that these impulses could not be controlled either by themselves or by anyone else. They felt sure that their drive aims could and would be gratified; reality contradiction did not seem to affect this conviction. Mark, at 13, was convinced that his mother wanted to have intercourse with him. One of the sources of this attitude was the absence of an adequate system of defenses, which meant that internal controls were insufficient; none of these children had reached the stage of developing a structured superego. External controls were also missing, in that the fathers of these children were all particularly unsuitable to serve as strong, protective objects for identification. Two fathers had died, two fathers had psychotic breakdowns, and two were absent in the army during their children's early years. The others seemed to play no positive role in the family, showing undue dependence on the mothers. Conversely, the mothers were all described as powerful, domineering women, who ruled their families more or less overtly.

There was also a high degree of parental collusion in the gratification of inappropriate wishes. Several of the children in this group were allowed into the parental bed until ages of 11 and 12; others were helped with toileting up to 7 or 8 years; most ruled the house with their tantrums and rages, and in two cases there was danger of the child causing serious harm to a sibling. Mark regularly ousted his father from the parental bed, to which father's response was a depressive withdrawal. When Mark began displaying an interest in girls in adolescence, his father became acutely anxious and then announced that he was homosexual, although this apparently resulted in no action. Throughout her childhood, as far back as she could remember, Mrs. S. spent long evenings lying on her parents' bed watching television while her father stroked her body. She reported her childhood notion that mother had relinquished father to her while keeping the other children for herself. Rubinfine (1965) has suggested that such parents are unable to limit and contain the child's aggression, a point amply confirmed by our material. When it was suggested to Albert's mother that firmness might help control his wild behavior, she refused on the grounds that she did not want to risk upsetting the boy; in his teens, when his father became annoyed at Albert's resentment of his claims on his wife, one solution proposed by the family was that Albert and his mother should move into a flat together, leaving the rest of the family behind.

Both the delusion of omnipotence and the libidinization of painful experience persist in the pathology of adult patients. For example, a neurotic professional woman who lived out her beating fantasy in numerous unsuitable relationships reported a dream of marrying her father. In her associations, she revealed that she still thought that she really could marry her father and that no one could stop her from fulfilling her wishes. A male graduate student with beating fantasies had undergone frequent enemas as a child. For many years in analysis he recalled the enemas with enjoyment and remembered his older sister looking on with what he imagined to be jealousy. He said he felt special because he was the only one in the family to enjoy this exclusive relationship with his mother. His wish for an enema from the analyst figured as a central transference theme; only after many years of work could he begin to acknowledge and experience the rage he felt at his mother's gross bodily intrusion. In his early adolescence his mother bought him some bright purple shorts, which he described as the token of their exclusive relationship. Only after working through his libidinization of the enemas could he also recall that he was teased by the other boys for wearing the "faggy" shorts.

TRANSITION TO LATENCY

Fantasies and anxieties about pain and suffering are universal, as is the beating wish (Novick and Novick, 1972). With some resolution of the oedipus complex and the formation of the superego, children move into the latency period. Only at this point did a transitory beating fantasy emerge in some of the girls in our sample. When it occurred, it clearly represented both oedipal strivings in regressed form and punishment for them, as Freud described. Gradually sexual excitement and masturbation were divorced from the fantasy and the wishes appeared in increasingly distanced forms. In our study we concluded that this transitory beating fantasy was a normal transitional component of postoedipal development in girls and may be more common than is generally supposed. Female patients who present a beating fantasy may have regressed in or out of treatment to this postoedipal moment in development. As described above in the case of Mrs. S., it is only with clinical criteria of persistence and centrality of the fantasy, as well as the quality of the transference relationship, that the differentiation between a transitory and a fixed fantasy can be made.

In contrast, the children who later developed a fixed beating fantasy had no latency period to consolidate ego development and spent those years either in the enactment of preoedipal and oedipal sadomasochistic impulses or under the restriction of crippling inhibitions and severe obsessional symptomatology. For example, a potentially intelligent and creative woman with a fixed beating fantasy who sought analysis originally because of repeated work failure reported that she stopped learning in her school years and spent her time preoccupied with fantasies of imminent destruction which she contained by ritualistic repetitions of magical phrases.

Puberty and Adolescence

The emergence of the fixed fantasy in the group of disturbed boys coincided with the onset of puberty, in all cases following the first emission. At 13 Mark reported a masturbation fantasy in which he first thought of undressing a girl in his class; the girl changed to an older woman and then, as his excitement mounted, the image changed to that of his mother. As he reached a climax the content shifted to his father walking in, holding him down and beating him on the buttocks. Mark, who was then as tall as his father, felt that he was "a Hitler" capable of killing his father. He not only wished to replace his father, but thought that his mother wanted him to do so. Pubertal changes in general give the stamp of reality to fantasies of gratifying infantile impulses. It was only because of the structural development fostered by years of analysis that the children in our sample could develop a fantasy outlet as an alternative to action. The capacity to contain impulses in fantasy represents an achievement. Less fortunate adolescents act out their impulses in self-injurious behavior or suicide.

Our children and adults used the *fixed* beating fantasy for important ego and superego functions which should have developed in latency, if these patients had been able to achieve a latency phase. These functions were control of anxiety, stabilization of the "representational world" (Sandler and Rosenblatt, 1962), and defense against direct drive discharge. The *transitory* beating fantasy found only in girls became progressively distanced from frightening oedipal wishes. The *fixed* beating fantasy, on the other hand, represented the most innocuous form of the wish; variations on the theme often involved more ominous fantasies of suicide, self-mutilation, and death. Abel had fantasies of being beaten by older boys, pop singers, and football players, but also masturbated with fantasies of having his penis and testicles burned or otherwise damaged. Further masturbation fantasies involved death and suicide; indeed, in late adolescence, some years after the termination of analysis, Abel attempted suicide. In the cases of Abel and the other boys with a fixed fantasy, we could see a diminution of anxiety when the beating fantasy was employed, whereas fantasies of death or mutilation soon became anxious preoccupations and led to feelings of overwhelming terror. One might say that in place of a fear of being destroyed or damaged, they created a pleasurable fantasy of being beaten, i.e., anxiety had become libidinized.

In the early phases of treatment of these children, it was often unclear who was standing for whom in the constant flux of externalizations, internalizations, and confusions with the object. In a brief sequence a child could become both the powerful attacking object and the victim of the attack. In the beating fantasy, however, there was a clear differentiation maintained between self and object. The subject was always the victim and the beater was invariably a person who figured in the child's real life, often the father or someone drawn from the class of father representatives. These characteristics may be seen in one boy's fantasy of being held down by two older boys from school and beaten on the buttocks. For the next two years, the fantasy remained basically unchanged, unlike the constantly elaborated imaginative productions of children with transitory beating fantasies, in which the characters were drawn from anywhere but real life. We would suggest that formation of the fixed fantasy not only required a modicum of stability of representations, but also seemed of itself to contribute to maintaining stability in the usual chaos of the representational world of these children.

Despite positive changes in these cases the "delusion of omnipotence" seemed unaltered. After 6 years of treatment Mark remained convinced that his death wishes would destroy the object. The work of Lamb (1976), Abelin (1975, 1980), and others has underscored the importance of the father in the preoedipal development of the child. Through each stage in the development of the children in the fixed beating fantasy sample, the fathers failed to perform their necessary functions. As R. Furman (1986) so clearly describes, the father's initial role is to protect and support the primacy of the mother-child relationship. Mark's father reacted to his wife's pregnancy with intense jealousy, confirming the mother's pathological fantasies about the effect of the new baby on the other family members. Mary's father retreated into a busy professional life during the pregnancy and her first year, emerging periodically only to criticize mother's handling of the baby. During the toddler phase, Furman describes the importance of the father as a source of additional love for the child and support for the adult ego of the mother. Mark's father was as messy and uncontrolled as his toddler son; rather than taking pride in and fostering Mark's emerging autonomy, he joined with his wife in externalizations of the devalued anal aspects of his personality.

By the time Mark reached puberty and his analysis had helped him to approach the possibility of oedipal level impulses, he had no loving, consistent parental relationship to draw on as an internal resource in his struggle to control his incestuous wishes. After each achievement, which he experienced as an aggressive attack on the object, he immediately had to find out whether the analyst was still alive. It is in relation to this "delusion of omnipotence," the continuing lack of internal and external controls, that one of the important functions of the beating fantasy could be seen. From the material of these children, the timing of the emergence of the fantasy, and the content of the fantasy, it was evident that the beater in the fantasy represented a wished-for, ideal father, a strong male who would limit and control the fulfillment of omnipotent, libidinal and destructive wishes. The fathers of all these patients were particularly unsuitable to serve as strong, protective objects for identification. In the fantasy the beater was a father or father representative who was always a powerful, assertive figure punishing the child, often to stop him from gratifying a forbidden wish. Mark's fantasy was of attempting to go to bed with a middle-aged woman visitor; but before he could do so, his father stopped him, held him down, and beat him. In reality his father was a passive, ineffectual man who did not stop him from entering his mother's bed whenever he wanted to. Thus instead of internalizing a representation of a strong father, to build a superego, and defend against unacceptable impulses by means of age-adequate mechanisms such as repression, reaction formation, displacement, and especially sublimation, these children used the beating fantasy to control and limit drive discharge and gratification of omnipotent wishes. The fixed beating fantasy functioned in place of a superego, which would normally be formed in latency.

We have seen a similar outcome, arrived at by a different path, in the females with fixed beating fantasies. The fathers of the girls continued and intensified their denigration of the mothers and actively involved themselves in overstimulating relationships with their daughers from the oedipal phase on, with the result that a component in the masochistic pathology of the females was intense bisexual conflict and severe penis envy. The girls, like the boys, were unable to internalize an autonomous superego. In addition, the denigrated mother was not used as a feminine ego ideal. Mary entered treatment looking like a boy and declared her three vows—not to have a boyfriend, not to marry, and not to have children.

TECHNICAL IMPLICATIONS

Freud wrote to Jung in 1909, "In my practice, I am chiefly concerned with the problem of repressed sadism in my patients; I regard it as the most frequent cause of the failure of therapy.

Revenge against the doctor combined with self-punishment. In general, sadism is becoming more and more important to me" (cited in Bergmann and Hartman, 1976, p. 33). In his last work, Freud still comments that we are "specially inadequate" (1940, p. 180) in dealing with masochistic patients. We may note that the Wolf-Man had a fixed beating fantasy and would have qualified for inclusion in our sample (Blum, 1974).

All of the children with fixed beating fantasies had many years of analysis. The change in the overt behavior and functioning of some was quite remarkable. Obvious manifestations of sado-masochistic relationships with peers or adults disappeared; they seemed to be coping well and even functioning quite independently. Frequently it was near termination that the child would first hint at and then disclose the existence of a beating fantasy. Analysis had fostered the development of certain ego functions, especially those necessary for the use of fantasy as a discharge channel, and had addressed some of the preoedipal determinants of the masochism. The formation of a beating fantasy at puberty was achieved on the basis of these gains. However, on follow-up, we found that some of these boys suffered psychotic breakdown in later adolescence, some attempted suicide, and others remained tied in a submissive, dependent relationship with an overpowering mother. Our findings on the various determinants of the fixed beating fantasy and the multiple ego functions it served suggest certain technical approaches which may improve the outcome of these cases.

For example, the fact that the beating fantasy served in lieu of important ego functions suggests that interpretation of the drive determinants will not be effective until concomitant work has been done on the ego pathology. Specifically, focus on the "delusion of omnipotence" would be important; if the patient could internalize and experience a capacity for controlling drive discharge, the necessity for a masochistic fantasy might diminish. Work could then turn to the determinants of the underlying masochism with special attention directed at the three aspects emphasized in this paper, i.e., the adaptive, defensive, and instinctual motives. The patient's masochistic behavior and fantasies would then be seen as a threefold attempt to (1) maintain a preoedipal object tie to his mother; (2) defend the object against his destructive wishes; and (3) participate in a sadomasochistic sexual relationship.

As noted earlier, Mark's mother reacted with increasing distress and ultimately depression to his adolescent moves toward separation. Extensive analysis of his omnipotent aggressive fantasies was not sufficient to help Mark separate from his mother without work on his denial of the reality of her preexisting problems around being left. When he saw her intense reaction to his brother's departure for college, he could not avoid recognizing her own hostile need to control those around her. The work could then return to his wishes to invite her control, thereby maintaining the narcissistically gratifying illusion that his mother clung to him out of love.

During the first two years of Mary's analysis, when she was 18 to 20 years old, she was completely dependent on her mother, who did her laundry, bought her clothes, cut her hair, and cooked for her. During this time much of the work focused on Mary's hurt and rage and her many ways of defending against the experience or expression of anger at her mother. The subsequent shift in her defense system, especially the infantile dependence, enabled her to become more active and self-sufficient. After an extended period of work, Mary managed to confront her mother over her intrusive behavior. Mother reacted by crying, and running away for several hours. Mary eventually moved to her own apartment and, when she first returned home for a weekend visit, her mother retreated to the attic and refused to come down to greet Mary. The accumulation of such incidents breached Mary's denial and she began to talk more in sessions about mother's "weirdness." When she turned to her father for reality confirmation, he did not validate her perceptions and support her healthy ego growth, but rather told her they must be involved in "some mother-daughter game." At that point she realized that the whole family had colluded for years to cover up mother's pathology. Mary moved then into a period of pleasure in her independent activity; she talked of "building a wall" between her and her mother, so that she could assign feelings to the appropriate person. She had earlier described her terror during electrical storms, but during this phase of treatment Mary realized that it was not she, but her mother who was so terrified. Mary herself actually enjoyed watching the lightning. Once this distinction had been made, it was much easier to work on Mary's contribution to the persisting infantile tie.

The ongoing preoedipal tie is the greatest stumbling block to progress. In order to break the tie the patient will have to become aware not only of his internal conflicts but also of his mother's pathology, especially her hostile opposition to progressive development. He will not only have to face his own destructive wishes but also relinquish his denial of his mother's hostility toward independence. Unless the preoedipal tie between mother and child can be broken, little change in the patient's underlying disturbance can be expected.

Work on the underlying motives must be accompanied by work on ego pathology, such as the persistence of omnipotent thinking and the inability to fuse drive impulses. For some time during the fourth year of Mary's analysis, material emerged which demonstrated the many ways she worked to maintain the delusion of the power of her wishes. If something she had wished for did not occur, she convinced herself that she had not wished her hardest. Habitually, on reaching the corner of the street, she looked at the stoplight, willing it to change color; when of course it did, she experienced a feeling of exultation in her power. This work prepared the way for material to emerge regarding another determinant of her experienced omnipotence. This was the lack of fusion of her aggressive impulses, which left them free to rage unchecked. Thus, any angry feeling in thought, fantasy, or dream instantaneously led to total bloody annihilation. For many years her dreams were filled with images of mutilation, horrible death, and destruction. After her love for her younger brother was acknowledged, she dreamed about a baby, which led to a fantasy of saying to her angry baby, "It's all right, I still love you."

In hindsight, looking at the timing of the emergence of the beating fantasy in the child sample and the follow-up data, it becomes apparent that some of the cases in the original group were terminated prematurely. The very achievements which contributed to the capacity for fantasy formation obscured the continued operation of masochistic pathology encapsulated in the beating fantasy. This attempt at a solution to needs from all levels of development could not stand up to the internal and external demands of life. Thus, indications for termination should be carefully scrutinized in these patients.

CONCLUSIONS

In elucidating a developmental line of masochism we have been working toward a definition of the term. Valenstein (Panel, 1981) noted that a discussion of masochism can easily "be obscured in a sea of words" (p. 674). Grossman (1986) surveyed the history of the concept and concluded that the term has only a restricted application. Maleson (1984) presents a broad definitional possibility which accepts existing usage and refers to all behavior, thoughts, fantasies, and symptoms or syndromes characterized by subjectively experienced pain or suffering which seems unnecessary, excessive, or self-induced. Unfortunately, this definition demands a judgment as to what is unnecessary or excessive pain. It also leads to the view that the choice of any experience or activity which may include pain, such as childbirth or self-sacrifice, is necessarily masochistic. We do not find any necessary relationship between feminine functions and masochism.

In addition to being too inclusive, this definition ignores the significant difference between a normal and a masochistic relationship to pain. For adaptive growth, a child must learn to tolerate pain within a certain range. Paradoxically, masochists who actively seek painful and humiliating experiences find ordinary levels of real pain intolerable.

But Maleson also suggests a narrow definition which would confine the label to states of physical or mental suffering in which a clear linkage to sexual, genital excitement is demonstrable. The experience of pain or suffering does not in itself warrant a conclusion that the behavior is masochistic, nor does the existence of genital excitement. We think it is possible, based on the work we have described in this paper, to come to a more satisfactory definition. Masochism is the active pursuit of psychic or physical pain, suffering, or humiliation in the service of adaptation, defense, and instinctual gratification at oral, anal, and phallic levels.

Masochism is a clinical concept, and the definition requires some concrete observational referents to be of any value. We are suggesting that the data base of the definition is the transference and counterreaction of the analytic situation. The patient's persistent search for pain or humiliation will be figured forth in the transference, often in subtle responses to interpretations. The counterreaction of the therapist may provide the first clue of an underlying masochistic fantasy in the patient. The therapist may feel the impulse to be sarcastic, impatient, or teasing. Less subtle reactions may take the form of being late, forgetting appointments, falling asleep, forced termination, etc. The epigenetic layering of masochism and its multiple functions emerge within the transference relationship, and must be dealt with in that context.

There has long been controversy over whether the determinants of masochism are preoedipal or oedipal, and whether the underlying conflicts primarily concern drive gratification or relate to maladaptive modes of coping with traumatic objects. These were questions posed in the 1984 Panel on masochism and depression. By examining the development of beating fantasies in particular, we have tried to throw light on the determinants of masochism in general. In our view, not only are derivatives of each phase discernible in masochism, but the pain-seeking behavior which starts in infancy alters and is altered by each subsequent phase, including the oedipal and postoedipal. Postoedipally, masochistic impulses are organized as conscious or unconscious fantasies which are fixed, resistant to modification by experience or analysis, serve multiple ego functions, and take the form, although not necessarily the content, of the beating fantasy. In the fantasies the subject is an innocent victim, who achieves through suffering reunion with the object, defense against aggressive destruction and loss of the object, avoidance of narcissistic pain, and instinctual gratification by fantasy participation in the oedipal situation. Suicidal pathology, masochistic perversions, certain forms of hypochondriasis and psychosomatic illness, and moral masochism have in common an _underlying fantasy structure_. In our view, this fantasy structure is the "essence of masochism" (Freud, 1919, p. 189).

BIBLIOGRAPHY

ABELIN, E. C. (1975). Some further observations and comments on the earliest role of the father. *Int. J. Psychoanal.*, 56:293–302.

––––– (1980). Triangulation, the role of the father and the origins of core gender identity during the rapprochement subphase. In *Rapprochement*, ed., R. F. Lux, S. Bach, & J. A. Burland. New York: Jason Aronson, pp. 151–169.

BAK, R. C. (1968). The phallic woman. *Psychoanal. Study Child*, 23:37–46.

BALINT, M. (1968). *The Basic Fault*. London: Tavistock Publications.

BERGMANN, M. & HARTMAN, F. R. (1976). *The Evolution of Psychoanalytic Technique*. New York: Basic Books.

BIEBER, I. (1966). Sadism and masochism. In *American Handbook of Psychiatry*, ed. S. Arieti. New York: Basic Books, pp. 256–270.

BLOS, P., JR. (1985). Intergenerational separation-individuation. *Psychoanal. Study Child*, 40:41–56.

BLUM, H. P. (1974). The borderline childhood of the Wolf-Man. *J. Amer. Psychoanal. Assn.*, 22:721–742.

BRINICH, P. M. (1984). Aggression in early childhood. *Psychoanal. Study Child*, 39:493–508.

CAIN, A. C. (1961). The presuperego "turning inward of aggression." *Psychoanal. Q.*, 30:171–208.

ESCALONA, S. K. (1968). *The Roots of Individuality*. London: Tavistock Publications.

FENICHEL, O. (1945). *The Psychoanalytic Theory of Neurosis*. New York: Norton.

FERBER, L. (1975). Beating fantasies. In *Masturbation from Infancy to Senescence*, ed. I. M. Marcus & J. J. Francis. New York: Int. Univ. Press, pp. 205–222.

FREUD, A. (1960). The child guidance clinic as a center of prophylaxis and enlightenment. *W.*, 5:281–300.

FREUD, S. (1905). Three essays on the theory of sexuality. *S.E.*, 7:125–243.

––––– (1915). Instincts and their vicissitudes. *S.E.*, 14:109–140.

––––– (1918). From the history of an infantile neurosis. *S.E.*, 17:3–123.

––––– (1919). 'A child is being beaten.' *S.E.*, 17:175–204.

––––– (1923). The ego and the id. *S.E.*, 19:3–66.

––––– (1924). The economic problem of masochism. *S.E.*, 19:157–170.

––––– (1940). An outline of psycho-analysis. *S.E.*, 23:141–207.

FURMAN, E. (1984). Some difficulties in assessing depression and suicide in childhood. In *Suicide in the Young*, ed. H. S. Sudak, A. B. Ford, & N. B. Rushforth. Boston: John Wright, pp. 245–258.

––––– (1985). On fusion, integration, and feeling good. *Psychoanal. Study Child*, 40:81–110.

FURMAN, R. (1986). The father-child relationship. In *What Nursery School Teachers Ask Us About*, ed. E. Furman. New York: Int. Univ. Press, pp. 21–34.

GLENN, J. (1984). A note on loss, pain and masochism in children. *J. Amer. Psychoanal. Assn.*, 32:63–73.

GROSSMAN, W. I. (1986). Notes on masochism. *Psychoanal. Q.*, 55:379–413.

LAMB, M. E. (1976). The role of the father. In *The Role of the Father in Child Development*, ed. M. E. Lamb. New York: John Wiley, pp. 1–63.

LICHTENBERG, J. (1984). Continuities and transformations between infancy and adolescence. In *Late Adolescence*, ed. D. D. Brockman. New York: Int. Univ. Press, pp. 7–27.

LITMAN, R. E. (1970). Sigmund Freud on suicide. In *The Psychology of Suicide*. New York: Jason Aronson, pp. 555–586.

LOEWENSTEIN, R. M. (1957). A contribution to the psychoanalytic theory of masochism. *J. Amer. Psychoanal. Assn.*, 5:197–234.

MALESON, F. G. (1984). The multiple meanings of masochism in psychoanalytic discourse. *J. Amer. Psychoanal. Assn.*, 32:325–356.

NIEDERLAND, W. G. (1958). Early auditory experiences, beating fantasies, and primal scene. *Psychoanal. Study Child*, 13:471–504.

NOVICK, J. (1980). Negative therapeutic motivation and negative therapeutic alliance. *Psychoanal. Study Child*, 35:299–320.

_____ (1984). Attempted suicide in adolescence. In *Suicide in the Young*, ed. H. S. Sudak, A. B. Ford, & N. B. Rushforth. Boston: John Wright, pp. 115–137.

_____ & NOVICK, K. K. (1972). Beating fantasies in children. *Int. J. Psychoanal.*, 53:237–242.

OLINICK, S. L. (1964). The negative therapeutic reaction. *Int. J. Psychoanal.*, 45:540–545.

ORGEL, S. (1974). Fusion with the victim and suicide. *Int. J. Psychoanal.*, 55:532–538.

PANEL (1981). Masochism: current concepts. N. Fischer, reporter. *J. Amer. Psychoanal. Assn.*, 29:673–688.

_____ (1984). The relation between masochism and depression. J. Caston, reporter. *J. Amer. Psychoanal. Assn.*, 32:603–614.

RUBINFINE, D. L. (1965). On beating fantasies. *Int. J. Psychoanal.*, 46:315–322.

SANDLER, J. & ROSENBLATT, B. (1962). The concept of the representational world. *Psychoanal. Study Child*, 17:128–145.

STERN, D. W. (1985). *The Interpersonal World of the Infant*. New York: Basic Books.

TRONICK, E. Z. & GIANINO, A. (1986). Interactive mismatch and repair. *Zero to Three*, 6:1–6.

WINNICOTT, D. W. (1960). The theory of the parent-infant relationship. In *The Maturational Processes and the Facilitating Environment*. New York: Int. Univ. Press, 1965, pp. 37–55.

Denial of Physical Illness in Adolescence
Collaboration of Patient, Family, and Physicians

LYNN WHISNANT REISER, M.D.

DENIAL PRESENTS A SPECIAL PROBLEM WHEN A PHYSICAL ILLNESS occurs along with other psychological or behavioral signs or symptoms.[1] In these cases a patient may emphasize a psychiatric disorder to defend against the anxiety of confronting the physical illness. When this denial is supported by those around the patient, in particular family and physicians, the patient's self-assertions are legitimized and possible physical causes further negated.

This is a case study of a 19-year-old college student (referred to here as Ann) who presented with an atypical eating disorder—but subsequently was found to have an intradural extra-medullary dorsal meningioma at T4. The patient first sought medical help 3 months after the onset of her eating disorder. Although she was evaluated medically and psychiatrically numerous times, her tumor was not diagnosed until 1½ years later when it had progressed almost to the point of total obstruction. The meningioma was removed; remission of symptoms both of the tumor and of anorexia nervosa followed.

Associate clinical professor, Department of Psychiatry, Yale University School of Medicine, New Haven, Conn.

1. Though puzzling, denial of serious physical illness is not uncommon. Its frequency in everyday life is exemplified in the CPR course manual (Effron, 1985, p. 6): "It is extremely important to realize that the victim has a natural tendency to deny that he may be having a heart attack."

This patient offers a particularly dramatic example of the problem of denial and negation. Close examination is instructive in suggesting warnings for physicians treating patients with simultaneous physical/psychological complaints.

The case raises several important questions about denial of physical illness by the patient, family, and members of the medical community in the face of obvious physical signs, symptoms, and complaints.

1. How did several internists and neurologists manage to avoid an organic diagnosis of Ann's condition?

2. How and why was this lack of organic diagnosis reinforced by her parents?

3. How and why was the denial of the physical illness so intense and sustained in this patient herself?

4. Why did her psychiatrist initially accept the diagnosis of anorexia nervosa as sufficient?

CASE HISTORY

To "seek more academic opportunity" Ann transferred into a university in the city where I work and was referred to me as a case of anorexia nervosa by her hometown psychiatrist. When she arrived, her medical care was taken over by a local internist and a complete medical workup was performed. The impression was "anorexia nervosa, probable hysterical gait disturbance— R/O atypical hypothyroidism." I began work with her with a diagnosis from her referring psychiatrist which had already been confirmed by several internists. She would give ample evidence of psychological distress.

Ann began psychotherapy with me in February. She had sought psychiatric treatment as a "last resort." Twice-a-week meetings were scheduled, but at first she frequently forgot or canceled sessions so that we met only 15 times between February and late April. These few sporadic meetings turned out to be more of an extended evaluation than a treatment. Still, these psychoanalytically informed interviews uncovered material which had been previously denied and unreported and so had been unavailable.

Ann's appearance was striking. Blond and attractive, she had grey eyes and an expressive mouth. Speaking like an actress and gesturing dramatically, she presented herself in a bold and vivid way. She dressed eccentrically, covering her emaciated body in voluminous but drab-colored clothing.

Ann was preoccupied with her "fat" bloated abdomen, disturbed bowel function, especially constipation; and pain in her arms and legs. She spent much of the time of her first visits with me expressing vague distress and sobbing. Only after my urging and persistent encouragement did she describe her life situation, history, and specific feelings.

A typical response (in answer to my question "When did your legs last feel strong?") consisted of Ann describing an incident at length: At home for Christmas break a year ago during her first semester, she decided to go jogging with her mother—this in spite of the fact that "Jogging is Mother's special time to be alone." Although her mother continued to jog at her usual steady rate, Ann felt compelled to race with her. "I hate to run, but in gym I always have to be first!" Ann dashed away. Arriving home, Mother found father and daughter enjoying a special Sunday breakfast that Ann had cooked. Ann's answer when I had attempted to focus on her physical state seemed to offer the symbolic meaning of the symptom, namely, that her leg weakness was related to competitive feelings with her mother.

For years, Ann had taken pride in always having a "flat tummy" no matter how chubby she had been. She was now distraught that she had failed to flatten her abdomen despite dieting. She reported that she weighed herself often, but she was unable to lose more weight.

In early March, she went home for spring break. On her return she noted that one of her adolescent sisters had developed an eating disorder. Her own symptoms had worsened markedly. She was particularly upset by edema in her legs, which felt weak and painful, and by her bowel dysfunction. Of her own accord she decided to stop her laxative and enema abuse and to follow the regimen suggested by her internist. She began to eat more regularly and to take vitamins. Having made this concession, after a few weeks she became even more alarmed when she failed to improve. I too was becoming increasingly uneasy as her physical condition worsened.

Initially I had asked that reports of her previous medical workups be sent to me; finally, I telephoned the pediatric neurologist who had evaluated Ann that past fall. He assured me that Ann did not have a neurological problem except as secondary to anorexia nervosa and that he was confident that Ann's problem was psychological. He described to me his own close relationship with Ann's family and asked me not to judge them too harshly or to blame them for her disorder. He characterized them as "basically caring parents who did the best they could."

I also had been in frequent telephone contact with the internist who was now seeing Ann monthly. She too viewed Ann as primarily psychologically impaired. For treatment she relied on reassurance and symptomatic interventions.

I began to augment my own understanding of her unusual constellation of symptoms by researching my medical texts about neurological conditions related to starvation—such as Beriberi. None fit Ann's case.

Ann now attended sessions more regularly and suddenly seemed determined to be a "good psychotherapy patient." While therapy sessions had previously been filled with sobs, cries for help, and dramatic expressions of desperation, she now focused on her efforts to control her appetite and to lose weight, or her "fat stomach" and her sense of worthlessness and self-hatred. She also became both explicit and revealing of her feelings and gave details of personal history.

Moreover, in these therapy sessions she also brought in dreams and new memories and was desperately eager to discuss them. Significantly, it was through associations to the dreams and memories that she revealed new details of her physical condition. For the first time she confessed she had been experiencing fecal incontinence beginning the previous September. She now described her incontinence vividly with bitterness and self-hatred in her voice, "I lost 'it' [her feces] on the way to the bathroom—I would force myself to pick it up with my bare hands—the bathroom is where I deserve to be." Punishing herself for lack of control and keeping her problem secret, sometimes she would continue to sit in the library covered with feces hidden under her coat. (Thus she repeatedly and dramatically emphasized her feelings rather than her physical condition.) This fecal incontinence had not been included in her medical reports. She had explained that she felt ashamed to complain of her incontinence to her physicians. Ann explained this loss of control by her abuse of laxatives. Soon afterward, during another of these sessions (late March), she revealed her history of urinary incontinence. In response to this new piece of medical history, I became more suspicious that there must be a primary neurological disorder, in addition to the anorexia nervosa and its side effects.

The way she presented this new key symptom was instructive. That particular day she had walked into my office for her session dripping wet, apologizing profusely and offering abjectly to stand or to sit on a newspaper. At last she sat down and explained that, walking with great effort to the office, she had felt an uncontrollable urge to urinate. She decided not to go to a nearby house to ask to use the bathroom or to squat in the street— instead she wet herself. She had spent the minutes prior to the session in the bathroom adjoining the waiting room washing herself and all her clothes. She embellished her account with a detailed and dramatic rendition of her fear of embarrassing me by intruding on my neighbors, or of spoiling my furniture, and ended it declaring how dirty and smelly she felt. I was puzzled by her appearance and explanation. I expressed this feeling and in the context of reacting to my puzzlement, she offered more history—the circumstances of her first menstrual period and a memory from her first grade in school of having to put up her hand to ask for permission to go to the bathroom and on one occasion having wet her pants when her raised hand was not recognized by the teacher.

She then stated (in answer to my question) that the first time she wet herself as an adult was in the beginning of her second year of college (about 6 months before we began work). A middle-aged, rather shy, and ineffectual professor had invited her to come to his apartment to work on a report. She was surprised to find herself the guest of honor at a romantic dinner. He asked her to come with him on vacation and to meet his parents. She turned down his proposal, but on the way home alone, filled with feelings about the "encounter," she found herself urgently needing to urinate and did so in the street under her cloak. She felt publicly embarrassed, humiliated, and ashamed.

Through her recounted associations, which also contained and elaborated the meaning of the symptom for her, Ann gave a history of increasingly severe urinary incontinence which led me to suspect that difficulties with bowel control must be due to loss of anal sphincter tone rather than dietary and laxative abuse. I began to suggest more medical workups; she countered with more elaborate and suggestive psychodynamic material.

In the session after she revealed her urinary incontinence, she reported dreaming that she had been shot by her sister and had blood pouring out of the holes in her chest and abdomen. The blood was both like menstrual blood and like urine pouring out uncontrollably. She remarked that she had had a "heavy menstrual flow like her mother," and severe menstrual cramps. She remembered in the dream she had been waiting to die and had asked, "When is the last sharp pain that comes before death?" Ann commented that she had not gotten her period for a year and a half and declared, "When I get it back, it will mean I'm all well. I don't want to get it now because I don't want things to go on like this."

Ann also stressed how regular and predictable her periods had been—declaring that she could tell the day before, then 15 minutes before exactly when the flow would begin. She contrasted this sense of control with her fear of being out of control of her first period. "I was in a new school the first week, I went to the bathroom just before cheerleader tryouts. A smart, prissy girl was in the next booth. I cried out, 'OH SHIT, I just got my period for the first time!!' I stuffed toilet paper in my panties and went to try out, worried that, when I did the splits, blood would be on the floor, but it was okay, I made cheerleader." This memory is of an earlier time when Ann was able to continue functioning at a high level despite physical discomfort and anxiety about bodily functions. It would be reassuring if her incontinence were something like menstruation over which she could gain a sense of control.

In associating to the thoughts of death in the dream, Ann

declared she would commit suicide if she knew she would never walk or dance easily again.

Ann remembered first missing her very predictable period under the stress of preparing to move again—to leave home for college. When the time to leave approached, Ann's period was late and she thought she was pregnant. She confided this to her mother and they "worried together." She got her period in the car on the day her father dropped her off at college, the afternoon she vowed to lose weight. Thus over and over, Ann explained the meaning to her of particular bodily functions, focusing on her lifelong struggle to control her body. Recounting these memories she attempted to convince herself (and me) that her current problem was no different.

Although Ann expressed memories and feelings she connected with her symptoms, this did not alleviate her symptoms and indeed they continued to get worse.

Since her return from spring vacation I had persistently suggested that she be hospitalized for further evaluation of her physical condition. She still clung to a conviction that all of these problems were psychological in origin but finally yielded to my suggestion. She insisted on finishing her exams first. Before they would agree to the hospitalization, her parents requested that I explain my rationale to their internist. Ann, her parents, and their medical consultants remained convinced that her problems were psychological. They consented to hospitalization on a psychiatric unit.

In early May, Ann entered a psychiatric evaluation unit. Neurological findings indicated a need for a myelogram. At this point her parents and their physicians back home telephoned the unit chief to object, questioning the usefulness of subjecting Ann to this painful and invasive test. However, subsequently consent was given and the myelogram showed a mass at T4. Surgery the next day revealed a benign, slow-growing tumor of a type of spinal cord meningioma which may well have been present for as long as 9 to 10 years. The tumor had recently reached the point of near total compression of the cord. This accounted for the exacerbation of Ann's symptoms during the spring.

Ann recovered rapidly after the surgery. A year later the only residual from the surgery was a numb area around the scar. Her eating disorder disappeared. She gained 50 pounds over the year, back to her weight in high school. Her menstrual periods started the following January. She returned to college and did well academically, although seeming less pressured. Ann did not return to psychotherapy. She could not bear to come back to my office; she feared she would have to face "it" all again and still felt unable to confront her memories and feelings. Two years later Ann referred a close friend to me for psychotherapy.

DISCUSSION

This case, while raising a number of questions, also suggests possible answers.

1. How could Ann's *physicians* have missed the diagnosis in the face of such obvious physical signs, symptoms, and complaints?

Ann had been under medical care since she first began to show signs of an eating disorder. She had been extensively worked up at two excellent medical centers by specialists in eating disorders, in addition to specialists in nutrition and a neurologist.

In May, a year before the tumor was diagnosed, because of her deteriorating physical condition, she had been evaluated at a university medical center by a specialist in internal medicine and nutrition. At that time he described:

> . . . a young woman with a history of a 45 pound weight loss over a six month period, amenorrhea for six to seven months, history of attempts of subterfuge with regard to eating, harsh self-imposed dietary restrictions, diarrhea, history of laxative abuse, binge eating and self-induced vomiting . . . emotional lability, compulsive overachieving, a feeling of being driven by her parents to be perfect. She complained of pain in her legs while walking and dancing and occasionally of falling.

On physical examination he noted lanugo hair and a trace of ankle edema. Diagnosis: anorexia nervosa.

The following November, she was referred to a pediatric neurologist, a close friend of the family, for evaluation of weakness in her legs. The neurologist's diagnostic impression was "non-specific weakness—a part of her general asthenia."

Reading the history, a diagnosis of physical illness seems apparent. Why did it take so long to establish?

For one thing, Ann's history was very consistent with the diagnosis of anorexia nervosa. Let us review her clinical course with this in mind.

Ann described herself as always healthy. During high school her physical health seemed robust. She exercised and practiced dancing relentlessly, valuing "gracefulness" above all, and she indeed did become an excellent dancer. She was an attractive girl and had taken great care in her grooming. Although she felt overweight (weight 145 pounds, height 5'6"), she was in such good physical shape that "no one noticed." She did not diet.

On the day her father dropped her off at college for the first time, she abruptly vowed to be thin and began to diet rigorously (remember that she was worried about being pregnant at that time). She then weighed 155 pounds. She lost weight rapidly and in November her menstrual periods stopped. She became increasingly isolated and focused on getting good grades, losing weight, and exercising, particularly dancing. By that Christmas vacation she had lost about 45 pounds. Her parents were concerned, for the first time, wondering if she was becoming anorectic.

Meanwhile, Ann experienced increasing weakness in her ankles and lower legs. By February of her freshman year she was unable to dance in a recital. By March of that year, midway through the second semester when she "felt her body was out of control," she cut her nails short and began to wear dark and voluminous concealing clothes.

Her parents increasingly worried about her rapid weight loss and her preoccupation with being fat. They were now convinced she had anorexia nervosa. At their insistent urging, she consulted two specialists in eating disorders before returning to her mother's therapist for once-a-week treatment. She commuted to her hometown to meet with him on and off for the year. She used these sessions to express emotion, silently sobbing or crying about her sense of isolation and despair.

Her school performance continued to be excellent. She majored in dance. In the second semester she took a psychology course and received honors for her research paper on anorexia nervosa.

She was referred in May to a specialist in internal medicine and nutrition (see above). He advised behavioral modification techniques to promote weight gain. That summer she began to binge eat and gained weight (from 78 pounds up to 110 pounds). She concurrently developed edema in her legs which she believed was related to the rapid weight gain.

Her internist noted that when he saw her the following October, her weight was 110 pounds; she was eating very little and felt pessimistic about the future, a clinical presentation in many ways compatible with the diagnosis of anorexia nervosa.

Furthermore, in addition to the obvious eating disorder, the physical syndrome associated with benign thoracic spinal meningioma is one which is often missed. A more detailed discussion of the medical difficulty with diagnosis and, in particular, the surprising coincidence of symptoms of anorexia nervosa and spinal cord meningioma is included in an earlier paper (Reiser and Swigar, 1984).

In this case, there are several other contributing factors. First was the diagnosis of "hysteria" suggested by several of her physicians. Here too she is typical of patients with spinal cord meningioma (Epstein et al., 1971). Her behavior suggested the *belle indifference* of the hysteric; for example, as her ability to walk was increasingly impaired, she still preferred to call out to passersby for help when she fell rather than use a cane or walker, or avoid walking long distances. Although she complained of feeling humiliated, she publicly and dramatically wept and moaned aloud with pain.

During our last session she commented matter-of-factly—and with a note of satisfaction as she manually lifted one leg over the other to settle herself into the chair—that she could now much better understand how to portray a crippled person. She conveyed uncertainty: was she even at that moment acting or experiencing physical difficulty?

Ann met all the criteria for a diagnosis "hysteria" as outlined by Murphy (1982). (She, of course, also met the *DMS III* diagnostic criteria for 'atypical eating disorder.") Murphy stresses the importance of not continuing redundant medical evaluation in the hysteric but in pursuing psychological therapy instead. This approach, of course, must have contributed to the action of Ann's internists and neurologists: they had a diagnosis (of hysteria and atypical eating disorder) and so turned her over to the psychiatrist.

Since Ann used her symptoms to demand special treatment, this secondary gain from her symptoms helped raise doubts about her actual disability. I myself spoke with her college Dean in order to verify her need for a first-floor room, one usually reserved for students with upper-class standing. (The Dean's demand that she "prove her inability to climb stairs" was in itself remarkable.)

An additional contributing factor for Ann surely was her "VIP status" which often leads to treatment failure. Weintraub (1964) noted several characteristics of what he termed "VIP status." This included either the patient being a prominent person or having a close relative who held status: Ann's father was a well-respected member of the academic community; and Ann's mother was a lawyer with an important political post.

Also important in Weintraub's description was the need of the patient or her family for the patient to be special (this certainly fits Ann's case) and the ability to bring pressure to bear for favored treatment (Ann's parents were personal friends of a number of prominent physicians).

Ann qualified as a VIP patient. Even the mode of referral to me exemplifies this. Before I met with Ann her family physician called me several times to describe her case in detail and to verify that I would see her immediately. He seemed eager to make certain that I would understand Ann and care for her properly. This, and the tone of the later calls from the other physicians who had treated her, emphasized Ann's specialness. Like other VIPs, Ann refused hospitalization except on her terms.

Certainly the attempts of her parents and their physician friends to obtain special treatment for Ann in the hospital are classic examples of VIP status serving to hinder rather than help treatment.

2. It is also puzzling how and why *her parents* were able to

deny or negate so persistently the physical components of her pathology. Without more extensive/intensive interviews with them it is impossible to do more than speculate.

I obtained the family history, much of it during the hospitalization, from Ann herself, Ann's family psychiatrist, and the hospital social worker who interviewed Ann's parents.

I met Ann's parents for the first and only time in the hospital cafeteria where they awaited the outcome of her surgery. Underscoring their reaction to my having suggested a physical basis for Ann's problems as miraculous was their response to my having recognized them as Ann's parents. They were overcome with wonder, even though I told them the nurses had given me a clear description of them.

An important factor in her parents' need to deny Ann's physical illness may have been her role in the family. Ann was the oldest of many siblings, a much wanted child. She had been "the perfect child." Her parents were intensely proud and possessive of her. Both parents viewed Ann as "special." They repeatedly described her as "creative, brilliant, dramatic, and beautiful." She was an A+ student and a leader at school and at home. In particular her father seems to have "glorified" her—he viewed her as "like him in every way."

It must have been difficult for either parent to acknowledge that there could be something seriously wrong with Ann. This attitude would facilitate their accepting the physicians' reassurances of psychological rather than physical impairment. Anorexia nervosa was a familiar, acceptable syndrome with treatment available.

3. Ann herself contributed to the difficulty in sorting out her diagnosis by her own inability to focus on her physical symptoms. Ann's tumor was characteristically a slow-growing one which may have been present for as long as 9 to 10 years. Its onset thus may date as far back as the time of her family's move when she was 12. She had difficulty in adjusting to this move and to the beginning of adolescence.

Ann had been a healthy "model" child without behavior problems. Ann's family moved every year until she was 6, but then lived in the same town until she was 12, when they moved to a new city. Ann resented the moves, had difficulty making friends and getting established in the new school. Her parents noted that she was "briefly unhappy." She also reached puberty around this time. Ann described herself as having been a fat child and a chubby young adolescent, teased and tormented about her weight.

Ann experienced the effects of the tumor as symbolically related to the physical changes of puberty, particularly menstruation. For example, just before beginning treatment with me, at an anniversary party given by Ann and her siblings for their parents, she decided to wear the special beautiful gown her mother bought her for the occasion. This was the first time in about 10 months she had "dressed up." She also took a laxative and during the party lost control of her bowels. To hide this, she collapsed on the floor in front of mother's best friend. When the friend expressed concern, Ann told her not to worry, that she'd just gotten her period. By this time Ann had not had a period for over a year.

The need to deal simultaneously with bodily changes of adolescence and subtle, but gradually worsening effects of the tumor led to a kind of psychological adaptation particular to a girl with Ann's natural endowment and in this culture.

Anorexia nervosa has been described as a response to sexual maturity and the related changes in the body—the patient struggling with her own body to control these changes, and to externalize the struggle. Bruch (1973) especially emphasized that patients with anorexia nervosa were out of touch with their own bodies and hypothesized that they never learned to monitor and understand feelings of hunger, satiety, etc. One might speculate that for Ann loss of control of her body with the progressive encroachment of the tumor—perhaps beginning coincidently with the changes of puberty—represented both punishment for forbidden oedipal strivings and at the same time an opportunity for continued childlike closeness and intimate involvement with both parents. Whether or not the tumor was already present at puberty, certainly in Ann's mind the two were related, expressed in her feelings about control and loss of control of body fluids, particularly menstrual blood.

Did the psychological stressors (move to a new school, breaking up with a boyfriend, leaving home for college, etc.) precipitate and exacerbate the physiological events—or did Ann, sensing the progressive loss of control of her body, utilize the psychologically meaningful events to express her awareness of her internal state and the symbolic meaning to her of her progressive loss of function?

On a deeper level Ann seemed to experience her physical symptoms metaphorically as punishments for forbidden wishes. Oedipal issues and conflicts were evident in her memories of racing with her mother and the story of the professor's invitation to dinner, with each victory followed by a punishment—loss of physical function. In a dream she associated the pain of the tumor with being shot and with menstrual blood. These sexualized images linked her fantasy of punishment for sexual wishes with her progressive physical disability. She seemed to justify her increasing pain as deserved punishment and thus used her real illness masochistically. Her eating disorder might be understood as compensation/justification for the punishment (progressive loss of motor and sensory function and pain) that she was experiencing.

Certainly her subsequent structuring of her life can be viewed as an effort to express, compensate for, and deny an awareness of increasing disability and sense of loss of control.

First athletic prowess and especially talent for dancing, which demanded strength in her legs and a sense of position of her body in space, were particularly suited to helping Ann learn to control her body, thus compensating for progressive loss of proprioception (with altered sensation from her nipples down) and altered vibration sense. This might be viewed as an overcompensation (Castelnuovo-Tedesco, 1981) which enabled her to tolerate/deny the defect.

Later, Ann's research in the widespread and available literature about anorexia nervosa and bulimia provided her with a "blueprint" for taming an unruly body and for expressing her need for others to help control her body. Knowledge of this syndrome may have combined with her acting talent to enable her to act like and be an anorectic in a very convincing way.

Ann achieved some sense of control by projecting her inner conflict outward—visible weight loss, refusal to eat, dramatic gait disturbance, symptoms which provoked people in the environment to reassure her by insisting that she could control her body. Frequent assurances from respected authorities, her parents and physicians, that there was nothing physically wrong, except when she was causing herself, served to exacerbate Ann's coping style. This resulted in her "feeling crazy" since her perception of the world was so different from what she was told. She presented herself in a bizarre, exhibitionistic, "crazy" way, wishing she could believe that her parents and doctors were right.

4. Finally, I wondered what kept me from recognizing immediately and clearly that Ann's distress had a physical etiology. At the first session, I had noticed that she moved awkwardly and often stumbled, lurching into the wall as she entered the office. Responding to her complaint about the long hill to my office and to her apparent difficulty, I observed that it would be possible to see a therapist closer to where she lived. She refused, saying, "No problem." In retrospect, my response, offering a practical solution rather than listening for the meaning of her statement, suggests that very early on I must have been uneasy about the nature of Ann's presentation but reluctant to pursue my observations.

First must have been my prior mind set: I had had several lengthy telephone conversations with her referring psychiatrist and was prepared to treat a patient with anorexia nervosa. Reinforcing this was my respect for medical authority: I knew that she had been extensively worked up in an excellent medical center and further that she had been examined and was being followed by an internist whose expertise I valued.

My current identification as a psychiatrist had led me to have some reluctance to step into other medical roles: had I gotten out my percussion hammer and done a neurological exam myself, the diagnosis might have been clarified sooner.

I think, however, I was more inclined to be tempted to join in the denial myself by several other factors. One was a wish for certainty—the relief at having a diagnosis of some sort and thus a plan for treatment rather than confronting the anxiety of seeing a patient deteriorate without a sufficient explanation. Not just Ann, but her parents, physicians, and I wished for a sense of control. Ann's presentation helped to encourage this. Paradoxically, Ann's exaggeration of her symptoms served to conceal them from her physicians and me. We repeatedly disregarded

the physical pathology hidden within the psychological embroi-
dery. Ann, an intelligent, sophisticated, well-read young woman, seemed to buttress the diagnosis of hysteria by offering a
psychological explanation for each deterioration in her physical
state. When she revealed another symptom in therapy, she embedded it in a meaningful symbolic context.

My own sense of helplessness as Ann's condition continued to
deteriorate also clouded the picture. I was aware of wishing that
someone else would help me out and that her internist would
find a cause and cure for her symptoms. Freud (1900) expressed
similar questions in his analysis of the dream of a patient, Irma,
who had consulted him, complaining of a number of physical
symptoms:

> *I was alarmed at the idea that I had missed an organic illness.* This
> . . . is a perpetual source of anxiety to a specialist whose practice
> is almost limited to neurotic patients and who is in the habit of
> attributing to hysteria a great number of symptoms which other
> physicians treat as organic. On the other hand, a faint doubt
> crept into my mind—from where, I could not tell—that my
> alarm was not entirely genuine. If Irma's pains had an organic
> basis, once again I could not be held responsible for curing
> them; my treatment only set out to get rid of *hysterical* pains. It
> occurred to me, in fact, that I was actually *wishing* that there had
> been a wrong diagnosis; for, if so, the blame for my lack of
> success would also have been got rid of [p. 109].

Like Freud, I felt concerned that I would be "passing the
buck." This too kept me from being more insistent earlier that
Ann's physical symptoms were not primarily psychological and
should be medically evaluated further.

CONCLUSION

A number of factors came together to make it especially difficult
to reach a correct diagnosis early in Ann's treatment: the kind of
tumor Ann had; her character structure which fit the diagnosis
of hysteria; her VIP status; the caring professionals' relationship
with her parents; her particular family history which sensitized
both parents to illness and loss; her role in the family as the
special child; and, in Ann herself, the coincidence of the tumor

with her adolescence; her use of overcompensation as a defense; and as part of this, her coincident eating disorder presenting many of the same symptoms and signs as the tumor.

However, even in such a complicated overdetermined case (and, in the end, what case isn't?), it is important to keep in mind several guidelines which may help to sort out the presence of an underlying physical illness from a primarily psychological disorder.

1. There must be a positive reason to make a psychological diagnosis. In Ann's case, there were criteria for hysteria and for anorexia nervosa, but they explained only some of her symptoms.

2. The psychiatrist must remain aware of his or her own medical knowledge about how syndromes present, rather than relying on other medical authority. It was the history of Ann's urinary incontinence that finally crystallized for me that there must be an underlying physical defect.

3. The patient's response to interpretation may help. Psychological symptoms "join in the dialogue" (Freud, 1918)—getting worse, better, or changing. Ann's symptoms—in spite of her understanding more about their history and meaning—continued to get worse.

4. A steady deterioration (not an occasional exacerbation) in the symptom picture (even more so if the deterioration is completely unrelated to interpretative interventions) is in itself significant.

5. Finally, it is essential to keep in mind the possibility that, contrary to the old medical adage "Occam's Razor" of attempting to find one syndrome to account for all the symptoms, the patient may have multiple illnesses. Ann, while rid of this physical impairment, may still carry psychological handicaps.

BIBLIOGRAPHY

BRUCH, H. (1973). *Eating Disorders.* New York: Basic Books.
CASTELNUOVO-TEDESCO, P. (1981). Psychological consequences of physical defect. *Int. Rev. Psychoanal.*, 8:145–154.
EFFRON, D. M. (1985). *Cardiopulmonary Resuscitation.* Tulsa: CPR Publishers.

EPSTEIN, B., EPSTEIN, J., & POSTEL, D. (1971). Tumors of the spinal cord simulating psychiatric disorders. *Dis. Nerv. Syst.,* 32:741–743.

FREUD, S. (1900). The interpretation of dreams. *S.E.,* 4 & 5.

_____ (1918). From the history of an infantile neurosis. *S.E.,* 17:3–123.

MURPHY, G. (1982). The clinical management of hysteria. *J. Amer. Med. Assn.,* 247:2559–2564.

REISER, L. W. & SWIGAR, M. (1984). Anorexia nervosa masking the diagnosis of spinal meningioma. *Gen. Hosp. Psychiat.,* 6:289–293.

WEINTRAUB, W. (1964). The VIP syndrome. *J. Nerv. Ment. Dis.,* 138:181–193.

Eating Her Words
Food Metaphor as Transitional Symptom in the Recovery of a Bulimic Patient

VICTORIA SHAHLY, M.A.

METAPHOR IS PURPORTEDLY CENTRAL TO BOTH THE EVOLUTION OF psychoanalytic theory (Edelson, 1983; Pederson-Krag, 1956) and the successful application of psychodynamic technique. While there is much philosophical debate regarding the legitimacy of metaphoric constructs in analytic theory formation (Edelson, 1983; Wurmser, 1977), the therapeutic efficacy of metaphor goes relatively unquestioned. Empirical validation of "metaphor-analysis" (Carveth, 1984) has been confined to unpublished doctoral dissertations, and even theoretical discussion of the subject is scarce (Billow, 1977; Carveth, 1984; Lenrow, 1966). Certainly, no study has documented the metaphoric process as it unfolds over the course of treatment. In this paper I attempt a brief overview of the literature on metaphor in the context of psychoanalysis and then more thoroughly examine the role of figurative language in the recovery process of a bulimic patient. I hypothesize that metaphor performs a particular function for patients with eating disorders and so provides an especially potent source of intervention.

Doctoral candidate in clinical psychology at University of California, Berkeley.

The preparation of this paper was supported by National Institutes of Health National Research Service Award MH17496 from the National Institute of Mental Health. I wish to thank Drs. Janet Adelman, Philip Cowan, Ravenna Helson, Sheldon Korchin, Georgine Marrott, Gerald Mendelsohn, and Abby Wolfson for helpful comments on an earlier version of this paper.

THEORETICAL AND CLINICAL OBSERVATIONS

The first detailed psychoanalytic account of metaphor was provided by Sharpe (1940), an ex-teacher of English literature. In her classic paper, she maintained that "A subterranean passage between mind and body underlies all analogy" (p. 156). Sharpe related the achievement of sphincter and urethral control to the contemporaneous acquisition of speech; physical discharge is substituted with linguistic discharge and "words themselves become the very substitutes for the bodily substances" (p. 157). Speech itself is then conceived as a metaphor, and metaphoric utterances are elevated to the status of an "ultimate speech" which directly connects present affective states with archaic psychophysical experience. The patient's spontaneously produced metaphors—although perhaps adopted from colloquial language—reveal much about the earliest incorporated environment, pregenital and oedipal development, and habitual level of instinctual tension; they are the "epitome of a forgotten experience" (p. 168). Sharpe reported that comments such as "I've wandered off the point and can't find it again" and "I'm glad you don't ram psycho-analytical theory down my throat" recall actual suckling experiences which were incorporated into the psychological constitution of the speaker. The analyst may solicit further associations to the metaphor or, preferably, interpret it.

Arlow (1979) argued that by listing sets of metaphors with universally constant meanings, Sharpe has separated them "from their dynamic context, with the end result that specific metaphorical expressions came to take on a uniform, standardized meaning with basic Kleinian concepts. . . . Thus, instead of expanding communication by way of metaphor, she contracted the metaphor into standardized, dictionary-type significations" (p. 370). Although Arlow proposes a more idiosyncratic interpretive approach, Carveth (1984) noted that he too was guilty of reaching conclusions uninformed by the patient's associations.

While Sharpe promoted metaphor as a means of understanding the repressed conflicts of neurotics, the next two decades of research focused instead on its potential for communicating with and treating severely disturbed patients. Ekstein and Wallerstein (1957) described the difficulties of working with borderline and psychotic children: fluctuations in ego states and primitive transferences and communication modes conspire to disrupt traditional therapeutic planning and technique. The "symbolic act as interpretation" was offered as a means of communicating with children who could not comprehend secondary process language. Later, Caruth and Ekstein (1966) presented a more formalized view of "interpretation within the metaphor"; what amounted earlier to an impulsive and intuitive physical gesture has here evolved into an essential "self-conscious, rational therapeutic technique" (p. 35). They maintain,

> The metaphor utilizes the primary-process material, manipulates it, as it were, but does not translate it or lift its meaning into the language of secondary process. The metaphor may be of particular value with the patient who is beginning to decathect any discourse which requires adaptation to reality. Like the dream, the metaphor enables the patient to maintain the necessary distance from content with the feeling that the meaning of the dream metaphor is ego-dystonic and not meant by him "really." Only gradually is the meaning accepted as part of the inner reality . . . the metaphor simultaneously maintains discontinuity by not forcing the conflict into direct consciousness, and yet, paradoxically, creates greater continuity by permitting insights that can be tolerated from the increased psychic distance which the metaphor facilitates [p. 36].

Caruth and Ekstein recommended that the therapist "use" only the patient's own spontaneously produced metaphors and observed that fluctuations in the patient's metaphoric competence were diagnostic of changes in ego function. A normal or neurotic individual may consciously select metaphors as a vicarious means of communicating surpressed content, "of simultaneously keeping and revealing a secret" (p. 38), or of saying something without actually saying it. The regressed borderline or schizophrenic patient becomes unable to differentiate between symbol and the object symbolized: "The 'as-if' quality of the more abstract meaning of the metaphor is lost and it becomes an immediate concrete experience" (p. 38). For such patients, acting out then serves as an expressive "action metaphor" (Ekstein, 1961). The therapist may establish contact using a similar symbolic act and then follow it immediately with a verbal metaphoric communication which may forestall further regression.

Cain and Maupin (1961) acknowledged the utility of the technique but cautioned that its intriguing creative aspects may encourage therapists to prolong its use beyond the point therapeutically indicated and that "wild" or awkwardly phrased metaphoric interpretations may compound the child's difficulties. They further worried that interpretation within the metaphor may arouse the paranoid trends which are omnipresent in borderlines and schizophrenics and so may actually undermine the therapeutic alliance. Caruth and Ekstein (1966) responded that the correctly chosen metaphor reassures the incipient paranoid that he is genuinely understood and will not be "forced to reveal or deal with anything except that which he himself selects" (p. 41). They seem overoptimistic, however, regarding the therapist's infallibility.

Aleksandrowicz (1962) adapted the metaphoric technique for the treatment of an adult schizophrenic. Consistent with Ekstein and Wallerstein, he observed that for such patients "words mean action and thoughts fuse with reality. . . . The metaphoric displacement may serve for him as a substitute for the normal person's (and the neurotic's) separation of thought and action. . . . The therapist, by entering the semantic world of the patient, transforms his autistic language into a private language of two people" (p. 98). Aleksandrowicz, however, extended the technique of "interpretation within the metaphor" to "response within the metaphor." By shifting his emphasis from simple acceptance and reassurance to the metaphor's affective content and then to its defensive function, he reported that he was able gradually to alter his patient's symbolic capacity and strengthen her ego function.

Working with a less disturbed woman, Reider (1972) reported that responding to his patient's metaphors with those of his own manufacture rather than with direct interpretation, as Sharpe recommended, "lent a fortunate distance. Moreover, it gave the patient a choice among the multivalent meanings of the metaphor to use as she wished. I believe it was, *inter alia*, this freedom of choice, a freedom towards activity, which enabled her to break through the repression" (p. 469). Reider maintained that his unconscious choice of metaphor informed him further about the patient's psychodynamics and was useful in understanding his own countertransference.

Stating the perspective more strongly, Poland (1986) remarked that when the analyst "limits himself to the patient's words, he may make new connections, yet he seriously risks a mirroring that promotes a *folie à deux*. . . . When he modifies the patient's words, he suggests new possibilities of understanding" (p. 257).

Rather than utilize the patient's own figurative expressions or respond to them with those of his own, Lenrow (1966) suggested that the therapist spontaneously introduce his metaphors into the treatment. Such metaphors demonstrate the therapist's flexibility, simplify events in terms of a concrete schema, permit a tactful "half-playful, half-serious" discussion of sensitive issues, and transfer easily to new situations. Reviewing Lenrow's assertions, Fine et al. (1973) agreed that such metaphor usage facilitates constructive behavior change. In later work, Pollio et al. (1977) refined their position by adding that metaphor serves to approximate repressed conflicts until they become conscious and more directly communicable.

Perhaps the most conservative approach was delineated by Voth (1970) who observed that patients increase their metaphor use when the transference relationship is particularly intense. Although such metaphors are symptom-equivalents, they are especially amenable to interpretation because resistance is particularly low at these times. They are therefore unusually important and, unless focused analytic work is contraindicated, Voth recommended that the therapist "interrupt the patient's flow of associations and ask him to associate to what he has just said" (p. 601).

Rather than delineate specific treatment techniques, more recent work emphasizes the role of metaphor in the formation of empathy and insight. Olinick (1976, 1978) maintained that the patient's verbal or action metaphors derive from primary and secondary process sources and so may constitute the analyst's principal means for achieving empathic "trial identifications" and thus insight. Similarly, Arlow (1979) wrote that the analyst's ability to resonate or empathize with his patient's inherently ambiguous metaphors is crucial to successful treatment and that "psychoanalysis is essentially a metaphorical enterprise. The patient addresses the analyst metaphorically, the analyst listens and understands in a corresponding manner" (p. 373f.). Noting that metaphor literally means "to carry over," he asserted that transference neurosis represents the patient's metaphorical misapprehension of his relationship with the analyst. Shengold (1981) further stipulated that "Analysis can be conceived of as a concentration on the characteristic metaphors of a patient: what and how they connect; how they are coordinated; what prevents or arrests the connective flow; how metaphor can be used for defensive purposes: the need to evoke the patient's awareness and responsibility for his metaphors, and especially for the passions attached to, or contained in, them" (p. 302).

Both Olinick (1976, 1978) and Shengold (1981) identified metaphor as a transitional phenomenon in Winnicott's sense, i.e., as a mediator between inner and outer reality, self and other, childhood and adult experience. This integrative aspect of metaphor is presumed to benefit the disintegrating egos of troubled patients.

Several recent authors have focused on the therapeutic effect which accompanies the "de-literalization" of a symptom and its consequent expression via metaphoric discourse. Wright (1976) asserted that a symptom is an "abortive," preverbal metaphor, while true metaphor is a "paradigm of integration within the ego" (p. 98). The translation of symptom or enactment into "the universe of things said" and symbolized via metaphorization frees it of its self-destructive impulsive quality and leads to understanding (p. 100). Thus, although the actual technique is not elaborated, "The undoing of a symptom is in part the creation of *metaphor* from symptom" (p. 98). Similarly, Linden (1985) agreed that "it may be the aim of therapy to undo such phenomena [as acting out] by converting them to metaphors" (p. 398).

From a deconstructionist perspective, Carveth (1984) commented that "the neurotic's problem is *not* that his thinking is metaphorical but rather that he is *possessed by* his metaphor . . . ; that he is *used by* it rather than *using* it critically in his thinking and acting . . . psychoanalysis (as "metaphor-analysis") is an exercise in becoming conscious and self-critical in our employment of the metaphors . . . we live by" (p. 512).

Grubrich-Simitis (1984) specified the treatment goal of psychoanalytic work with children of Holocaust survivors as overcoming the "concretism" to which they are prone and restoring metaphoric competence. She theorized that through "the use of metaphor, aggressive drive impulses can find a compromise outlet, which does not really endanger subject or object, i.e., without anything literally destructive or perhaps murderous occurring . . . the capacity for metaphorization seems to be one of the most effective means at the ego's disposal in its battle to tame and regulate the drives" (p. 305f.).

Interestingly, these most current references to metaphor reiterate a general point made by Freud in 1914: that psychoanalytic treatment aims to "divert into the work of recollection any impulse which the patient wants to discharge in action" (p. 153).

EMPIRICAL RESEARCH

The empirical studies of metaphor use in psychotherapy are confined to recent doctoral dissertations, perhaps unpublished because of the unspectacular nature of the findings. In brief, major difficulties operationalizing metaphoric and literal utterances, empathy, insight, and therapeutic outcome conspired to yield inconsistent, questionable findings. Still, the studies roughly indicate that both the patient's own metaphors and therapist-generated metaphors facilitate the emergence of useful material and maximize interpretive possibilities. This latter finding implies that metaphor allows the therapist to exploit the "principle of multiple appeal" (Hartmann, 1951), i.e., simultaneously to access the multiple determinants of a given conflict. Gore's (1977) finding that creative metaphor use by patients either represented or reflected successful sublimation of impulses is consistent with the clinical observations of Wright (1976), Linden (1985), and Grubrich-Simitis (1984). Unfortunately, no study investigated the natural history of metaphor use throughout the therapeutic process.

410   *Victoria Shahly*

FIGURES AND FIGURATIVE LANGUAGE

"The ego is first and foremost a bodily ego"
Freud (1923, p. 26)

Several authors have addressed the fundamental relationship between body and figurative expression. Freud (1923) recognized that an artifact of ego development was a pervasive tendency to organize and describe experience metaphorically in somatic terms. Speaking of the function of judgment, he (1925) said, "Expressed in the language of the oldest—the oral—instinctual impulses, the judgement is: 'I should like to eat this', or 'I should like to spit it out'; . . . the original pleasure-ego wants to introject into itself everything that is good and to eject from itself everything that is bad" (p. 237). As discussed earlier, Sharpe (1940) also reported that early physical experience predated and conditioned later metaphysical expressions. Lewin (1971) suggested that the evolution of the ego from the primitive body ego itself entails a metaphorization of sorts and that the ego is therefore primarily a metaphoric structure. Accordingly, he reasoned that figures of speech originate in the body or body image.

More recently, Ritvo (1984) remarked:

> The body ego lends itself to the plastic representation of ideation and unconscious fantasy. The mental processes serving these transformations are rooted in the same human endowments and capacities which underlie symbolization and figurative expression. With the development of verbal language, figures of speech, e.g., metaphors, become possible, providing the psyche with a rich storehouse of potential imagery for the representation of psychic processes and contents. The earliest figures of speech use the body as metaphor [p. 450].

Ritvo further noted that as eating relates to the earliest experiences of gratification and frustration, it is often conscripted to express ambivalence regarding loving and hating, and aggression and fear of punishment. His psychoanalysis of several late adolescents with eating disorders revealed that

> Food, eating, and the body image were employed to an unusual degree in the concrete, symbolic, and metaphorical expressions

of ideation and unconscious fantasy. Curiously, they were all immersed in literary interests; several of them were gifted writers and poets, so that figurative, metaphorical expression played a large part in their daily lives [p. 455].

CASE PRESENTATION

I also observed a similar reliance on body- and food-related metaphor by a bulimic woman, a sometime poet whom I shall call Sarah. It is my contention, however, that such metaphor usage was not simply diagnostic of this patient's oral-dependent conflicts but was instrumental in her recovery.

Sarah was seen by me once weekly for 30 sessions of individual psychodynamic psychotherapy at a university outpatient clinic. Her treatment was unfortunately discontinued at the end of the academic year due to the clinic's closure. She was an attractive, well-groomed young woman of average weight who was separating from her third husband. Although she lived alone with her young son, she visited her parents almost daily; they had paid for her two previous brief psychotherapies and her son's private schooling. Acutely aware of her lack of college education, Sarah was a successful and articulate personnel manager whose hobbies tended toward intellectual pursuits such as going to the opera and writing poetry. Despite her obvious verbal fluency and familiarity with the lay literature on bulimia, she twice misspelled the syndrome "bullimia" on the intake information sheet, a slip which soon proved to have dynamic significance. Sarah was warm, witty, habitually apologetic, invariably prompt, and somewhat overcompliant. Her transference was of the oral, introjective sort described by Greenson (1967): she hungrily "drank in" my every word, constantly solicited "feedback," perceived silence as a desertion, and dreaded separations. Her presenting complaints were bulimia, of 1½ years duration, and chronic depression.

Although the bulimia proper had begun immediately after separating from her third husband, Sarah reported a preoccupation with food since adolescence. She described her father as an authoritative, perfectionistic, unemotional man, a "stick" whose career took him away from the family 6 months of every year. Her mother, a "loud Jewish American Princess," would "nurture herself" during his absence by constant "noshing." Upon the father's return, violent arguments would ensue between the parents regarding the mother's weight gain. The father frequently threatened to leave the family at which point the mother would "egg him on" or counter with a similar threat. Dinnertime was consequently a "constant battle," a situation which was compounded by Sarah's brother's refusal to "clean his plate"; the mother was remonstrated for eating too much, the brother for eating too little, and Sarah kept her plate and "my conscious clean" but never asked for seconds. In her family, people would literally "cry over spilled milk." She attributed her notion that to have a surplus of food was "criminal" to her mother's selfish overindulgence which threatened the family unity and to her father's penuriousness. Even more decisive, however, she claimed were her maternal uncle's concentration camp experiences: "I always felt guilty for having when others didn't. Mother was in the U.S. during a blackout; she waited it out on a bag of sugar. Now she always stocks up on food, just in case. I was constantly told how bad things were. I was lucky, had things easy when they had to suffer so. Holocaust stories were told to us constantly. My uncle lived through the camps. Mother wouldn't talk about it, would sugar coat it or shut it out. But my uncle would talk. . . . I thought of the bombs a lot."

Other inconsistencies permeated Sarah's family life. Her father was affectionate before she reached puberty, but opprobrious afterward. Attributing his discomfiture to her svelte figure, Sarah reported that she "almost" wanted to be fat. She recounted a trip to the beach with her family. She and her mother both wore shorts and Sarah was dismayed by the cellulite and varicosities on her mother's legs. Her father pointedly complimented Sarah on the thinness of her own legs and, although she never liked to be "second banana," she became acutely aware of her mother's hurt. Sarah felt "starved for affection" and also that she must "starve for" her father's affection, but coincidently felt that doing so would risk her mother's love. Sarah's mother was also consistently unpredictable. "One minute she'd be hugging me and the next minute she'd be screeching at me for something I couldn't anticipate." Such lability made Sarah grit her teeth to choke back her fury and "walk on eggshells."

Sarah's great fear of abandonment fueled her tireless efforts to be "especially good, a real good egg" so as not to precipitate further disruptions. As a child, she would very deliberately "suffer in silence, to eat it, so to speak." Even as an adult, whereas her family would figuratively explode at the dinner table, she would remain calm but later literally disgorge her food in private. After all, she could only "swallow" so much. She felt that she must "cushion" people from her anger, that she must not "blow up" or they would retaliate by firing or leaving her. Similarly, she must not display strong preferences, she must seem content with "life's leftovers." She must never impose her desires on others, "shove things down someone else's throat." To retain her family's sympathy and attention (especially important following her marital separation), she felt she must remain "fragile as an egg." And here we come to the meaning of "bullimia." Sarah suspected that she was really "as strong as a bull," that she was "bullish," a "bully"—in fact, a person manager. Fearing that her displays of anger would have irrevocable consequences, that "like Humpty-Dumpty" she would never be able to set things aright, she used bulimia to keep herself weak and exhausted. The illness prompted her parents' solicitude: they paid her therapy bills, inquired after her progress and well-being, and frequently relieved her of her maternal duties. Late in the therapy, Sarah concluded that bulimia kept her dependent on her parents or "spoon-fed." She was "fed up" with her "childish" behavior and earnestly wanted to change.

DISCUSSION

That Sarah relied heavily upon food- and body-related metaphors is apparent from this brief sketch. More informative, however, is the *sequence* in which the metaphors and bulimic symptoms manifested themselves during treatment. For brevity, only the oral-passive/aggressive determinants of her bulimia will be discussed in detail; oedipal and narcissistic contributions, although significant, will not be emphasized.

The first 4 weeks were marked by almost exclusively concrete references to bulimia. Sarah attributed her "disease" to a bio-chemical aberration and requested a trial of mipramine. She focused on the details of her caloric intake and her family's dietary habits. On several occasions, she reported that she was "always hungry," but did not relate this to inadequate affection or her feelings that she "should earn more money, have a better job. I can't be happy where I am." Emotional upsets were directly converted into somatic complaints (e.g., "I felt so bad I came home and threw up," and "Thinking of babies makes my stom-ach turn"), but this too was curiously dissociated from bulimia. Only once, during week 3, did Sarah allude to the possible psy-chodynamic significance of her compulsive eating behavior, say-ing, "I just stuffed my anger. I've been thinking just recently about how if I didn't 'stuff it' so often, I wouldn't have to stuff food." She binged and purged approximately five times weekly during this phase.

Weeks 5 through 7 were characterized by progressively exten-sive food/body metaphors. Although Sarah still maintained that her anger was hormonally conditioned and reported that an unpleasant movie made her "sick to her stomach," she also rec-ognized that she had a tendency "to blow things out of propor-tion" and noted that when she indulged herself in substitute gratifications, she "didn't need to binge." Her more psychologi-cal appraisal of her conflicts led to significant dysphoria: "I feel worse than I did before treatment. Then I was just *binging*. Now I'm *thinking* about these things instead. I *feel* such anger." Her bulimic episodes dropped to four and then to only three times a week.

During week 8, Sarah made no references to bulimia as a physiological entity and reported no somatic conversions. Rather, she achieved the major insight that "deep down I sus-pect I'm as strong as a bull. When I'm bulimic, I'm exhausted, sleepy." She was vaguely aware of the secondary gain involved, namely, that her bulimia-induced passivity maintained her de-pendent relations with her parents. She reported having no bulimic symptoms during this time.

Sarah became quite panicked by the implications of her in-sight and subsequently regressed to her literal-minded ap-proach in the following two weeks. She denied that there was "anything to that bully stuff." Hunger again implied physical hunger and her symptoms merely "came down to just controlling my urges to eat, regulating my caloric intake." She became "phobic of being fat" and revived her interest in medications and laboratory tests. Anxiety again "hit" her in the stomach. She binged and purged daily with great violence.

During weeks 11 through 13, Sarah was able to recover her psychological acumen of the eighth week. She remembered that as a child she was a notorious "bully" and that her "bullishness" alienated her peers. Being helpless was seen as a precondition of intimacy in her family as well. She recognized dependent urges as the source of her anger with me for not instituting pharmacotherapy; she felt as if I weren't "feeding" her. She commented, "I don't have the compulsion to lose 30 pounds anymore." Bulimic episodes dropped to four and then three per week.

Another "regression" to concretism followed these observations in week 14. Although concerned that "the scale won't be balanced—that I might get more than I give"—and fearful of people's reaction to her as she could be "such a bully," Sarah never connected her images of scales and bullies to bulimia. She was once more preoccupied with weight gain and literal hunger and reported about four unusually violent purges for that week.

Sarah's metaphor usage was consistently highest during weeks 15 through 22, especially crucial sessions. She expressed her feelings that she must "contain my anger, but sometimes like with food there's too much and I explode"; that as a child she must be perfect or risk abandonment, a realistic fear with her father's frequent absences. She noted that bulimia "consumes" time and prevents her from independent endeavors. To the word "strong," she associated her grandmother, a woman "strong and selfish" to the point of literally witholding food from her children. Sarah admitted that she too might be pushy, might "shove my weight around," might devour or destroy those around her and, as with Humpty-Dumpty, be unable to reconstitute them. She explicitly recognized the symbolic, metaphoric nature of the bulimia (e.g., "When I'm hungry now I try to *figure* out what I *really* want") and that it had many layers of meaning "like so many layers of fat." Her now mild bulimic episodes dropped to three times per week and then stabilized at approximately one to two times weekly.

Sarah gradually curtailed her metaphor use throughout the remainder of the sessions. Significantly, however, there was no corresponding recurrence of concretisms or exacerbation of her bulimic symptoms. During week 27, she reported, "I feel I've made an incredible breakthrough; I used to literally feel hungry." She had progressed from her initial concrete conceptions of bulimia and high somatization to an intermediate stage of metaphors with concrete food/body referents and little somatization, and finally into an entirely abstract phase where food and bodily functions were largely irrelevant.

THE ROLE OF THERAPY

Sarah's previous, unsuccessful, behaviorally oriented therapies conceived of her symptoms in concretistic ways which merely reinforced her own prodigious somatic defenses. I introduced psychodynamic formulations which either made such functional equivalents untenable or unnecessary. Recognition of the psychogenetic components of her symptom permitted Sarah to "reconstruct" her bulimia in symbolic terms. She spontaneously transferred her interest in literal food to a preoccupation with food metaphors: she came to "eat her words" instead of food. Periodically, she reacted against the individuation which recovery implied by regressing from her metaphysical stance to her original physical expressions, ones which incidentally paralleled the rudimentary "body ego" and concrete operational abilities of the dependent child. At such times, I acted to "de-literalize" the now frank bulimia by reconnecting physical symptom with the corresponding affect and psychic conflict. In Freud's (1914) words, I set "about a perpetual struggle with the patient to keep all the impulses which [s]he would like to carry into action within the boundaries of [her] mind" (p. 163). Such de-literalization sometimes took the form of simple empathic statements where concern was shifted away from soma and onto emotional state. At other times, I would interpret the meaning of a concrete symptom by reintroducing Sarah's own metaphors or closely related images. The concrete food referents of such metaphors seemed to serve to establish contact with the patient; the abstract implication of the metaphor then conveyed the "deep," psychological meaning. Near the end of treatment, Sarah had dissociated her conflict almost entirely from food and demonstrated exclusively the well-integrated ego functions and formal operations of the adult. At the same time, she became progressively detached from her parents: her daily visits were reduced to weekly visits augmented by occasional phone calls. She refused parental financial support and relied more heavily on formal childcare.

It is important to note that both a decrease in concretisms and an increase in metaphors generally *preceded* the remittence of bulimic symptoms. Such a lagged response suggests that the de-literalization of bulimia actually contributed to Sarah's improvement rather than merely reflected her behavior change *ex post facto.* In other words, food and body metaphors most likely mark/facilitate the conceptual shift which initiates recovery.

Because of Sarah's characterological overcompliance, the question of transference cure is relevant. Unfortunately Sarah has since relocated and is unavailable for follow-up. Although the stability of her improvement is of course important, my aim is not to demonstrate the ultimate efficacy of food metaphor, but merely to document its utility as a transitional phenomenon, i.e., as a means of mediating between primitive, concrete expressions of conflict and more sophisticated conceptual forms which are more accessible to consciousness and interpretation. As bulimia has physically damaging effects (most notably, electrolyte imbalance), such de-literalization can be vital. Whether the psychodynamic "formula" was permanently "digested" or whether it too at some point will be "spit out" is undetermined. A maintenance course of therapy could certainly be instituted to prevent relapse.

METAPHOR: ITS SPECIAL IMPORTANCE TO BULIMIA

Several qualities of metaphor make it especially "palatable" to patients with eating disorders and suitable for use in intervention efforts. Most simply, metaphor entails a compromise formation similar to that represented by the bulimic symptom. Bulimia is above all a means of "eating" food without actually eating it. Analogously metaphor, as Ekstein and Wallerstein observed, is a way of "saying" something without actually saying it. Sarah's use of food metaphors permitted her to "have" her bulimia without actually having it, or in her terms to "eat her cake and have it too." Although one might worry that such a figurative substitution is specious, as noted earlier, it both circumvents the dangerous physical sequelae of the literal symptom and permits a gradual transition to abstract, psychodynamic formulations. Converting the physical discharge of impulses into the work of recollection and reflection is the cornerstone of analytic therapy (Freud, 1914). Furthermore, Carveth (1984) states that "it is hard to conceive of any model of psychoanalytic cure other than as a shift from relatively pathological to relatively normal compromise formations" (p. 520).

The capacity of metaphor to expand the expressive possibilities of language is perhaps particularly appealing to patients such as Sarah with a family history of Holocaust survival. The emphasis upon limited resources, especially food, in such families is well documented (Bergmann and Jucovy, 1982; Grubrich-Simitis, 1984). To make a single word or image "serve" to express multiple meanings is analogous to the economical distribution of food during wartime. Sarah's use of the word "egg" exemplifies this. Eggs connoted humiliation ("egg on the face"), anxiety ("walking on eggshells"), aggression ("egged on," the Humpty-Dumpty image), emotional vulnerability ("fragile as an egg," "cracking up," "thin-shelled"), and docility ("a good egg"). From a therapeutic vantage, reflection on such a parsimonious use of language highlights for the patient her guilt surrounding "having." Less speculatively, the therapist's elaboration of the various elements of the image permits, as Pollio et al. (1977) suggest, an efficient means of calling attention to the multiple determinants of the central conflict.

Several writers have observed that because metaphor denotes one thing by describing another, it implies a "similarity in the midst of difference" (Isenberg, 1963; also Arvanitakis, 1982; Billow, 1977); "there are *two* phenomena being compared that are *not* alike in all respects, and that the two phenomena being contrasted are *not* absolutely antithetical" (Carveth, 1984, p.

513). Bruch (1973) maintains that eating disorders arise when there is discrepant "feedback" regarding feeding behavior. Even more crucial, however, is the patient's coincident failure to individuate. Patients with eating disorders suffer from "*the basic delusion of not having an identity of their own,* of not even owning their body and its sensations, with the *specific inability of recognizing hunger as a sign of nutritional need*" (p. 50).

Sarah certainly feared to separate from her parents; she believed that she must remain identical to them by being a nondescript, passive "good egg" or else destroy them. She insured her continued dependency via the childlike mechanism of somatic conversion. The more developmentally advanced metaphors to which Sarah "graduated" asserted that things can be both similar *and* different; or, in this context, that one can be both close to one's family *and* an autonomous adult. (Carveth has well described the intimate relation between the two binary opposites: metaphorical similarity/difference and familial symbiosis/separation.) As noted earlier, the translation of the original physical discharge into a "figurative" metaphor was apparently a sublimation of some merit. The success of the metaphor may have been enhanced by the "similarity-in-difference" inherent in metaphoric structure and which reiterates the quasi-detachment required by separation-individuation. This aspect of metaphor, combined with the "intimate separation" (Stone, 1961) of the therapist-patient relationship, may provide an unusually powerful model of individuation for patients with eating disorders.

SUMMARY

The earliest psychoanalytic references to figurative language recognized the fundamental relationship between body and metaphor. Current work reemphasizes the association between the somatic discharge of impulses and their metaphoric expression. Bulimic patients are particularly resistant to psychodynamic intervention because of the "constant ready availability of their own bodies for the representation and expression of psychic conflict" (Ritvo, 1984, p. 455). Metaphor, however, seems especially appealing to bulimics. Perhaps this is because the compromise-formation structure of metaphor parallels the structure of the bulimic conflict, the economy of expression permitted by metaphor is congruent with the patient's own concern with self-abnegation and greed, and the metaphor models a similarity-in-difference analogous to separation-individuation. This study proposes that the concrete referents of food and body metaphors provide a therapeutic bridge from physical discharge to metaphysical understanding and so "tip the scale" in favor of recovery.

BIBLIOGRAPHY

ALEKSANDROWICZ, D. R. (1962). The meaning of metaphor. *Bull. Menninger Clin.*, 26:92–101.

ARLOW, J. A. (1979). Metaphor and the psychoanalytic situation. *Psychoanal. Q.*, 48:363–385.

ARVANITAKIS, K. (1982). Aristotle's *Poetics. Amer. Imago*, 39:255–268.

BERGMANN, M. & JUCOVY, M. E., eds. (1982). *Generations of the Holocaust.* New York: Basic Books.

BILLOW, R. M. (1977). Metaphor. *Psychol. Bull.*, 84:81–92.

BRUCH, H. (1973). *Eating Disorders.* New York: Basic Books.

CAIN, A. C. & MAUPIN, B. M. (1961). Interpretation within the metaphor. *Bull. Menninger Clin.*, 25:307–311.

CARUTH, E. & EKSTEIN, R. (1966). Interpretation within the metaphor. *J. Amer. Acad. Child Psychiat.*, 5:35–45.

CARVETH, D. L. (1984). The analyst's metaphors. *Psychoanal. & Contemp. Thought*, 7:491–560.

EDELSON, J. T. (1983). Freud's use of metaphor. *Psychoanal. Study Child*, 38:17–59.

EKSTEIN, R. (1961). Cross-sectional views of the psychotherapeutic process with an adolescent recovering from a schizophrenic episode. *Amer. J. Orthopsychiat.*, 31:757–775.

———— & WALLERSTEIN, J. (1957). Choice of interpretation in the treatment of borderline and psychotic children. *Bull. Menninger Clin.*, 21:199–207.

FINE, H. J., POLLIO, H. R., & SIMPKINSON, C. H. (1973). Figurative language, metaphor and psychotherapy. *Psychotherapy*, 10:87–91.

FREUD, S. (1914). Recollection, repetition and working through. *S.E.*, 12:145–156.

———— (1923). The ego and the id. *S.E.*, 19:3–66.

———— (1925). Negation. *S.E.*, 19:235–239.

GORE, N. S. (1977). Psychological Functions of Metaphor. Doctoral dissertation, University of Michigan.

GREENSON, R. R. (1967). *The Technique and Practice of Psychoanalysis.* New York: Int. Univ. Press.

GRUBRICH-SIMITIS, I. (1984). From concretism to metaphor. *Psychoanal. Study Child*, 39:301–319.

HARTMANN, H. (1951). Technical implications of ego psychology. *Psychoanal. Q.*, 20:31–43.

ISENBERG, A. (1963). On defining metaphor. *J. Philos.*, 60:609–622.

LENROW, P. B. (1966). Uses of metaphor in facilitating constructive behavior change. *Psychotherapy*, 3:145–148.

LEWIN, B. D. (1971). Metaphor, mind and manikin. *Psychoanal. Q.*, 40:6–39.

LINDEN, J. (1985). Insight through metaphor in psychotherapy and creativity. *Psychoanal. & Contemp. Thought*, 8:375–406.

OLINICK, S. L. (1976). Empathy and metaphoric correspondences. *Annu. Psychoanal.*, 4:93–100.

——— (1978). Paradox and metaphor. *Int. J. Psychoanal. Psychother.*, 7:533–561.

PEDERSON-KRAG, G. (1956). The use of metaphor in analytical thinking. *Psychoanal. Q.*, 25:66–71.

POLAND, W. S. (1986). The analyst's words. *Psychoanal. Q.*, 55:244–272.

POLLIO, H. R., BARLOW, J. M., FINE, H. J., & POLLIO, M. R. (1977). *Psychology and the Poetics of Growth*. Hillsdale, N.J.: Erlbaum.

REIDER, N. (1972). Metaphor as interpretation. *Int. J. Psychoanal.*, 53:463–469.

RITVO, S. (1984). The image and uses of the body in psychic conflict. *Psychoanal. Study Child*, 39:449–469.

SHARPE, E. F. (1940). Psycho-physical problems revealed in language. In *Collected Papers on Psychoanalysis*. New York: Brunner/Mazel, 1950, pp. 155–169.

SHENGOLD, L. (1981). Insight as metaphor. *Psychoanal. Study Child*, 36:289–306.

STONE, L. (1961). *The Psychoanalytic Situation*. New York: Int. Univ. Press.

VOTH, H. M. (1970). The analysis of metaphor. *J. Amer. Psychoanal. Assn.*, 18:599–621.

WRIGHT, K. J. T. (1976). Metaphor and symptom. *Int. Rev. Psychoanal.*, 3:97–109.

WURMSER, L. (1977). A defense of the use of metaphor in analytic theory formation. *Psychoanal. Q.*, 46:466–498.

FREUD AND THEORY
BUILDING

Freud and the Father Complex

PETER BLOS, Ph.D.

IN STUDYING ADOLESCENCE FROM MANY ANGLES, I RECOGNIZED gradually but ever more clearly the boy's father complex—more precisely, the father complex of the son—and its influence on his personality formation. This discussion of the father complex is devoted to the male gender, a restriction that is based on my opinion that boys and girls pursue their own particular and specific lines of development early in life. They certainly cannot be viewed as mirror images in which we see the male as the original or standard bodily model. This early Freudian schema of infantile psychic development has received many decisive corrections, the results of systematic, observational infant studies. My own adolescent research has contributed its share to delimit and describe the particular stages of adolescent male and female development. Since I intend to submit to you in what follows some corrections of the classic Freudian theory, I wish to let you know in advance that I shall return to Freud, the scientist, and to Freud, the son and man, as they both were affected by the father complex. I shall then attempt to apply my corrections of Freud's developmental schema of early object relations to a review of

---

Sigmund Freud Lecture, May 6th, 1986, University of Vienna. Translated into English by the author.

In order to view this lecture in the light of its local importance, it must be stated that it was not given for an exclusively psychoanalytic audience but was to mark a cultural event. The paper was to state and explain the importance of Sigmund Freud for the history of Austria and the city of Vienna. The lecture was given under the auspices of the Sigmund Freud Society, the University of Vienna, and the City of Vienna. The occasion was given special dignity and momentum by the attendance of the President of Austria, some civic leaders, as well as deans from various academic departments.

some critical episodes in Freud's life which I believe still remain insufficiently understood.

We are familiar with the psychoanalytic postulate according to which the oedipus complex determines the fate of individual object relations. In fact, the oedipus complex has acquired over time such universal familiarity that we can now find these two words in every standard dictionary as well as in the established parlance of educated Western adults. What might require mentioning is the specificity of the revival of the oedipus complex in adolescence, when the relationship between the three persons— child, father, mother—appears dramatically in all possible permutations of their infantile emotional modalities (in the extreme: love and hate) but with a distinctive difference. This I intend to illuminate in discussing the boy's father complex and its influence on adolescent development. We are familiar with the fact that the infantile, triangular or triadic object relations reach their critical, conflictual apex in adolescence when the expression of genital sexuality as well as the emotional detachment from the parents have reached a maturational imperative. Both characterize adolescence and make the most pressing demands on the adaptive capacity of the maturing individual in his effort to bring about his departure from childhood and his entry into the antechambers of adulthood, called late adolescence or postadolescence.

The failures in emotional adaptation which we observe in many adolescents have interested me over the years. I slowly became convinced that the oedipus complex in its classical definition offers us only a limited clarification of the proverbial adolescent crisis. My clinical experience convinced me that the rivalry feelings of the male adolescent with his father, the expressions of competition, oppositionalism, and defiance, in action and thought, which are directed against the father, have to be largely comprehended as the result of an incomplete detachment from the early father and his protective presence in the boy's life—a presence either actual, construed, or wished for. Here we have to remind ourselves that the infantile attachment to the father passes through an emotional revitalization upon the arrival of puberty, i.e., with the onset of sexual maturation.

The role or function of the early father was that of a rescuer or savior at the time when the small child normally makes his determined effort to gain independence from the first and exclusive caretaking person, usually the mother. At this juncture the father attachment offers an indispensable and irreplaceable help to the infant's effort to resist the regressive pull to total maternal dependency, thus enabling the child to give free rein to the innate strivings of physiological and psychological progression, i.e., maturation. We find the roots of the boy's father complex at this point in the boy's development. The reverberations of this complex are never totally extinguished in the life of any man; they remain active and alive from "the cradle to the grave." We can hardly overrate their contribution to the process of growing up, of being a grownup, and of growing old. The resolution of the boy's paternal attachment is normally left incomplete at the end of early childhood because developmental pressures of a somatic, cognitive, and social nature outweigh the completion of this task of infancy. Normally, the irresistible beckoning of the latency period wins out. In adolescence, the interrupted processes of psychological growth must be taken up again because they cannot tolerate further delay when the irrevocable termination of psychological childhood is in sight.

The boy's extinguished yearning for the comforting comradeship with father turns into a frightening prospect at adolescence, when the regressive pull to the state of dependency on the paternal savior grows in intensity, especially in case he becomes resurrected as the little boy's idealized hero. This psychic constellation is experienced by the adolescent as an intolerable conflict. I have frequently made the observation that the boy's adolescent revolt against his father asserts itself with more boundless violence, the more profound the son's early father attachment had been and the more unaltered this attachment (usually successfully repressed) had remained in the boy's emotional life. Regardless of how successfully—or shall we say, how normally— the decline of the early father attachment proceeded over time, the tendency to idealization represents a lifelong problem for every man.

The irresistible turn of the pubertal boy to the female is to him the clear and definitive confirmation of his maleness. It is commonly observed either in his tender, affectionate, and adoring feelings for her or, on the other hand, in a precautious and sudden plunge into a total emotional and sexual engulfment by his juvenile love experience. This is an old and well-known story to which I intend to give some additional details. My work with male adolescents has convincingly demonstrated to me that the early adolescent sexual urgencies of which I speak here serve primarily to bring about the emotional distancing from the early father. The attainment of this libidinal detachment has to be achieved by the son in that crucial epoch of adolescence, before his sexual maturity can be fitted harmoniously into the widely roaming life of adult object relations.

Adolescence is the period in which the infantile remnants of the male father complex must be settled with finality—for better or for worse. I speak here about an infantile isogender attachment emotion in which we do not yet recognize the exclusive and typical features of the oedipus complex, such as rivalry, jealousy, envy, competition, aggression, and the wish to dislodge the paternal troublemaker for good. Of course, intimations of these emotions can be detected early in infancy. However, we recognize in the expression of these affects, even in asocial and delinquent forms of adolescent behavior, an effort by the growing child to liberate himself from an oppressive, confining, and restrictive dependency on one or the other or both parents. The infantile trend toward autonomy is always juxtaposed to a passive dependency wish, to a self-sufficient dual unity or a merger into oneness. After the completion of the psychological separation process, higher forms of differentiated object relations appear.

I speak here specifically of two infantile phases in object relations which are contrasted by essential differences. The earlier modality of object relations—the dyadic one—is exclusively experienced in the interaction between two partners, while the oedipal or triadic one comprises implicitly the interaction between three partners. I came to recognize that the focal determinant in the developmental disturbances of the male adolescent lies in the libidinal, positive attachment emotion of the boy to the father of his early childhood.

I have already pointed out what lent the original urgency to this attachment, namely, the need of the growing child to distance himself from the central female careperson, usually the mother. This developmental forward striving is introduced and supported by an innate biological growth process. I mention only locomotion, the capacity of sphincter control, the acquisition of language, of causal thinking, of the internalization of experience. Such maturational achievements lead, in a synergic fashion, to the typically human mental structuralization of symbolic thought and memory. These biologically initiated phenomena of psychic maturation and development are decisively supported in the male child by his emotional turn to the father, in whom he has suddenly discovered a mighty comrade in his budding self-affirmation, autonomy, and sense of identity (identification). The acquisition of this newly discovered caretaking person effectively supports the little boy in his gigantic effort to resist the alluring powers of the infantile, symbiotic mother. Within this emotional area of early father attachment lie the roots of the father complex. This complex is reanimated by the sexual maturation at puberty, and with it the need arises for the support and guidance by a male comrade and friend, cast into all kinds of concretizations or abstractions of the father imago. The sense of yearning implicit in this crossroads state easily turns into the threat of a return to the original father attachment which once in the dim past had enabled the male child to leave the "realm of the mothers" as Goethe (Faust, Part II) referred to this mysterious, archaic netherland of mankind. This realm became, under the influence of the boy's sexual maturation, the realm of the female with all its original temptations, fears, and apprehensions.

The effort to avert the danger of regression, inherent in the adolescent stage, is recognizable in the urgent adolescent striving toward freedom, independence, and self-determination. These years are marked by hero worship and hero search. The ensuing externalizations of internalized ideals are cast into personalities of the contemporary world and represent, at this youthful stage of life, the scouts and guides of a self-chosen safari into an unknown and unpredictable future, outside the direct and narrow influence of a broad historical family tradition to which we usually refer as "upbringing" or "background." Such transformations acquire slowly but firmly a lasting direc-

tion and structure; then the task of adolescence has been fulfilled and an individual's character has acquired its irreversible nature: adulthood has declared its presence; it is here to stay.

My work with adolescents has convincingly demonstrated to
me that the father complex of early male development and the
oedipus complex which follows it play roles of equal significance.
Both phases influence synergically the development and formation of the male personality and both require equal attention as
well as etiological acknowledgment in every kind of psychotherapeutic endeavor. I have learned from my work with male
adolescents that the unresolved dyadic father attachment represents a basic pathogenic structure which prevents the oedipus
complex from reaching its full maturation. Even though we can
no longer say that "the nucleus of the neurosis" is to be found in
the oedipus complex, we can state with certainty that the dyadic
pathogenic residues are subjected to a definitive organization
(neurotic or otherwise) with the ascendancy of the oedipal constellation, i.e., the oedipus complex.

We have never questioned that the unique roles of the father—dyadic and triadic—are not as significant and indispensable for the boy's further development as is the preceding caretaking and organizing presence of the early mother. The specific
modalities of these object relations influence the formation of
every personality in either growth-promoting or growth-inhibit-
ing trends. Our clinical observations always show fluctuating
combinations of both which are finally cast into enduring personality structures at the termination of adolescence. Both
trends throw their light and shadow on the life of every man or
every father whose life obviously begins with being a son. Both
trends show their equally irrepressible antagonistic, i.e., hostile
as well as tender and loving emotions throughout life. The never-ending consequences of the early father experience are easily
recognizable in the male friendships of adolescents and adult
men. To view this kind of relationship under the general de-
nominator of repressed homosexuality reduces the complex tex-
ture of human relationships to a pitiful simplification.

I have now reached the point in my exposition where I intend
to shift the focus of attention and relate what has been said to the
life of the man whom we honor today. The title of my talk

permits me to speak either about the father complex in psycho-analytic theory or about Freud's father complex in particular; both intentions were on my mind.

We know from Freud's writings that he always turned his interest to the smallest detail of expression, just in case it might contain something to be concealed or to be exposed. He thus succeeded in gaining access to the carefully guarded secrets and mysterious workings of the human mind. This process of obser-vation is intimately related to the psychoanalytic treatment of mental disturbances. Such often ignored details of expression to which I refer can easily be demonstrated in the field of language (e.g., slips of the tongue), in the field of motor activity (e.g., misplacing of an object), or in the field of mental functioning (e.g., forgetting, overlooking). These phenomena are called parapraxes.

It is therefore an especially significant surprise that the "mas-ter of interpretation" ignored a significant part of the Oedipus myth, while he placed another into the center of his theory of the neurosis. He designated a part of the oedipal drama to represent a universal and fateful experience in human life. I am not the first who noticed Freud's partial and discriminative use of the Oedipus myth. That part of the myth which Freud ignored is the crime of infanticide which the father committed when his son was born. The Oedipus tragedy was set into motion by a father who was afraid of his son with whom he became prematurely rivalrous. This father was King Laios. It was the father who exposed his small son to certain death, when he turned him over to a shepherd with the order to abandon him in the wilderness. The infidelity of fatherhood drove Oedipus, when he had reached manhood, back to his family in order to take by force his birthright, unlawfully withheld from him by his father. This emotional constellation of mutual, jealous competition, mutual idealization, aggrandizement, and distorted perceptions as they reigned between father and son was described in the complete text of the Oedipus myth. When such love-hate attachments are acted out in the lives of both male partners, the implicit conflicts represent a typical emotional constellation in the father-son and son-father relationship which I have observed regularly in my work with disturbed male adolescents and men. I came to assign to this particular son-father impasse a universal significance. My clinical experience forced me to recognize in the father complex of the male a normal stage in the boy's emotional development which precedes the oedipus complex, initiates it, and, indeed, is preconditional to its formation. This is to say, the formation of the oedipus complex is predicated on the resolution of the dyadic father complex.

This comment has brought me to the threshold of my thoughts about Freud's father complex and its influence on psychoanalytic theory building. We are well informed from Freud's writings and letters that there existed an intense emotional relationship between Sigmund and father Jakob which lasted with undiminished strength from earliest childhood to the adult life of the son. We have good reasons to assume that Sigmund thought of himself as "the declared favourite of the dreaded father."[1] He says of his father in a letter to Fliess (November 2, 1896): "I valued him highly and understood him very well indeed, and with his peculiar mixture of deep wisdom and imaginative light-heartedness he meant a great deal in my life." His father was a man who pleased him tremendously; being and remaining his preferred son was a powerful motivating force in many areas of his life. The son compared his father in his physical appearance to a popular hero of the times, Garibaldi. Freud (1900) wrote: "I remember how like Garibaldi he had looked on his deathbed" (p. 447). Quite objectively, the photographic portrait of the father bore a resemblance to the colorful leader of the Italian Resorgimento.

The above references are based on Freud's letters to Wilhelm Fliess and relevant passages in his writings. They allow us to

---

1. This statement is made on the basis of an inference; the quotation is lifted from *Moses and Monotheism* (1939, p. 106), more specifically from a reference to the Jewish legend of Joseph and his brethren. The reference has been considered by Freud scholars as an autobiographical remark. Both sons had a father named Jacob and both men were rewarded fame and wealth as the interpreters of dreams. With reference to the Strachey translation of the passage just mentioned, it should be explained that the original German word for the English translation into "favourite" is *Liebling;* literally translated it means "the most loved one" and is therefore a word which refers to an intensely libidinized relationship, commonly used as an endearing appellation to a beloved one of any age, quite similar in this respect to the English word "darling."

abstract from them a description of a stage in the development of Freud's father complex in statu nascendi. "The feared father"—in conjunction with the loved and loving parent—compounded the wish to prolong the infantile state of being the "declared favourite." This was to be realized by doing whatever needs to be done in order to fulfill the father's expectations which—no doubt—became identical with those of his son. This kind of bond between son and father is always strengthened and solidified by a mutual emotional reciprocity. Such libidinal transactions of infantile emotions finally become relegated by the process of growing up to the internal realm of the adult ego ideal. However, should the influence of adolescence in terms of the expectable transformations in psychic structure prove incapable of transmuting infantile idealizing object relations, then we can expect that the uniquely dyadic attachment emotions of son to father will extend their reverberations into the life of manhood.

In terms of a developmental perspective, the dyadic constellation just outlined contains elements of castration anxiety and castration wishes. We discern in these contradictory strivings a progressive and regressive propensity of basic "ambitendency" (Mahler et al., 1975) which is so characteristic of the dyadic phase. The dyadic father attachment of the boy and its dynamic function in male identity formation should be kept distinct and separate from the typical oedipal entanglements of son and father and their particular impact on male psychic structure formation. While congruities and similarities between both stages exist, I do not hesitate to say that the observable as well as the inferred differences are of great significance for etiological and prognostic considerations. This suggests that we view the two phase-specific son-father relationships—dyadic and triadic-oedipal—as two phenomena sui generis.

We might entertain the thought that a significant contribution to the defense mechanism of denial derives from the son's usual dyadic father idealization. This developmentally essential experience of the young child temporarily impedes the growth of the reality principle. Should this fallibility remain uncorrected during progressive development, the reactive turn to idealization in the face of danger becomes an anachronistic protection against anxiety and conflict. Under such circumstances every external or internal danger might evoke a denial, based on infantile idealization and observable in an overvaluation of the object and the self. Such distortions can assume dangerous proportions and, indeed, can threaten psychic integrity. What has once served, in the dyadic phase, as a means for psychological survival and a precondition for progressive development has been turned—under the influence of the dyadic fixation—into a developmental impediment. This could hardly be different since the perceptions of the inner and outer world as they are transacted by the ego are disjointed fragments of a distorted judgment which labors under the influence of a dyadic fixation.

The never-corrected idealization of the infantile object and, consequently, the induced, defensive overrating of the self or other endanger synergically the ego's reality testing or data processing. Over time in the individual's life, these hazards make their specific contribution to the adaptive failures and disturbances in object relations with which we are thoroughly acquainted from our therapeutic work. Furthermore, the consequences of the reality distortions of which I speak here, as well as the never completely abandoned use of infantile denial, can readily be observed in group psychology. For example, when the inhabitants of a country find themselves endangered and threatened by hostile forces, the tendency asserts itself to overrate catastrophically the powers of their government and their armed forces. Politicians have always known how to turn this human tendency to their advantage by either exaggerating the evil and ruthless powers of the enemy or by fabricating a potential adversary of inscrutable might.

The assumption of a deeply rooted dyadic father attachment in Freud's life encourages me to draw some conclusions which are suggested and supported by my clinical research on adolescence and its developmental conceptualizations. In broad outlines I assume that Freud's father attachment was never subjected to a sufficient or lasting resolution during his adolescence, namely, at that period in life when the final step in the resolution of the male father complex is normally transacted. We encounter emotional reverberations of the father attachment in displaced form in the life of the man Freud. I have only to point to his exclusive, possessive, and passionate friendships with men who were his scientific colleagues. Two such friendships played a fateful role in his life. One friendship was with Wilhelm Fliess, an older colleague and father figure; the other with Carl Jung, a younger colleague, so to say a scientific son whom the master wished to declare the prince royal in the realm of psychoanalysis. In this attempt Freud tried to accomplish what King Laios denied his son Oedipus. Freud repeated in this act of scientific fathership what his own father had expected from him, namely, to fulfill his wish to accomplish great things in his life and give reality to a tradition of expected fame. The father's mandate silently dominated Freud's life until he experienced during the fourth decade of his life a profound psychological crisis which was precipitated by the death of his father in 1896.

The ambivalent father attachment became manifest when the father became mortally ill and the son left the city to take an extended vacation of two months; and again, when he arrived too late at the funeral because he was detained at the barber (Letter to Fliess, November 2, 1896). These and similar emotional turbulences initiated Freud's self-analysis which led him to the creation of his magnum opus, *The Interpretation of Dreams*. He wrote in the foreword to the second edition (1908) that this work was "my reaction to my father's death—that is to say, to the most important event, the most poignant loss, of a man's life" (p. xxii). A sentence of such apodictic and affirmative singularity, overloaded with superlatives, cannot fail to raise the question why Freud had ignored the role of the father in the Oedipus myth, especially since he came to discover the "oedipus complex"[2] during the two years following his father's death when he formulated it as a universal psychological crisis in human life.

Freud's personal crisis which, as we shall see, became scientifically significant for the future of psychoanalytic theory building led him to doubt the momentous discovery he had made in the treatment of hysteria. He came to realize that the predicated, pathogenic experience of sexual seduction by the father in early

---

2. The first reference to the oedipus complex—not yet called with these words but clearly illustrated in his comments on the Hamlet tragedy—is to be found in a letter to Fliess of October 15, 1897.

childhood did not represent the universal condition sine qua
non of hysteria. Freud arrived at the conviction that the childhood remembrances of seduction which his female hysterics reported to him with such astounding regularity were, in many
cases, fantasies; as such they evoked pathological reactions as
severe as those founded on experiences in real life. This conceptual demarcation between an experiential world that is related,
on the one hand, to an inner life and, on the other, to the im-
pingement of reality, and the implicit theoretical differentiation
between the specific influences derived from these two worlds of
experience upon the causation of psychic illness, ushered in the
scientific advances of psychoanalysis in the twentieth century.
This demarcation was epitomized by Freud's mounting concentration on the inner world of wish fulfillment, namely, on his
dream research which followed the death of his father.

The fact that the crisis in Freud's personal life was unquestionably related to the death of his father has faced every Freud
biographer with the task of throwing some light upon the sequence of events during the years 1896 to 1898. We know that
Freud's father expected great things from his son; these expectations had settled like fateful obligations within Freud's moral
conscience. This mandate aggravated his psychic task to loosen
and transcend the father attachment, rooted in a never sufficiently abandoned dyadic father idealization. The attempted
resolution of the father fixation seemed to have been channeled
into the son's passionate and single-minded striving to reveal the
mysterious origins and workings of psychic illness. His work
reveals in historical perspective the personal conflicts which
played a significant role in determining his professional life. We
are well acquainted with the creative coupling of several tasks
and their mastery; such joined strivings are summarized under
the concept of motivation; one striving is objective and goal-
directed and the other is personal and emotionally biased. The
life histories of creative thinkers and inventors have granted us
glimpses here and there into these arcane and overdetermined
workings of the mind.

Returning to the theme of my presentation, I would say that
Freud's father idealization suffered a catastrophic shock at his
father's death, as is normally the case in the initial phase of

mourning. The fact that Freud's life crisis and the death of his father are interrelated has led Freud biographers to various conclusions and suppositions.

I have reported above that in the years preceding the crisis Freud had presented to the psychiatric community his seduction theory of hysteria. This theory was briskly rejected by his academic colleagues and made a subject of ridicule, e.g., "as a scientific fairytale" (Krafft-Ebing). Thus, the discovery which Freud expected to be a breakthrough in the comprehension and treatment of emotional illness turned into an occasion of contempt and isolation from the academic world. This turn of events liquidated the son's wish to present to his father the gift of fame and distinction as expected by him. The theory of infantile seduction would oblige the son to subject his personal and intimate life with his own father to an objective scrutiny, in order to comprehend its influence on his own emotional development and present state of mind. The argumentation of some Freud biographers was predicated on the inference that an inhibition arose in the mind of the originator of the seduction theory which in essence protested: no, my father has never done improper things. The motto *de mortuis nil nisi bonum* forced the son, in mourning after his father's death, to sacrifice his seduction theory by publicly declaring it invalid. This step was considered by Freud biographers as a compromise, shaped under the influence of a life-long unresolved ambivalence conflict and forced into an acute state by the mounting work of mourning. So much for the Freud biographers whose argumentation I intend to refute. We all know that Freud had based the revocation on his realization that the seduction theory, as formulated, could not stand up in the light of his clincal judgment.

I should remind you at this point of some comments made earlier in my presentation, namely, that the normal resolution of the tender, passive, imitating father attachment takes its concluding and definitive steps in adolescence. I draw the conclusion from the crisis which Freud experienced in his 40s (1896–98) that his self-analysis following the death of his father facilitated, even though it was a developmentally anachronistic or delayed move, the resolution of his father complex—at least as far as he could take it at that time.

In contrast to the widely accepted opinion that the revocation of the seduction theory was issued under the forceful directive of an infantile inhibition and a subordination to the father imago, it is my opinion that the liquidation of the controversial theory points to other determinants. One of them is to be found in his striving toward the liberation from his dependency on the father imago and the liberation from the need or mandate to fulfill his father's wish to possess a famous, triumphant son. Fame was to come from his epochal discoveries in the world of the mind, comparable only to the revolutionary discoveries of a Columbus or Galileo in the world of space. Freud demonstrated, as I see it, a remarkable and admirable courage when he turned the critical comments of his adversaries against himself, declaring his seduction theory a "scientific fairy tale." But, alas, such devastating words ex cathedra had no place for Freud in the field of science. Consequently, he could not let the problem come to naught at this point but subjected his clinical experience with his hysteric patients to a searching critique. This he did without hesitating to face squarely his past misjudgments and begin a renewed appraisal of the power of fantasy in the life of the human mind.

Freud's letters and writings do not contain a wealth of material illuminating his father complex, but there is little doubt about the influence of his self-analysis upon his growing detachment from the father imago. In this context it is of special interest to consult one letter to Wilhelm Fliess in which Freud informs his paternal friend, as the first one, of the revocation of his seduction theory. The author of the letter tells his friend that he is astonished, almost bewildered, that no sense of shame and no depressed mood are evoked in him by the inescapable realization that the seduction theory which he had so proudly pronounced to the world had proved to be wrong. On the contrary, the burial of the great discovery which had once filled him with immense pride now evoked in him a "sense of victory," based on the conviction that he had misapplied clinical data to his theory of psychopathology. He told his friend that the self-critique and the revocation were the "result of honest and vigorous, intellectual work" of which he rightfully felt proud. This famous letter of September 21, 1897 ends with a sentence the content of which—in the context of such a momentous communication—sounds so totally unexpected and puzzling, that no reader of this letter can help being perplexed; yet, till today no convincing explanation has been advanced. After Freud had reported to Fliess in greatest detail the radical extirpation of his seduction theory and with it the loss of "an everlasting fame" and of "an assured wealth," there suddenly came to his mind the words of a fragmentary story. The words read: "Rebekka, you can take off your wedding-gown, you're not a bride any longer!"[3]

It is the opinion of several Freud biographers, one of many being Max Schur (1972), that the mysterious sentence intends to say that Freud felt like a bride who got herself into trouble and had to give up her wedding. The reference of "the little story" that "came to his mind" to the revocation of the seduction theory seems rather obvious. In contrast, other biographers (e.g., Krüll, 1986) assume that Freud committed in his revocation an irrational act which was directed by the unconscious intent to abandon this aspect of his theory because it might lead to the discovery of a seduction in his own childhood and to the revelation of erotic tendencies in his father (perhaps perversions or other secrets) which had influenced his own emotional development. What generally and invariably is typical for the hysteric also should be applicable to Freud. But why—so we ask ourselves—the female identification with a dissolved betrothal and the forced return to the state of a sexually noncommittal, premarital autonomy? "No bridal gown for you any longer." After all, enough stories exist in which men had to renounce their conquests. We are reminded here that Rebekka was the name of Jakob Freud's mysterious second wife whose actual existence has remained dubious to this very day. I refrain here from speculating on such an unverified conjecture.

In this crucial letter I believe that Freud informed Fliess of the successful detachment from his infantile father imago, a task with which he had struggled since the death of his father. I suggest that in the letter to his friend, Freud tells of his liberation from the oppressive father idealization and father fixation. He

3. The original text of the letter reads: "not a *kalle* any longer." *Kalle* is Hebrew for "bride."

gives convincing expression to this psychological event by describing with clarity his sense of pride, triumph, and courage which accompanied the revocation. I arrived at this interpretation on the basis of my clinical experience which has taught me that a son's subordination of his life's work, ambition, dedication, and achievement to the libidinized expectations of his father are experienced by the son as a submissive and passive adaptation. The effort to surmount this never quite ego-syntonic position of a boy's active-passive balance in the mastery of self and environment reaches a crucial impasse at the closure of adolescence. At that juncture this unresolved imbalance frequently merges with associative identity fragments of a feminine self representation. If this emerging conflict cannot be contained or resolved, an abnormal psychic accommodation will take its course. It is not uncommon that the resolution of the father complex reaches its final stage during a man's mature years. In my clinical work I frequently observed that the death of a father occurring during a man's mature years can evoke a profound emotional crisis. Such vehement interruptions of a manageable and successful course of life, when investigated, frequently lead to the interference by a revitalized father complex. What brings such cases to our attention are, however, acute and noisy problems of the present-day life under which the father complex lies silently buried. It remains the task of analysis to unearth it and bring it to a resolution before the work of analysis can be declared completed. Should a delayed mastery of the father complex be reached at an advanced age (with or without therapeutic assistance), then new possibilities open their doors in a man's life, relative to perception, to action, to reflection, to thought, and to novel emotional experiences. This I tried to explicate in the discussion of Freud's midlife crisis.

BIBLIOGRAPHY

Blos, P. (1962). *On Adolescence.* New York: Free Press.
Freud, S. (1900). The interpretation of dreams, *S.E.*, 4 & 5.
———— (1939). Moses and monotheism. *S.E.*, 23:3–137.

———— (1950). *The Origins of Psychoanalysis.* New York: Basic Books, 1954.
KRÜLL, M. (1986). *Freud and His Father.* New York: Norton.
MAHLER, M. S., PINE, F., & BERGMAN, A. (1975). *The Psychological Birth of the Human Infant.* New York: Basic Books.
SCHUR, M. (1972). *Freud: Living and Dying.* New York: Int. Univ. Press.

Freud's Seduction Theory

EMANUEL E. GARCIA, M.D.

RECENTLY MUCH ATTENTION HAS BEEN FOCUSED ON FREUD'S SO-called seduction theory of the etiology of neurosis (Masson, 1984). While both critics and admirers of Freud seem to agree on its importance in the development of psychoanalysis, strikingly divergent interpretations of the seduction theory have emerged. Thus, a review of the establishment and evolution of the seduction theory in Freud's work should prove useful.

Because Freud's scientific publications serve as the definitive embodiment of his theoretical formulations, they—and not his private correspondence or other personal material—consequently form the basis for the investigation that follows.

THE SEDUCTION THEORY ACCORDING TO FREUD

The seduction theory of the etiology of hysteria and obsessional neurosis was set forth by Freud in three papers, all appearing in 1896. As with any hypothesis *in statu nascendi*, inconsistencies of presentation may be detected; however, in the case of the seduction theory the inconsistencies that occur do not vitiate its core. They concern ancillary aspects, as we shall see. Nevertheless, contrary to the impression left by Masson (1984), the seduction theory was not without its deficiencies. Despite Freud's persuasive eloquence and conviction, some portions of his argument are noticeably weak.

It will be valuable to preface this examination of the seduction theory by referring to Freud's own comprehensive and lucid

Resident in psychiatry at the Institute of Pennsylvania Hospital, Philadelphia.

I wish to acknowledge my indebtedness to the late Harold Feldman.

discussion of the different types of etiological influences, which he grouped into three classes, namely, (1) preconditions, (2) concurrent causes, and (3) specific causes.

Preconditions and specific causes are both indispensable for the production of the disorder; but while preconditions also figure in the etiology of other, different disorders, specific causes "appear only in the aetiology of the disorder for which they are specific" (Freud, 1896a, p. 147). This is an important point because the discovery of merely a single case in which a previously postulated specific cause does *not* occur necessarily invalidates the postulate, thus demoting the ostensible specific cause to the status of concurrent cause, i.e., something which *might* contribute but which is *not* indispensable to the production of the disorder.[1]

What, then, did Freud regard as the specific cause of the neuroses? In "Heredity," citing 13 fully analyzed cases, Freud wrote, "I was obliged to see that at bottom the same thing was present in all the cases submitted to analysis—the action of an agent which must be accepted as the specific cause of hysteria. *This agent is indeed a memory relating to sexual life*" (p. 151f.; my italics). Then, a few sentences later, Freud proclaimed, "*A passive sexual experience before puberty;* this, then, is the specific aetiology of hysteria" (p. 152). Are there two causes of hysteria? Is a contradiction implicit in these statements?

I have deliberately chosen to present these two claims in such a fashion to highlight an important point. After having referred to the "memory relating to sexual life" as the specific cause of hysteria, Freud went on to describe its content: "*a precocious experience of sexual relations with actual excitement of the genitals, resulting from sexual abuse committed by another person*" (p. 152), the postulated event having taken place before puberty (specifically, before the ages of 8 to 10). With his reference to a memory, that is, to a *psychic phenomenon*, Freud unquestionably placed the etiology of hysteria in the psychological realm, where indeed his emphasis had been in 1894. However, he could account for the formation of this psychic phenomenon only by assuming that it

---

1. I am indebted to K. R. Eissler (1985) for reemphasizing the importance of this very basic and general rule about scientific hypotheses.

was a reproduction of actual events or, more accurately, of the perception of those events when they occurred.

Consider the existence of a psychic scene, which we shall regard as the specific cause of a hysteria. How can this scene come to be created? It might indeed be the pristine, undistorted psychic representation of an actual extrapsychic event. Or it might not be identical to any extrapsychic event, in which case it can only be a psychic creation of sorts, the result of rearrangements, reassemblings, distortions, and colorings of extrapsychic events, running the gamut from full-blown fantasy, with but a passing or meager homage to actual events, to the mental representation that is but the slightest modification of the perception of an actual experience. (Here I am assuming the capability of an undistorted perception of events at the time of their occurrence, for the purpose of simplifying our discussion.)

In 1896 Freud had essentially identified the psychic scene—let us label it "Z"—as the specific cause of hysteria. But because he could account for the formation of Z only by the first of the possibilities outlined in the preceding paragraph, he made the understandable assumption that Z was a memory. In other words, the psychic scene was equivalent to an actual event, which we shall label "A." This assumption, which implied the extraordinarily restricted view of the child's mind and its capabilities prevalent at the turn of the century, represented a tight coupling of Z to A. Thus the apparent contradiction alluded to above is resolved. The invocation of Z simultaneously required that of A. It would be totally in keeping with Freud's view to refer to Z and A as the postulated proximal and distal causes of neurosis.

In this same paper Freud (1896a) also offered an explanation of the etiology of obsessional neurosis, which differed from that of hysteria. In hysteria he found a passive sexual experience "submitted to with indifference or with a small degree of annoyance or fright. In obsessional neurosis it is a question on the other hand, of an event which has given *pleasure,* of an act of aggression inspired by desire (in the case of a boy) or of a participation in sexual relations accompanied by enjoyment (in the case of a little girl)" (p. 155). Thus, in obsessional neurosis, both the nature of the inferred sexual experiences and the content of the psychic scenes *are different from* those of hysteria. The defensive formations characterizing obsessional neurosis center upon an active subject—active in either perpetrating acts of sexual aggression or experiencing sexual relations pleasurably. The self-reproaches that later turn into obsessional ideas are reproaches against the material contained in the psychic scenes portraying such active participation.

Although Freud postulated a previous seduction, undergone passively, which was necessary to have produced such "unnatural" sexual precocity, in fact the analysis of obsessional neuroses uncovered a core that consisted *not* of the postulated "initial" seduction of the presumably passive child, but of the nonpassive sexual pleasure *as represented in the psyche*. (It is worth noting that Freud stated that 3 of his cases were "pure" obsessional neuroses at this time.) The only common etiological element shared by hysteria and obsessional neuroses was, strictly speaking, purely psychological. With his assumption of an initial passive seduction in the etiology of obsessional neuroses, Freud found himself forced to struggle with the dilemma of the "choice" of neuroses, i.e., explaining why one child would respond to seduction by becoming hysterical, and another by seducing in turn and thence to develop obsessions.

In the papers that followed Freud stressed further the psychological aspect of the etiology of the neuroses: "it is not the experiences themselves which act traumatically [neurosogenically] but their revival as a *memory* after the subject has entered on sexual maturity" (1896b, p. 164). In a footnote he commented on the much stronger effect of the memory versus that of the experience upon which it had ostensibly been based, concluding, interestingly enough, that such an inversion of the typical state of affairs "seems to contain the psychological precondition for the occurrence of a repression" (p. 167). Again, he took pains to clarify the etiological influences by stating that "the defence neuroses are indirect consequences of sexual noxae which have occurred before the advent of sexual maturity—are consequences, that is, *of the psychical memory-traces* of those noxae" (p. 168; my italics).

Freud continued with an even more cogent depiction of the psychical factor in "The Aetiology of Hysteria," where he wrote:

But we must not fail to lay special emphasis on one conclusion to which analytic work . . . has unexpectedly led. We have learned that *no hysterical symptom can arise from a real experience alone, but that in every case the memory of earlier experiences awakened in association to it plays a part in causing the symptom.* If—as I believe—this proposition holds good *without exception,* it furthermore shows us the basis on which a psychological theory of hysteria must be built [p. 197].

Freud (1896c) asserted that "*hysterical symptoms are derivatives of memories which are operating unconsciously*" (p. 212). However, Freud deferred discussion of how a purely psychological phenomenon—a scene or memory, if you will—can produce such an enormous pathogenic effect, while the actual experience fails to produce any at the time of its occurrence.

We have now reached the point where we must ask ourselves a host of questions, e.g., what was the nature of the sexual experience, the "memory" of which acted as specific cause of the neuroses? Who committed the "assaults"? And how did Freud suppose children to have reacted to these experiences? I shall trace Freud's answers sequentially.

THE NATURE OF THE SEXUAL EXPERIENCE

The event of which the subject has retained an unconscious memory is *a precocious experience of sexual relations with actual excitement of the genitals, resulting from sexual abuse committed by another person;* and *the period of life* at which this fatal event takes place is *earliest youth*—the years up to the age of eight or ten, before the child has reached sexual maturity [1896a, p. 152].
. . . *these sexual traumas must have occurred in early childhood (before puberty), and their content must consist of an actual irritation of the genitals (of processes resembling copulation)* [1896b, p. 163].

Sexual experiences in childhood consisting in stimulation of the genitals, coitus-like acts, and so on, must therefore be recognized, in the last analysis, as being the traumas which lead to a hysterical reaction to events at puberty and to the development of hysterical symptoms [1896c, p. 206].

In the third paper, however, Freud appeared to expand the range of such sexual activities beyond genital stimulation, thus departing from the earlier two papers: "these infantile sexual scenes . . . include all the abuses known to debauched and impotent persons, among whom the buccal cavity and the rectum are misused for sexual purposes" (p. 214). It remains unclear whether Freud attached much significance to the extragenital processes, that is, whether he included them as distal causes of neurosis in his theoretical formulation.[2]

WHO COMMITTED THE ASSAULTS?

Freud reported that in a majority of the cases presented in the two earlier papers (7 out of 13), sexual relations between *children,* usually brother and sister, in many cases continuing until puberty, constituted the distal etiologic events. In the remaining 6 cases, adults were deemed guilty of the "brutal assaults," and an unspecified few cases revealed combinations of the two. Freud accounted for the male child's seduction of his slightly younger sister by assuming that he "had been abused by someone of the female sex, so that his libido was prematurely aroused, and then, a few years later, he had committed an act of sexual aggression against his sister, in which he repeated precisely the same procedures to which he himself had been subjected" (p. 165). To support this claim Freud gave an example illustrating how brother, sister, and "somewhat older male cousin" each fell ill, presumably with neuroses, ultimately initiated by a female governess who had seduced the male cousin, who himself consequently seduced his slightly younger male cousin (Freud did not describe the sexual processes here), who in turn seduced his own sister. The evidence Freud presents to uphold his assumption seems scant and somewhat strained; certainly it carries none of the conviction that imbues his psychological account of neurosogenesis.

Of the adult perpetrators of the seductions, Freud enumerated nursemaids, governesses, domestic servants, and teachers. However, he failed to mention the fathers of female patients who were so often revealed to be the culprits (see Strachey's note, p. 164).

2. Judging from Freud's later references, extragenital processes did *not* possess specific etiologic importance, in contrast to direct genital stimulation.

In "The Aetiology of Hysteria," by which time Freud had analyzed 18 cases, he specified that 6 of the 18 were males, 12 females—and that the cases were either pure hysteria or mixed hysteria-obsessional neurosis (contradicting his earlier claim of 3 pure obsessional neuroses).[3] Here, however, Freud grouped the sexual experiences into three classes: (1) isolated assaults by adult strangers, mostly practiced on females; (2) "love relationships" lasting for years with familiar adults—"a nursery maid or governess or tutor, or, unhappily all too often, a close relative" (p. 208); and (3) sexual relations between two children of opposite sex, usually brothers and sisters, continuing often *beyond* puberty. Freud asserted that in most cases two or more "aetiologies" together had been discovered. Nowhere did Freud explicitly inculpate a child's parents.

Citing instances for which he was "sometimes" able to prove that in the child-child relations the boy had been previously seduced by a female adult, Freud concluded by asserting that adults were invariably the agents laying the foundation for neurosis. But his language betrayed the sparsity of evidence when he wrote, "*I am inclined to suppose* that children cannot find their way to acts of sexual aggression unless they have been seduced previously" (p. 208; my italics).

THE SEDUCTION EXPERIENCED

Freud seems surprisingly inconsistent in his descriptions of the responses of the children to the neurosogenic sexual experiences. He referred to them on the one hand as brutal assaults, abuses, grave sexual injuries, disgusting practices, acts of sexual aggression, noxae and traumas. On the other hand he wrote that these very same grave injuries and traumas were "submitted to with indifference or with a small degree of annoyance or fright" (p. 155). Furthermore, although he often made reference to these experiences as traumas, Freud repeatedly took pains to emphasize that they themselves failed to act traumatically—that "their revival as a *memory*" did instead (p. 164). If, as Freud asserted, the inferred sexual experience was indeed "innocuous

3. See Freud (1896a, p. 155). See also p. 446 above.

at the time it happened" (p. 213), how could it operate traumatically? Once more we are led to the realm of the psychological, where the apparent contradictions can be resolved only through an inference that these experiences become traumatic through the agency of their assumed psychical representations, since they "could after all only exert a psychical effect through their *memory-traces*" (p. 202). Thus, strictly speaking, it is only in the psychological sphere that Freud's footing was firm, specifically in the attribution to psychic scenes (rather than the sexual experiences themselves) of traumatic power and thus neurosogenesis.

With respect to *physical* trauma, Freud conceded that none actually resulted. Even when the assaults were committed by adult strangers, Freud wrote that they "knew how to avoid inflicting gross, mechanical injury" (p. 208).

SUMMARY

In retrospect, Freud may perhaps be justifiably accused of an unwarranted boldness in not restricting his etiologic claims to the realm where the evidence was far and away the strongest, namely, the psychological. A more circumspect investigator might have contented himself with revealing that in all of the analyses conducted reports of sexual experiences apparently occurring during early childhood had arisen; and that these psychic scenes were of crucial importance in the development of the neuroses, at the very center of symptom formation. He would clearly have labeled the assumption that these scenes constituted accurate representations of actual events as speculative, especially considering that reasonable confirmation of the occurrence of such events was obtained for only two cases (1896c, p. 206), and that patients reported having had "no feeling of remembering the scenes" (p. 204).[4]

Freud, in accordance with the times, was hampered by a lim-

---

4. But I do not think it would have been unreasonable, even for the most cautious of researchers, to have inferred sexual motive forces stemming from early childhood to be the determinants of the psychological phenomena which, after all, could not arise from thin air.

ited understanding of the sexual life and the mental capabilities of children. They seemed incapable of fantasy: either they received impressions passively (as, for example, hysterics-to-be), or they operated as mindless automata, mimicking adults' behavior (obsessives-to-be). And, hand in hand, they seemed incapable of autonomously motivated sexuality.

Nevertheless, Freud succeeded in masterfully establishing the importance of psychic scenes concerning infantile sexual experiences in the creation of neuroses, a discovery whose validity he never repudiated.[5] He also reaffirmed and reemphasized his earlier adumbration of the concept of psychical conflict: "the outbreak of hysteria may almost invariably be traced to a *psychical conflict* arising through an incompatible idea setting in action a *defence* on the part of the ego and calling up a demand for repression" (p. 210f.).

Freud was well aware of the immediate significance of the psychic reality of these scenes and of the power of the "sexual motive forces" at work in the neuroses he was treating. The seduction theory, when broken into its components to be analyzed, reveals itself to be primarily a psychological theory insofar as specific etiology is concerned. Indeed, we perceive in it the basic ingredients of Freud's later, more mature understanding of neurosogenesis, namely, psychic scenes of infantile sexuality.

There are difficulties and inconsistencies, to be sure—for example, in Freud's postulating previous seductions to account for sexual relations between children, despite acknowledging his ability to demonstrate adequate evidence only "sometimes" (p. 208), and in his attempts to explain the distal etiologic component of obsessional neurosis. However, as far as neurosogenesis goes, they are relatively inconsequential. The abandonment of the seduction theory merely represented Freud's uncoupling of Z and A, the so-called proximal and distal causes, thus implying a much-expanded conception of how a neurosogenic psychic scene could come about.

---

5. Although in the *Studies on Hysteria* Freud was cognizant of a sexual factor in the etiology of hysteria, he did not deem it to be invariably present. See Breuer and Freud (1893–95, pp. 257–262); Strachey's introduction (p. xxvf.); and Freud (1910a, p. 40).

"The Aetiology of Hysteria" Revisited

"The Aetiology of Hysteria," Freud's last and perhaps most powerful public account of the seduction theory, is a curious and intriguing work. In Masson's (1984) eyes, the paper represented a singular act of courage on Freud's part, wherein its author set forth the truth about the abuse of children in the face of a hostile medical audience. So highly does Masson regard it, that he has reprinted its text in his book and urges the reader to peruse it as a preface to his own material.

While I would not dispute the power, eloquence, and courageousness of the paper, a reexamination shows that it is much more than a mere enunciation of the seduction theory. It is pregnant with incipient ideas that would occupy Freud far into the future. Freud was ultimately not to be diverted from psychological exploration. The evidence of Freud's psychological preoccupations is abundant, but he may have attempted to skirt the frontiers that beckoned.

Freud clearly states that the mere occurrence of infantile sexual experiences is not sufficient to account for the development of a neurosis—a psychological factor as well is essential, namely, the unconscious psychic presence of the scenes. However, he "prudently" avoids a discussion of just how "those experiences produce conscious or unconscious memories—whether that is conditioned by the content of the experiences, or by the time at which they occur, or by later influences" (p. 211). In other words, he refrains from investigating the dynamic process ultimately responsible for neurosogenesis, a matter he doubtless foresaw as highly complex. Linked with this issue is that of why one individual with a history of infantile sexual experiences would succumb to a neurosis, while another with a nearly identical one would not—a problem which, on the level of theoretical generalization, would remain unsolved for a lifetime.

Similarly, Freud defers discussion of two other "purely psychological" problems: (1) how an unconscious memory of an experience innocuous at the time of its occurrence could be posthumously neurosogenic; and (2) why one person would develop hysteria, and another an obsessional neurosis (the "choice" of neuroses). He refers the reader to the "future *psychology of the neuroses*" (p. 219).

In rebutting an anticipated objection that the infantile sexual experiences might be so widespread as to detract from any specific etiologic significance, Freud rightly pointed out that "The area of occurrence of an aetiological factor may be freely allowed to be wider than that of its effect, but it must not be narrower" (p. 209). Then, in a passage that bolsters the view of a psychological core of the seduction theory and presages his future perspective on etiology, Freud "admits" that the almost universal occurrence of infantile sexual activity would render its demonstration without significance; and he proceeds to emphasize that "the aetiological pretensions of the infantile scenes rest . . . above all, on the evidence of there being associative and logical ties between those scenes and the hysterical symptoms" (p. 210). In other words, Freud is telling us in as decisive a manner as possible that what is of primary importance in neurosogenesis is the *current* operation of psychic scenes—not the assumed experiences of which they were allegedly reproductions, and which might well have been the lot of many nonneurotics. The distal etiologic component, it seems, has become a *precondition:* the proximal is the actual specific cause. Furthermore, with what may seem to the reader to be a wearisome regularity, Freud proposes not to enter upon an inquiry into the other factors "which the 'specific aetiology' of hysteria still needs in order actually to produce the neurosis" (p. 210).

In setting forth the specific etiology of hysteria Freud had done no more than establish the presence of unconscious scenes of infantile sexuality, whose content necessitates a defense designed to keep them from reaching consciousness, i.e., the neurosis. To explain the formation of these scenes he was constrained to invoke the actual occurrence of what they pictured. However, the assumed distal causative component was significant only in its ability to produce the current psychic constellation that served as actual, operative, neurosogenic agent.

To risk repetition, the psychological factor by rights occupied the central place in the seduction theory, and was considered so by Freud despite his trumpeting of the distal agent's role. For the sake of argument, however, let us make the assumption that the very heart of the seduction theory was indeed the demonstration of the sexual abuse of children by adults. If we grant, as Freud was willing to do, that persons who never came to develop a neurosis underwent the same infantile experiences that characterized the history of neurotics, then we are compelled to investigate those additional factors that were responsible for producing the neuroses in these others. Second, if we recognize the existence of an unconscious psychic constellation to which the symptoms of a neurosis are linked and upon which they are dependent, neither the assumption of the occurrence of a seduction nor the assumption that the scene is fantasy would diminish its power. The psychic reality of the patient remains to be dealt with. An apt illustration of this can be found in Freud's case of the Wolf-Man. Freud was never able to establish whether or not the Wolf-Man's primal scene represented an actual childhood event or contained fantastic elements, a "failure" which had no significance for the understanding of his neurosis (1918, p. 97).

In "The Aetiology of Hysteria," most, if not all, of the questions that intrigued Freud belonged properly to the realm of psychology, as he so often declares. For despite his bold demonstration of a *caput Nili* of neuropathology, i.e., his trumpeting of the assumed distal etiologic component, Freud had reached a cul-de-sac. The secrets of the neuroses and of human nature lay in the domain of psychology, not neuropathology. In this sense, the neuropathological issue was plainly and simply a dead end. The path left open to Freud proceeded in a completely different direction; it would lead ultimately to a less simplistic view of childhood sexuality and its mental consequences, and to an unrivaled psychology of man.

Why Freud was diverted from this path,[6] even if momentarily, to make proclamations about neuropathology is not pertinent to this study; but it is a topic which might bear interesting fruit in the hands of an investigator of genius.

---

6. Not without reluctance, apparently. For instance, Freud found it necessary to remind himself and the reader not to be distracted from the etiologic discussion by the astonishing fact that "hysterical symptoms can only arise with the co-operation of memories" (p. 197).

The seduction theory, in its insistence on the operation of infantile sexual forces, as inferred from their psychological representations, made a remarkable contribution—a contribution which must not be overshadowed by Freud's assumption that only seduction could generate these forces.

FREUD'S LATER VIEWS ON SEDUCTION

Before proceeding to analyze Freud's own account of his refutation of the seduction theory, I must clarify his subsequent views on seduction. Although he discarded the belief that *in all cases* the psychic scenes at the center of a neurosis were simply the unaltered reproductions of actual events, Freud never denied either the occurrence of seductions or their potential neurosogenic character. For example, in "Three Essays on the Theory of Sexuality" (1905b) Freud wrote: "Thus the sexual abuse of children is found with uncanny frequency among school teachers and child attendants, simply because they have the best opportunity for it" (p. 148). Elsewhere he wrote, "Phantasies of being seduced are of particular interest, because so often they are not phantasies but real memories" (1916–17, p. 370). And he clearly labeled seduction a "common" phenomenon (1931, p. 232; 1940, p. 187), though he specified that the "sexual abuse of children by adults" and children's "seduction by other children" were not universal experiences (1940, p. 187).

Of irrefutable importance is the central role of an actual seduction in one of his famous case histories, that of the Wolf-Man. It is evident that Freud not only made numerous references but attached considerable significance to the Wolf-Man's seduction by his sister. He stated clearly that the Wolf-Man's "seduction by his sister was certainly not a phantasy" (p. 21), but was in fact "an indisputable reality" (p. 97). We will speak later of the effects Freud attributed to this seduction: but let us content ourselves for the moment with directing the reader to the many passages where the seduction is discussed (see pp. 20f., 27, 47, 56, 61, 68, 94, 97, 108f.), and by remarking that Part III of the case history is notably entitled "The Seduction."[7]

_____

7. It is difficult to reconcile Masson's picture of a man who denied the

In 1896 Freud believed that infantile sexuality was the consequence of either the passive experiencing of sexual acts at another's hands, or the active perpetration of sexual acts, in imitation of those to which one had earlier been subjected. As Freud's appreciation of the mental life of children expanded, seduction would come no longer to have such an exclusive role. He discovered that seduction was not the only path to the arousal of a child's sexual life—that indeed infantile sexuality arose from "internal causes" as well. Concomitantly Freud began to credit children with a far more complex mental capacity by recognizing their ability to wish, invent, and fantasize, as well as to record. Naturally these mental processes were grounded in actual experiences, but no longer would Freud's view be so restrictive as to require that a psychic scene formed in childhood need be the impression of an identical extrapsychic experience.

In this new context seduction retained an important, albeit not exclusive, role, and Freud (1931) clearly attributed to it a number of "extensive and lasting consequences" for the sexual life of the child and the psychological character of the adult (p. 232).

Specifically, Freud found that seduction could cause the initial appearance of true genital sensations in the child (1905a, p. 57n.; 1933, p. 120); lead to genital masturbation (1905b, pp. 190, 220; 1917, p. 353; 1940, p. 276) and perversions (1905b, 191f.; 1916–17, p. 209); hasten sexual development, resulting in precocious sexual maturity (1910b, p. 131f.; 1931, p. 242); cause the premature fixation of libido (1922, p. 231); create a behavioral pattern of repeatedly provoking similar acts (1939, p. 75f.); diminish a child's educability (1905b, p. 234); and even interrupt or bring to an end the period of latency (1905b, p. 234).

To the Wolf-Man's seduction Freud attributed his patient's passive sexual aim (1918, pp. 27, 94, 108; 1926, p. 107), his hostility toward women (1918, p. 68), and in general both the encouragement of his sexual development as well as its disturbance and diversion (1918, p. 108).

---

importance of external reality, specifically, of seduction, with the writer who has made the statements quoted above, and who has emphatically drawn our attention, in great detail, to the role of a sexual seduction in the development of his patient's neurosis—all well after he is presumed to have abandoned the seduction theory.

Freud included seduction among the trio of traumas commonly present in the history of neurotics—witnessing parental intercourse, being threatened with castration, and suffering a seduction by an adult. He emphasized the "material reality" of the seductions, which "is often established incontestably through enquiries from older members of the patient's family" (1916–17, p. 368f.). He obviously continued to attribute to seduction an important role in the etiology of the neuroses (1925, p. 34f.).

In summary, we see that throughout his career Freud never doubted either the occurrence of childhood sexual abuse or its significance for the psychological development of an individual. Furthermore, Freud attached much weight to experiences others dismissed as trivial, e.g., the mere *observation* of parental intercourse (1916–17, p. 369), and the hygienic ministrations of mothers (1931, p. 232; 1933, p. 120; 1940, p. 188). Freud was even sensitive to the abusive nature of affectionate games played by parents and other adults with children (1913a, p. 287; 1918, pp. 32, 106). Surely someone as keenly aware of such activities would not disregard the traumatic effects of an actual assault— as Freud's writings undeniably demonstrate over the course of his life.

From Seduction to Spontaneous Sexuality

Throughout this paper I have referred to the etiologic theory of the neuroses propounded by Freud in 1896 as the "seduction theory," albeit reluctantly. Such a designation has the disadvantage of imparting undue emphasis on the secondarily evoked, distal, etiologic component while slighting the fundamental psychological aspects of the theory. I employ the term only for the sake of convenience.

As we have seen, more than seduction formed Freud's early etiologic theory; but even so astute and authoritative a historian as Ernest Jones (1953) fell into the awkward error of proclaiming that Freud had built his entire theory of hysteria on seductions (p. 265), despite simultaneously offering abundant evidence to the contrary (pp. 278–283).

In his now-notorious letter of September 21, 1897 to Fliess, Freud explicitly underscored the points so amply demonstrated in his papers of 1896. After referring to developments which necessitated a revision of a portion of the seduction theory, he wrote, "In this collapse of everything valuable, *the psychological alone has remained untouched*" (1985, p. 266, my italics). Nevertheless, this aspect seems to have received very little attention from historians.[8]

Freud explicitly referred to the seduction theory and the path that led to its revision in several papers. His accounts seem to vary occasionally in details, but in general they provide a consistent and understandable picture. Of paramount importance was the discovery which, in one blow, effectively demolished any etiologic pretensions Freud had reserved for the necessity of an actual seduction in neurosogenesis. He had been able to demonstrate, in *at least one case* of neurosis, that a seduction had *not* occurred—a "contradiction in definitely ascertainable circumstances" (1914, p. 17) of the assumption that the psychic scenes of seduction recounted by patients were *always* representations of actual events.

Now one might wonder how Freud could determine with any accuracy whether or not something had actually occurred in the relatively far past of a patient's life, contending that hard evidence would have been impossible to obtain. As is the case for all historical events not directly witnessed, the question is one of probabilities. There is no reason to conclude that Freud was any more or less accurate in his assessment of probabilities than before. Following the same method of gathering data, Freud had simply encountered a case in which, as far as he could determine, seduction had not taken place, but a neurosis had nevertheless developed. Seductions, therefore, must not be absolutely necessary to the formation of the psychic scenes responsible for neurosogenesis.

In his most lucid account of the revision of his etiologic views, Freud (1914) explained:

> If hysterical subjects trace back their symptoms to traumas that are fictitious, then the new fact which emerges is precisely that they create such scenes in *phantasy*, and this psychical reality requires to be taken into account alongside practical reality.

8. I hope I will be forgiven this incursion into Freud's private correspondence, which I have made only to underscore a point already well established.

This reflection was soon followed by the discovery that these phantasies were intended to cover up the autoerotic activity of the first years of childhood, to embellish it and raise it to a higher plane. And now, from behind the phantasies, the whole range of a child's sexual life came to light [p. 17f.].

In 1896 Freud's understanding of childhood was limited, by no means encompassing the notion of spontaneous infantile sexuality. He came eventually to realize, as described above, that far from being sexually passive children were active sexual creatures of formidable mental capacity.

The first public intimation of this change can be found in the 1898 essay, "Sexuality in the Aetiology of the Neuroses." Here Freud reiterated some basic points made in the papers of 1896 concerning the importance of childhood sexual experiences in neurosogenesis. Although Strachey considered the paper to contain "little more than a restatement of Freud's earlier views on the aetiology of the neuroses" (p. 262), one cannot help noting a few substantial differences. For example, Freud made the truly remarkable statement that "We do wrong to ignore the sexual life of children entirely; in my experience, children are capable of every psychical sexual activity, and many somatic sexual ones as well" (p. 280).

Notwithstanding the qualifying comments that followed, e.g., that the human species in general strives to avoid sexuality in childhood, and that childhood sexual experiences are bound to be pathogenic, this marked a definite departure from views held in 1896. Freud had taken a considerable step in exhibiting such an appreciation for the psychical capabilities of children—a step that brought him nearer to the ideas about infantile sexuality which would eventually find expression in "Three Essays." Furthermore, Freud refrained from employing the terms "seduction," "traumas," "assaults," and the like; he referred instead simply to "the sexual experiences of childhood," reiterating that "the manifestations of the psychoneuroses arose from the deferred action of unconscious psychical traces" of these experiences (p. 281).

The next reference, chronologically, to the etiologic role of seduction occurs, fittingly enough, in the work which Jones calls one of Freud's "two mightiest achievements" (p. 267): "Three

Essays on the Theory of Sexuality." In treating the "accidental external contingencies" that affect sexual activity, e.g., seduction, Freud (1905b) wrote:

> I cannot admit that in my paper on 'The Aetiology of Hysteria' I exaggerated the frequency or importance of that influence, though I did not then know that persons who remain normal may have had the same experiences in their childhood, and though I consequently overrated the importance of seduction in comparison with the factors of sexual constitution and development. Obviously seduction is not required in order to arouse a child's sexual life; that can also come about spontaneously from internal causes [p. 190f.].

It is worth noting again that Freud took pains to give seduction its due, expressly reemphasizing its significance for the 18 analyses he had conducted when he wrote "The Aetiology of Hysteria." It is also worth observing that in "Three Essays," where he indeed proposed the universality of infantile sexuality, Freud intimated that the problem of neurotic etiology could not be fully explained by invoking such a universal phenomenon: constitutional and developmental factors warranted consideration.

Freud's first full description of his path from seduction to spontaneous infantile sexuality was provided in the paper, "My Views on the Part Played by Sexuality in the Aetiology of the Neuroses" (1906). Since it does not differ from the later account quoted above ("On the History"), there is no need for repetition; however, I will have occasion to take into consideration certain details shortly.

We also have the opportunity to resolve an apparent paradox cited by Masson (1984) who notes Freud's claim in "Three Essays" not to have exaggerated the frequency or importance of seduction in 1896, and compares it to Freud's remarks in "My Views" about having overestimated the frequency of seductions.

The context, however, in which the latter statement is made renders its meaning clear and dissolves any ostensible contradiction. Freud (1906) wrote:

> At that time my material was still scanty, and it happened by chance to include a disproportionately large number of cases in which sexual seduction by an adult or by older children played

the chief part in the history of the patient's childhood. I thus over-estimated the frequency of such events (though in other respects they were not open to doubt) [p. 274].

Here Freud still acknowledges the occurrence and etiologic importance of seduction in the cases he had analyzed in 1896; his overestimation lay in extrapolating from his own small sample of cases to *all* cases of neurosis. Indeed, in "The Aetiology of Hysteria" Freud was prepared for the possibility that the nineteenth case could very well invalidate his postulate (see 1896c; p. 200).[9]

In the same paper he rejected outright his earlier attempt at solving the problem of the choice of neuroses, and reemphasized the roles of constitution and heredity in neurosogenesis, correcting his earlier prejudice for accidental influences. He reported the "realization that infantile sexual activity (whether spontaneous or provoked) prescribes the direction that will be taken by later sexual life after maturity" (p. 274), and in his newer etiologic schema replaced "infantile sexual traumas" with the "infantilism of sexuality" (p. 275). Evincing a marked shift of etiologic perspective, he said, "Thus it was no longer a question of what sexual experiences a particular individual had had in his childhood, but rather of his reaction to those experiences—of whether he had reacted to them by 'repression' or not" (p. 276f.).

The sphere of etiologic influences was broadened to include "everything which can act in a detrimental manner upon the processes serving the sexual function" (p. 279). Nevertheless, he was at pains to stress the ideas of 1896 that remained valid, calling the significance of infantile sexual experiences in the etiology of neuroses, which he had established in 1896, one of the cornerstones of psychoanalysis, and asserting that "whatever modifications my views on the aetiology of the psychoneuroses have passed through, there are two positions which I have never

9. In two later accounts, Freud gave the impression that the reports of most of his female patients in 1896 who claimed to have been seduced by their fathers were not true. This is at odds with the statements quoted above, but I suspect that Freud may have been making a general comment referable to the female patients he had seen over a long period of time rather than to the subset of patients he had analyzed when the 1896 papers were written. See Freud (1925, p. 34) and (1933, p. 120).

repudiated or abandoned—the importance of sexuality and of infantilism" (p. 277f.).[10] The frequently cited "abandonment" of the seduction theory is a dramatization of a gradual process of revision involving only a certain portion of the theory. There was never anything approaching a wholesale repudiation.

In addition to the two major works cited above (1906, 1914), the other substantial account of the revision of the seduction theory is contained in "An Autobiograpical Study" (1925). However, in several other works Freud touches briefly on relevant aspects of the topic (see 1905b, p. 190f.; 1916–17, pp. 368–71; 1923, p. 244; 1931, p. 238; 1933, p. 120; 1940, pp. 187ff.). Not only are a number of interesting points raised, but occasionally Freud can be perplexing; therefore it should prove worthwhile to examine some issues.

PSYCHICAL VERSUS EXTERNAL REALITY

After recognizing that hysterics could fantasize the sexual traumas uncovered in the analyses, Freud (1914) was led to the conclusion that "psychical reality requires to be taken into account alongside practical reality" (p. 17f.). In "Two Encyclopaedia Articles" (1923), he stated that fantasy "carried more weight in neurosis than did external reality" (p. 244): and in 1925 Freud wrote that "as far as the neurosis was concerned psychical reality was of more importance than material reality" (p. 34).

A key to this confusing parade of statements is provided by Freud in the *Introductory Lectures on Psycho-Analysis,* where he discussed fantasy, psychical reality, and external reality and, referring to the infantile scenes brought up by the patient in analysis, wrote: "It will be a long time before he [the patient] can take in our proposal that we should equate phantasy and reality and not bother to begin with whether the childhood experiences under examination are the one or the other . . . and we gradu-

10. To call attention to the importance of the contributions of the 1896 theory is not to say that it was a completely adequate, immutable theory. It is instructive to compare it to the vastly more complex, yet still admittedly inadequate "classical" etiologic formula described by A. Freud (1965, p. 150) many years later.

ally learn to understand that *in the world of the neuroses it is psychical reality which is the decisive kind*" (p. 368).

The discovery that some of the traumatic scenes related by hysterics had not actually occurred in no way detracted from their psychic significance. If we return to our schema where psychic scene Z assumed primary importance in neurosogenesis, we see simply that Freud had come to recognize that A was not the sole path to Z. Fantasy, in however slight a degree, was implicated in the alternative route, which we shall label "B." Thus A and B became partners of equal status—their importance lying essentially in their capacity to generate the relevant psychic scenes (Z) at the core of a neurosis.[11] Freud's statement that fantasy carried more weight than external reality becomes intelligible if we assume he used the term "fantasy" as the equivalent of "psychic reality" or "psychic scenes." An example of such usage may be found in the following: "A phantasy of being seduced when no seduction has occurred is usually employed by a child to screen the autoerotic period of his sexual activity" (1916–17, p. 370). Although Freud was no stranger to the notion of psychical reality in 1896, he had not yet grasped the fact that in its utter preeminence it could also differ markedly in content from actual experiences. Either A *or* B could lead to Z.

Additionally, whether or not Freud came to believe that most seductions were fantasized is irrelevant in the face of the psychic power he attributed to the scenes. Far from representing a denigration of individual worth, the appropriate valuation of psychical reality reflects the highest respect for the individual.

THE SCENES OF SEDUCTION

What of the traumatic scenes themselves? How did they arise and what did they represent?

---

11. See Freud (1900): "Real and imaginary events appear in dreams at first sight of equal validity; and that is so not only in dreams but in the production of more important psychical structures" (p. 288). Note also: "Neurotics . . . are only affected by what is thought with intensity and pictured with emotion, whereas agreement with external reality is a matter of no importance" (1913b, p. 86).

In all of the pertinent accounts, with the exception of "An Autobiographical Study," Freud (1916–17) states that the seduction scenes—"*when no seduction has occurred*" (p. 370; my italics)—constituted fantasies that served as attempts to cover up memories of autoerotic infantile sexuality. Once the analyses penetrated this defensive screen, the whole rich realm of spontaneous infantile sexuality could be brought to light.

It is of interest to note in this context that Freud believed the seduction fantasies *not* to have arisen, at least in the form in which they appeared, during the period of childhood to which they purportedly referred. These "imaginary memories" were "mostly produced during the years of puberty" (1906, p. 274). To spare himself shame about childhood masturbation the individual retrospectively fantasizes "a desired object into these earliest times" (1916–17, p. 370).

This last statement alludes to the seduction scenes as manifestations of the oedipus complex, a point explicitly made by Freud (1925 and 1933, p. 120). Bear in mind, however, that Freud's reference to the oedipus complex had to do *only* with his female patients who regularly produced scenes in which their fathers figured as seducers.[12] In the cases of his male patients and in the instances where siblings or other children played the seducer's role, Freud apparently did *not* consider the seduction scenes to be expressions of the oedipus complex; at any rate, he made no mention whatsoever of such a function. Thus, in addition to their role in screening autoerotic infantile activities, the seduction scenes (when they represented *fantasies* and not actual seductions), in some cases at least, expressed wishes that presumably were associated with those activities.

Now that the topics of retrospective fantasies and screening have been raised, a brief digression is in order. In 1899 Freud published a remarkable paper entitled "Screen Memories," which leaves no doubt that by this point he had discarded his earlier assumption that seduction scenes or other childhood "memories" consisted simply of resurrected images that had

---

12. In the 1933 paper, Strachey calls our attention to the fact that nowhere in the pertinent publications of 1896 did Freud specifically mention the fathers of his female patients as seducers (p. 120f.).

been formed during the period to which their content belonged, as the immediate consequence of an experience's impression. What one recollected about childhood is instead a worked-over version of the memory traces laid at the time, which remain unknown in their original form. Thus the distinction between screen memories, which Freud demonstrated as reconstructions, and other memories from childhood became blurred. Freud (1899) concluded:

> It may indeed be questioned whether we have any memories at all *from* our childhood: memories *relating to* our childhood may be all that we possess. Our childhood memories show us our earliest years not as they were but as they appeared at the later periods when the memories were aroused. In these periods of arousal, the childhood memories did not, as people are accustomed to say, *emerge;* they were *formed* at that time. And a number of motives, with no concern for historical accuracy, had a part in forming them, as well as in the selection of the memories themselves [p. 322].

Nevertheless, with respect to these issues as they related to the oedipus complex, Freud (1916–17) wrote:

> But it would be a vain effort to seek to explain the whole Oedipus complex by retrospective phantasying and to attach it to later times. Its infantile core and more or less of its accessories remain as they were confirmed by the direct observation of children [p. 336].

Freud had still more to say about the seduction fantasies of his female patients. Behind the figure of the father lurked that of the child's mother. It was she who, by dint of her role in caring for her child's hygienic needs, unavoidably aroused strong genital sensations. She thus inevitably became the child's first seducer, providing the realistic grounding for the subsequent seduction scenes (Freud, 1931, pp. 232, 238; 1933, p. 120; 1940, p. 188). As Freud stated, "The fact that the mother thus unavoidably initiates the child into the phallic phase is, I think, the reason why, in phantasies of later years, the father so regularly appears as the sexual seducer. When the girl turns away from her mother, she also makes over to her father her introduction into sexual life" (1931, p. 238).

SUMMARY

Freud attributed to the seduction scenes their screening and oedipal functions only when it seemed clear that the seductions as reported had not actually occurred (although even the fact of their occurrence would not necessarily preclude these operations).

Recognition of the oedipus complex in the subset of female patients claiming to have been seduced by their fathers was preceded by Freud's establishment that the seduction scenes could be fantasies, and by his discovery that as fantasies they served a defensive screen covering up autoerotic infantile sexuality, the exploration of which led to the discovery of the oedipus complex.

The reason why adherence to the seduction theory of 1896 would have had "grave consequences" or proved "fatal" to psychoanalysis had nothing to do with belief or disbelief per se in the occurrence of childhood seductions. Rather, it concerned its potential for preventing the psychoanalytic investigation of infantile sexuality. With respect to the consequences of having freed himself from the restrictive assumptions about childhood under which he labored in 1896, Freud was clear and consistent throughout his life. The matter is summarized particularly well in 1925: "When the mistake had been cleared up, the path to the study of the sexual life of children lay open. It thus became possible to apply psycho-analysis to another field of science and to use its data as a means of discovering a new piece of biological knowledge" (p. 35).

It seems inevitable that Freud, adhering to the impartial evaluation of data appearing in free association, would not have been long in reaching the realm of infantile sexuality even if he had not become convinced that some of the seduction scenes had been fantasies. After all, seduction continued to retain a share, though humbler, to be sure, in the etiology of neuroses; but it was subsumed under the more general heading of childhood sexual activities. When seduction took place, it did so in the context of the development and natural history of these infantile sexual phenomena. Seduction and spontaneous sexuality are not mutually exclusive: they can and do indeed coexist.

Freud's journey of discovery, in retrospect, appears eminently reasonable. And his comportment as an investigator can serve as a model for any scientist. When confronted by data that were in disagreement with prevailing assumptions, he accommodated his views to fit the facts, rather than vice versa. Little more can be asked of a man of science; indeed, for most it proves an insurmountable task.

As the science of psychoanalysis developed, the "histopathologic" specificity that marked Freud's early search for the etiology of neuroses gave way to a deeper and broader perspective. In the last years of his life Freud implicated a combination of constitutional and accidental factors, along with biological, cultural, and phylogenetic influences, leaving it "for the science of the future to bring these still isolated data together into a new understanding" (1940, p. 186).

BIBLIOGRAPHY

BREUER, J. & FREUD, S. (1893–95). Studies on hysteria. *S.E.*, 2:1–305.

EISSLER, K. R. (1985). Personal communication.

FREUD, A. (1965). Normality and pathology in childhood. *W.*, 6.

FREUD, S. (1894). The neuro-psychoses of defence. *S.E.*, 3:45–61.

———— (1896a). Heredity and the aetiology of the neuroses. *S.E.*, 3:141–156.

———— (1896b). Further remarks on the neuro-psychoses of defence. *S.E.*, 3:162–185.

———— (1896c). The aetiology of hysteria. *S.E.*, 3:191–221.

———— (1898). Sexuality in the aetiology of the neuroses. *S.E.*, 3:263–285.

———— (1899). Screen memories. *S.E.*, 3:303–322.

———— (1900). The interpretation of dreams. *S.E.*, 4 & 5.

———— (1905a). Fragment of an analysis of a case of hysteria. *S.E.*, 7:7–122.

———— (1905b). Three essays on the theory of sexuality. *S.E.*, 7:135–243.

———— (1906). My views on the part played by sexuality in the aetiology of the neuroses. *S.E.*, 7:271–279.

———— (1910a). Five lectures on psycho-analysis. *S.E.*, 11:7–55.

———— (1910b). Leonardo da Vinci and a memory of his childhood. *S.E.*, 11:63–137.

———— (1913a). The occurrence in dreams of material from fairy tales. *S.E.*, 12:281–287.

———— (1913b). Totem and taboo. *S.E.*, 13:1–161.

———— (1914). On the history of the psycho-analytic movement. *S.E.*, 14:7–66.

———— (1916–17). Introductory lectures on psycho-analysis. *S.E.*, 15 & 16.

_____ (1918). From the history of an infantile neurosis. *S.E.*, 17:7–122.

_____ (1922). Some neurotic mechanisms in jealousy, paranoia and homosexuality. *S.E.*, 18:221–232.

_____ (1923). Two encyclopaedia articles. *S.E.*, 18:235–259.

_____ (1925). An autobiographical study. *S.E.*, 20:7–74.

_____ (1926). Inhibitions, symptoms and anxiety. *S.E.*, 20:87–172.

_____ (1931). Female sexuality. *S.E.*, 21:225–243.

_____ (1933). New introductory lectures on psycho-analysis. *S.E.*, 22:5–182.

_____ (1939). Moses and monotheism. *S.E.*, 23:7–137.

_____ (1940). An outline of psycho-analysis. *S.E.*, 23:144–207.

_____ (1985). *The Complete Letters of Sigmund Freud to Wilhelm Fliess, 1887–1904*, ed. J. M. Masson. Cambridge, Mass: Harvard Univ. Press.

JONES, E. (1953). *The Life and Work of Sigmund Freud*, vol. 1. New York: Basic Books.

MASSON, J. M. (1984). *The Assault on Truth*. New York: Farrar, Straus & Giroux.

A Menagerie of Illustrations from Sigmund Freud's Boyhood

LAWRENCE M. GINSBURG, J.D. AND
SYBIL A. GINSBURG, M.D.

> What someone thinks he remembers from his child-
> hood is not a matter of indifference; as a rule the re-
> sidual memories—which he himself does not under-
> stand—cloak priceless pieces of evidence about the
> most important features in his mental development.
> —FREUD (1910, P. 84)

THE ILLUSTRATIONS REPRODUCED HERE WERE FIRST PUBLISHED BE-
fore Sigmund Freud's teen-age years. According to Ernest Jones
(1953), he "remembered very little of the early period between
the ages of three and seven" and reputedly remarked: "They
were hard times and not worth remembering" (p. 15). Two of
the four memories which Freud, in later life, did attribute to this
four-year period (1859–63) involved pictorial imagery and its
vibrant imprint upon his persona even after coming of age. This
paper documents how such visual stimuli from Freud's preadolescent period were stockpiled and reanimated in subsequent memories and mental attitudes.

As a result of his own self-analysis, Freud realized that pages
of animallike prints often furnish a crucial starting point in reconstructing childhood pathology. Both of the examples re-

Lawrence M. Ginsburg is a member of the New York bar. Sybil A. Ginsburg
is a member of the Psychoanalytic Association of New York and the Western
New York Psychoanalytic Society. She is clinical assistant professor of psychiatry at the State University of New York Health Science Center (Syracuse, New
York).

ported by him (1913) centered around associations to folklore popularized by the brothers Grimm. The second of the two examples was presented as the Wolf-Man's "first anxiety dream" when he "was three, four, or at most five years old" (p. 284). Using illustrations to "Little Red Riding Hood" and "The Wolf and the Seven Little Goats," Freud was able to analyze his patient's dream "by the fact that the anxiety-animal was not an object easily accessible to observation (such as a horse or dog), but was known to him only from stories and picture-books" (p. 286).

1. The Bird-beaked Figures Dream

The Philippson's Bible (1858–59) which Freud began studying in 1863 or 1864 was illustrated with a variety of animals in both naturalistic settings and hybridized with human figures as Egyptian deities (see fig. 1).[1] Readers of *The Interpretation of Dreams* were invited by its author, over a third of a century later, to accompany him while he traced the unconscious determinants of an emotionally charged dream to eye-catching illustrations visualized during his boyhood:[2]

> It is dozens of years since I myself had a true anxiety-dream. But I remember one from my seventh or eighth year, which I submitted to interpretation some thirty years later. It was a very vivid one, and in it I saw *my beloved mother, with a peculiarly peaceful, sleeping expression on her features, being carried into the room by two (or three) people with birds' beaks and laid upon the bed.* I awoke in

---

1. In 1891, Freud's father sent him a volume of the Philippson's Bible as a birthday gift with an inscription, quoted by Ernest Jones (1953), which in part stated: "It was in the seventh year of your age that the spirit of God began to move you to learning. I would say the spirit of God speaketh to you: 'Read in My book; there will be opened to thee sources of knowledge and of the intellect.' It is the Book of Books. . . . Since then I have preserved the same Bible. Now, on your thirty-fifth birthday I have brought it out from its retirement and I send it to you as a token of love from your old father" (p. 19).

2. Jack J. Spector (1973) has cited an 1885 letter which Freud wrote from Paris to Martha Bernays about the obelisk from Luxor in the Place de la Concorde "with the prettiest bird's heads [Vogelkupfen]" as adult evidence of "his constant interest in such curious mongrel figures as those depicted in the Bible" (p. 60).

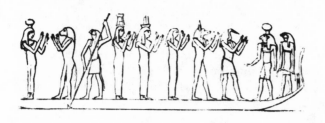

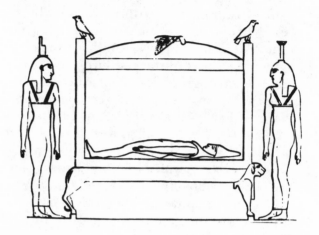

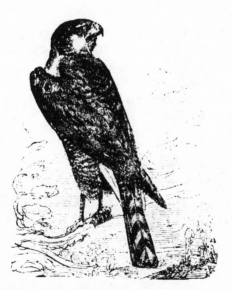

Figure 1. A composite of engravings from Philippson's Bible illustrating Freud's last "true anxiety dream" from *The Aesthetics of Freud* by Jack J. Spector. Copyright (c) 1973 by Praeger Publishers. Reprinted by permission of CBS College Publishing.

tears and screaming, and interrupted my parents' sleep. The strangely draped and unnaturally tall figures with birds' beaks were derived from the illustrations to Philippson's Bible [Freud, 1900, p. 583].

Eva M. Rosenfeld (1956) came to the conclusion that "One part of this dream belongs to Freud alone: his love of beauty expressed in his love and interest in art. It must have been this love of the beautiful and powerful which helped him to repress the frightening aspect of the god-birds" (p. 104).

In the monograph on Leonardo da Vinci, Freud (1910) quoted a "memory" or fantasy recorded by his subject as follows: "It seems that I was always destined to be so deeply concerned with vultures, for I recall as one of my very earliest memories that while I was in my cradle a vulture came down to me, and opened my mouth with its tail, and struck me many times with its tail against my lips" (p. 82). He then proceeded to analyze Leonardo's "vulture phantasy" in terms of its latent content at much greater length than the "birds' beaks" anxiety-dream of his own childhood.

Freud's retrospective autobiographical dream and his discussion of a fantasy or screen memory of Leonardo da Vinci both focus on parallel wildlife symbols.[3] In each instance, the phallic sadism becomes manifest in the choice of image.[4] In the "birds' beak" dream, Freud is the aggressor expressing a latency-aged boy's oedipal drives toward his mother. In Leonardo's "memory," a homosexual theme asserts itself wherein he is the passive victim with lips vulnerable to penetration by the vulture.

2. WILHELM BUSCH

Exactly when the work of Wilhelm Busch initially seized the young Freud's imagination is uncertain.[5] During 1859, while he

3. Addressing Jung on October 17, 1909, Freud wrote: "I have had an inspiration since my return. The riddle of Leonardo da Vinci's character has suddenly become clear to me. That would be a first step in the realm of biography" (McGuire, 1974, p. 255).

4. Michelangelo's *Moses* was another "horn-headed" work of art which commanded the adult Freud's attention.

5. In 1920, Freud observed that after fifty years, he still possessed only one of the books "that had survived from his boyhood" (p. 265).

was presumably learning to read, a serialized composition by
Busch appeared in the humorous and satirical weekly *Fliegende
Blätter* ("Flying Leaves" or "Loose Broadsides").[6] Its complete
title was "Naturgeschichtliches Alphabet für grössere Kinder
und solche, die es werden wollen" ("An Alphabet of Natural
History for Big Children and Those Who Wish to Become
Same"). In a letter written to Carl G. Jung almost a half century
later (McGuire, 1974, p. 339), Freud quoted the contrasting
verses (consolidated in fig. 2) with almost flawless accuracy.
Their most recent translation into English has been rendered as
follows:

> The ass is stupid, hence his name.
> The elephant is not to blame.
>
> The onion is the Hebrew's fare;
> The zebra lives both here and there.

A footnote at the end of the foregoing passage contains the
observation that Freud's reference was to "Busch's famous Abc."
His holographic notation suggests that what he remembered
came from the *A-B-C Buch aus dem Thierreich in Reimen und
Bildern* ("A-B-C Book of the Animal Kingdom in Rhymes and
Pictures"). The illustrations in this 1862 publication were all in
color.

Graphic art found in publications intended for children has
proven valuable in helping biographers re-create the cultural
context in which their subject's intellect developed. A number of
valid questions are manifested by the blatantly anti-Semitic "pic-
togram" at the bottom of figure 2. A theory which had already
been postulated by Freud (1905) offers the following rationale:

> The jokes made about Jews by foreigners are for the most part
> brutal comic stories in which a joke is made unnecessary by the
> fact that Jews are regarded by foreigners as comic figures. The
> Jewish jokes which originate from Jews admit this too; but they
> know their real faults as well as the connection between them
> and their good qualities, and the share which the subject has in

6. Publications embellished with graphic art intended for children were
gaining popularity as Freud's immediate family traveled from his place of birth
to Leipzig and a year later to Vienna. Distribution of the folk press upon
passenger trains and at railroad depots en route was promoted throughout
German-speaking Europe.

E

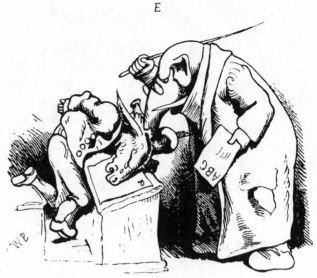

Der **Esel** ist ein dummes Tier,
Der **Elefant** kann nichts dafür.

Z

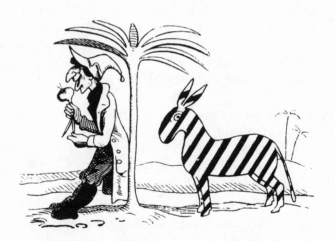

Die **Zwiebel** ist der Juden Speise,
Das **Zebra** trifft man stellenweise.

Figure 2. A composite of the "E" and "Z" illustrations from Wilhelm Busch's "Naturgeschichtliches Alphabet für grössere Kinder und Solche, die es werden wollen." Reproduced from *Wilhelm Busch, Sämtliche Werke,* edited by Otto Noldeke (1943).

the person found fault with creates the subjective determinant (usually so hard to arrive at) of the joke-work [p. 111f.].

What remains perplexing, however, is Freud's need to highlight such an anti-Semitic caricature in his private correspondence with Jung.

The components of figure 3 constitute the last two frames of *Die beiden Enten und der Frosch* ("The Two Ducks and the Frog").[7] It originally appeared in 1861 in the *Münchener Bilderbogen* ("Picture Sheets from Munich") and again in the 1867 book *Schnaken und Schnurren* ("Drolleries and Farces"). Comparison of the side-by-side translation with the version below seems to substantiate an exaggeration in Freud's German rendition of "three long weeks."

The text of Freud's July 1, 1907 letter to Jung reveals the extent to which his associational network centered upon books and animal imagery from "our friend Busch":

> I have read your student's paper with great interest and respect for her formulations of the questions of individual psychology. Naturally I find your ideas and your cool-headedness throughout. It is quite true, I believe, that attitude toward the examiner is a primary factor in determining the content of the reactions. This would be the best way of effecting "studies in transference." For the fun of it, I examined myself by letting myself react to the stimulus-words she uses in her paper. It worked very well, and I was able to explain the strangest answers. A disturbing mistake was that, while I was copying one word my reaction to it was affected by the following word. For instance, I reacted to *Buch—Buschklepper*, then to *Frosch—Busch*. Then of course it all became clear to me. *Frosch* had co-determined my reaction to *Buch* by reminding me of our friend Busch.
>
> > "For six long weeks the frog was ill,
> > But now he's smoking with a will."
>
> Yesterday I had my first good day after several weeks of dyspepsia. Before that I had been reacting exclusively to per-

---

7. The translator-editor's Afterword for the concluding frame included the following commentary: "*But now—praise be!—he's back to smoking:* When Busch himself fell ill, the harbinger of returning health was always his resumption of his inveterate smoking. And, he doubtless said, 'Gott sei Dank!' himself on such occasions."

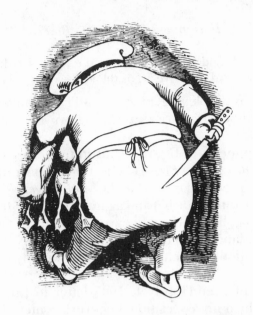

The cook, attracted by the row,
Grabs both and laughs: "I've got
   you now!"

Da kommt der Koch herbei
   sogleich
Und lacht: ,,Hehe, jetzt hab' ich
   euch!"

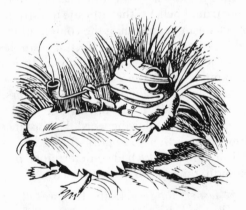

The frog was sick three weeks—
   no joking!—
But now—praise be!—he's back to
   smoking.

Drei Wochen war der Frosch so
   krank!
Jetzt raucht er wieder, Gott sei
   Dank!

Figure 3. Illustrations from Wilhelm Busch's "Die beiden Enten und der Frosch." Reproduced from *Max and Moritz*, edited and translated by H. Arthur Klein. Copyright (c) 1962 by Dover Publications. Reprinted by permission of Dover Publications.

sonal libido-complexes, often in a very obscure and artificial way. The "Klepper" comes from the kleptomania in Gross's book [McGuire, 1974, p. 69f.].

Shared imagery became one of the elements in Freud's transference to Jung and vice versa.[8] The pleasure derived by each of them in including such "visual shorthand" in their correspondence with one another is self-evident. What has been excerpted above provides vivid examples of Freud's propensity for identifying word-roots with various thematic representations.

Freud's proclivity for certain satirical artwork was perhaps an adult outgrowth[9] of his boyhood interests in pictorial stimuli expressive of erotically aggressive drives. Richard F. Sterba (1982) has remarked about his mentor's appetite for the work of "Wilhelm Busch, also an excellent draftsman, who illustrated his own verses with very funny drawings. Freud enjoyed the

---

8. Other references to Busch are found in Freud's July 7, 1909 letter and an undated letter believed to have been written to Jung in mid-1910 as well as Jung's November 22, 1909 letter to Freud. The Wolf-Man, in his recollections of Freud, stated that "Freud also fully appreciated humorists, and greatly admired Wilhelm Busch" (Gardiner, 1971, p. 146). Addressing his former classmate Wilhelm Knoepfmacher, Freud wrote: "During these holidays I have moved into another laboratory, where I am preparing myself for my real profession: 'flaying of animals and torturing of human beings,' and I find myself more and more in favor of the former" (see E. Freud, 1960, p. 6f.). According to George Rosen (1972), the clause following the colon "echoes the phrase 'To tease people, to torture animals' (*Menschen necken, Tiere quälen*) from the preface to *Max und Moritz* by the German humorist Wilhelm Busch (1832–1908)" (p. 23, n. 4).

9. Jack J. Spector (1973) inventoried Busch's output which finally came to rest in Freud's London study as follows: "a group of four Wilhelm Busch drawings: a donkey looking at an artist painting; a fish spitting at a fly; a rhinoceros staring at a Negro; and a chick breaking out of an egg, beside which the date '1 Jan. 1894' was written. Busch was a childhood favorite of Freud's, and his skeptical humor probably affected certain aspects of the psychoanalyst's views on art and the artist. Freud's pessimism, evolved in a climate that also produced Nietzsche's philosophy, found a comforting and amusing parallel in the superb humor of Busch, whose cartoons were known to every German child of the late 1860's and 1870's. Busch's dissection of a pretentiously pious woman (Die fromme Helene) and of an unfulfilled artist (Der Maler Klecksel) whose desires swell to abnormal dimensions, amusingly pre-figure the sharp observations of the disillusionizing Freud" (p. 17).

slapstick descriptions and illustrations of mishaps that Busch's fictitious characters suffered either by accident or through two mischievous boys, 'Max and Moritz,' or by other malicious persons. The delight at the damage or injury inflicted on others by Busch's characters is so often referred to in Freud's books and papers that one cannot help assuming that Freud enjoyed them thoroughly" (p. 74).

3. Friedrich Tschudi's *Animal Life in the Alpine World*

Freud's eldest son referenced a book awarded his father, for academic excellence, about "a study of animal life in the Alps by the Swiss writer, Tschudy" (M. Freud, 1957, p. 21). *Das Thierleben der Alpenwelt* (Tschudi, 1865) with its illustrations were successively viewed by both father and son during their early or preadolescent years and in turn "assumed heirloom status" among subsequent descendants. One such illustration (fig. 4) provides a divergent panorama of striking pictorial models. The left hemisphere of this title page portrays the centered, thus visually dominant world of harsh naturalism. Counterbalanced beyond a precipitous chasm and alongside the right margin, the artist gradually leads the viewer's eye to contrasting perspectives which bespeak harmony and tranquility. Harry Trosman (1985) has characterized the social value of the artist according to Freud as follows: "Not only was the artist the keeper of a wildlife preserve, 'who allows his erotic and ambitious wishes full play,' he also 'finds the way back to realty,' and he moulds 'his phantasies into truths of a new kind, which are valued by men as precious'" (p. 137).

The artistry in figure 5 seems to resemble the stylistic genre of Norman Rockwell a century later on the opposite side of the Atlantic. One is prompted to inquire about Freud's early contact with pet dogs. In his son's words, "My family, and father emphatically so, had unconsciously become dog-lovers. Yet neither father nor mother had kept dogs in their youth" (M. Freud, 1957, p. 190). The canines which the senior Freud adopted during the sixth decade of his life were Chows. With regard to another member of the same breed, Martin Freud noted, "When Marie Bonaparte wrote a book about her favourite Chow, Topsy, father was so delighted with it

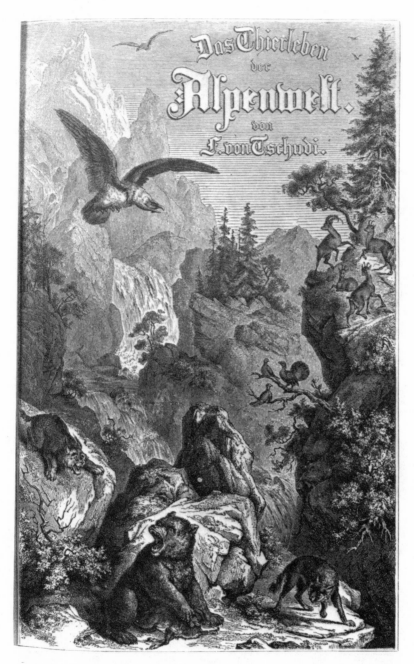

Figure 4.   Title page reproduced from Friedrich Tschudi's *Das Thierleben der Alpenwelt* (1865).

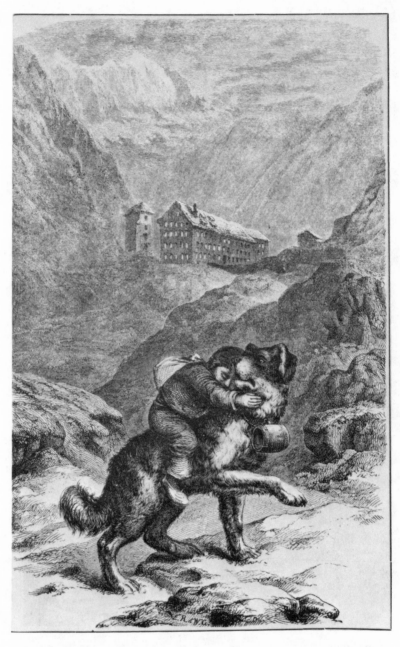

Figure 5.   Illustration reproduced from Friedrich Tschudi's *Das Thierleben der Alpenwelt* (1865).

that, helped by Anna, he translated the little book into German. It was published in 1939 by Albert de Lange of Amsterdam with Anna and Sigmund Freud mentioned as its translators" (p. 203). In elaborating upon the entire household's respect for the sensibility of their dogs, it is asserted that *Jofi*, "the dearest friend of father's later years," was his "favourite and never left him, not even when he treated patients" (p. 190).

4. ALFRED E. BREHM'S *ANIMAL LIFE WITH ILLUSTRATIONS*

According to Freud's older sister (Bernays, 1940), he won another book prize at age 11. She remembered the title as "a famous *History of Animal Life*" (p. 336). It has been further identified as "the popular *Life of Animals*" by Alfred E. Brehm (Knoepfmacher, 1979, p. 289). A "popular" series of Brehm's major work was edited by Friedrich Schodler (1868–70). The English translations cited by Bernays and Knoepfmacher suggest that Freud could have been the recipient of Volume I soon after its publication during either the last four months of his eleventh year or the first eight months of his twelfth year.

The use of animals as a vehicle for the expression of human conflict undoubtedly nurtured the "mind's eye" of the young Freud. A graphic example, rich in erotic and aggressive symbols (fig. 6), by Friedrich Specht captioned "The Common Porcupine" depicts the artist's subject "with spines erect ready to defend itself . . . because of the threatening appearance of the Snake in the foreground" (Peschuel-Loesche and Haacke, 1895, p. 355). The significance of porcupines upon the structuring of Freud's psychoanalytic thought has been examined elsewhere (Ginsburg, 1985).

5. THE BOTANICAL MONOGRAPH DREAM

I shall only quote enough of the dream to indicate the source we are looking for: . . . *I had written a* MONOGRAPH *on a certain* (indistinct) *species of plant. Source:* That morning I had seen a *monograph* on the genus Cyclamen in the window of a book-shop. . . . *The book lay before me and I was at the moment turning over a folded coloured plate. Bound up in each copy there was a dried specimen of the*

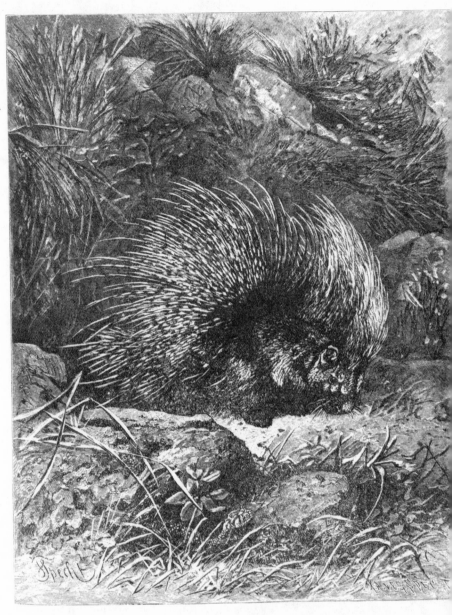

Figure 6.   Illustration for Alfred E. Brehm's *Illustrirtes Thierleben*. Reproduced from Brehm's *Life of Animals* (Chicago, 1895). Courtesy of Cornell University Libraries.

plant, as though it had been taken from a herbarium [Freud, 1900, p. 165 and p. 169].

In his dream interpretation, Freud (1900) associated to a screen memory dating back to 1861 or early 1862. He described it as follows:

> It had once amused my father to hand over a book with *coloured plates* (an account of a journey through Persia) for me and my eldest sister to destroy. Not easy to justify from the educational point of view! I had been five years old at the time and my sister not yet three; and the picture of the two of us blissfully pulling the book to pieces (leaf by leaf, like an *artichoke*, I found myself saying) was almost the only plastic memory that I retained from that period of my life. Then, when I became a student, I had developed a passion for collecting and owning books, which was analogous to my liking for learning out of monographs: a *favourite hobby*. (The idea of *'favourite'* had already appeared in connection with cyclamens and artichokes.) I had become a *bookworm*. I had always from the time I first began to think about myself, referred this first passion of mine back to the childhood memory I have mentioned. Or rather, I had recognized that my childhood scene was a 'screen memory' for my later bibliophile propensities [Cf. my paper on screen memories]. [p. 172f.].

Many clues to important aspects of Freud's personality are undoubtedly buried in the analysis of his screen memory about "a book with *coloured plates*." Uncamouflaged, as a strategem with which he credited himself at a precocious age for gaining intellectual mastery and power, is the mobilization of knowledge via book ownership.

Freud then declined to pursue the dream interpretation any further.[10] The analytic reader was left to hypothesize about the childhood passions with which his *"favourite hobby"* of book collection was linked. For our purposes, it seems fair to conclude that he was aware of his libidinization of the illustrations viewed by him as a youth and their indelible imprint upon his erotic-aggressive drive development.

---

10. His next paragraph began as follows: "For reasons with which we are not concerned, I shall not pursue the interpretation of this dream any further, but will merely indicate the direction in which it lay" (p. 173).

CONCLUSION

The precise details from a small sample of the animated illustrations which absorbed Freud during his own childhood have been resurrected in this paper for further study. An Alpine bestiary, a St. Bernard dog, a donkey and an elephant, two ducks and a frog, a falcon, a porcupine versus a snake, a zebra as well as assorted Egyptian "god-birds," and a dormant "book-worm" emerge from the shrouded object world of Freud's early life.

Anna Freud (1966) contrasted two developmental prototypes and their progression toward adolescence:

> Some boys love to read about discoveries and adventures or to study numbers and proportions or to devour descriptions of strange animals and objects, while others confine their attention to machinery, from the simplest to the most complicated form. The point which these two types usually have in common is that the object in which they are interested must be a concrete one, not the product of fantasy like the fairy tales and fables enjoyed in early childhood, but something which has an actual physical existence. When the prepubertal period begins, a tendency for the concrete interests of the latency period to give place to abstractions becomes more and more marked [p. 159].

She subsequently elaborated upon the epic nature of animal imagery in the fantasy life of children:

> I must say I was fascinated at the time by animal fantasies, and I always regretted that we didn't make more of a collection of them, because they are really marvelous. . . . Now it's television monsters, space creatures, whereas at that time it was what the children saw in the circus and heard about in their fairy stories. They had different sources [Sandler and A. Freud, 1985, p. 328f.].

When one reads her father's writings, the reader senses how the residue of illustrations which he viewed continued to come alive for him and assert themselves in his daily life.[11]

---

11. During his adult years, Freud often referred to certain emotional reactions associated almost contemporaneously with particular illustrations which he had pondered. One such review was contained in a letter to his fiancée on August 23, 1883 (E. Freud, 1960, pp. 44–47) after contemplating an illustra-

BIBLIOGRAPHY

BERNAYS, A. F. (1940). My brother, Sigmund Freud. *Amer. Mercury*, 51:335–342.

BREHM, A. E. (1864–65). *Illustriertes Thierleben.* Hildburghausen: Bibliographisches Institut.

BUSCH, W. (1859). Naturgeschichtliches Alphabet für grössere Kinder und solche, die es werden wollen. *Fliegende Blätter*, no. 784, p. 12f.; no. 785, p. 20f.; no. 786, p. 29f.

———— (1865). *Max and Moritz.* New York: Dover.

FREUD, A. (1936). The ego and the mechanisms of defense. *W.*, 2.

FREUD, E. L., ed. (1960). *Letters of Sigmund Freud.* New York: Basic Books.

FREUD, M. (1957). *Glory Reflected.* London: Angus & Robertson.

FREUD, S. (1900). The interpretation of dreams. *S.E.*, 4 & 5.

———— (1905). Jokes and their relation to the unconscious. *S.E.*, 8.

———— (1910). Leonardo da Vinci and a memory of his childhood. *S.E.*, 11:59–137.

———— (1913). The occurrence in dreams of material from fairy tales. *S.E.*, 12:279–287.

———— (1920). A note on the prehistory of the technique of analysis. *S.E.*, 18:263–265.

GARDINER, M., ed. (1971). *The Wolf-Man by the Wolf-Man.* New York: Basic Books.

GINSBURG, L. M. (1985). The imprint of Sigmund Freud's interest in porcupines upon the psychoanalytic study of group constructs. *Psychoanal. Contemp. Thought*, 8:515–528.

JONES, E. (1953). *Sigmund Freud,* vol. 1. New York: Basic Books.

KNOEPFMACHER, H. (1979). Sigmund Freud in high school. *Amer. Imago*, 36:287–299.

McGUIRE, W., ed. (1974). *The Freud/Jung Letters* (1906–1914). Princeton, N.J.: Princeton Univ. Press.

NOLDEKE, O., ed. (1943). *Wilhelm Busch, Sämtliche Werke.* Munich: Braun & Schneider.

PESCHUEL-LOESCHE, E. & HAACKE, W., eds. (1895). *The Animals of the World.* Chicago: Marquis.

PHILIPPSON, L. (1858–59). *Die Israelitische Bibel.* Leipzig: Baumgartner's Buchhandlung.

---

tion by Gustave Dore published in a late nineteenth-century edition of Cervantes' *Don Quixote.* Another appears in a passage about the content of his "Open-air Closet" dream which he connected to an illustration by Jules Garnier published in *Rabelais et l'Oeuvre* during the same period *The Interpretation of Dreams* was in final preparation. It was identified by him as among those illustrations which he had "on the previous evening before going to sleep . . . been turning over" (1900, p. 469).

ROSEN, G. (1972). Freud and medicine in Vienna. In *Freud,* ed. J. Miller. Boston: Little, Brown, pp. 21–39.

ROSENFELD, E. M. (1956). Dream and vision. *Int. J. Psychoanal.,* 37:97–105.

SANDLER, J. & FREUD, A. (1985). *The Analysis of Defense.* New York: Int. Univ. Press.

SPECTOR, J. J. (1973). *The Aesthetics of Freud.* New York: Praeger.

STERBA, R. F. (1982). *Reminiscences of a Viennese Psychoanalyst.* Detroit: Wayne State Univ. Press.

TROSMAN, H. (1985). *Freud and the Imaginative World.* Hillsdale, N.J.: Analytic Press.

TSCHUDI, F. (1865). *Das Thierleben der Alpenwelt.* Leipzig: J. J. Weber.

APPLIED PSYCHOANALYSIS

Ancient Mariner, Pilot's Boy
A Note on the Creativity of
Samuel Coleridge

EUGENE J. MAHON, M.D.

> In looking at objects of nature . . . at yonder moon dim
> glimmering through the dewy window pane, I seem
> rather to be seeking, as it were asking, a symbolical
> language for something within me that forever and
> already exists, than observing anything new. Even
> when that latter is the case yet still I have always an
> obscure feeling, as if that new phenomenon were a
> dim awakening of a forgotten or hidden truth of my
> inner nature.
> —COLERIDGE AS QUOTED BY CLARK (1981, P. 11)

> But I do not think "The Rime of the Ancient Mariner"
> was for Coleridge an escape from reality: I think it was
> reality, I think he was on the ship and made the voyage
> and felt and knew it all.
> —WOLFE (1932, P. 322)

WHEN COLERIDGE DIED IN 1834 CHARLES LAMB REMARKED, "NEVER saw I his likeness nor probably the world can see again." And a few years later, John Stuart Mill said of him, "The class of thinkers has scarcely yet arisen by whom he is to be judged." This is high praise indeed for a man who lived most of his life in misery, was addicted to opium, suffered from loneliness, depression, and sleeplessness most of his life, and who wrote of

Assistant clinical professor of psychiatry, Columbia University, College of
Physicians and Surgeons, and a member of the faculty (child analysis and adult
analysis) at Columbia University Center for Psychoanalytic Training and
Research.

himself, "I am loving and kindhearted and cannot do wrong with impunity but O I am very weak—from my infancy have been so—and I exist for the moment," and who wrote his own epitaph:

> Stop, Christian passer-by—Stop child of God
> and read with gentle breast. Beneath this sod
> a poet lies or that which once seemed he.
> O lift one thought in prayer for S.T.C.
> that he who many a year with toil of breath
> found death in life may here find life in death
> mercy for praise—to be forgiven for fame
> he asked and hoped through Christ. Do thou the same
> [p. 216].

Samuel Taylor Coleridge has been a source of endless fascination for the literary critic and applied psychoanalyst for practically two centuries. This is not surprising since the "sage of Highgate," as he came to be called later in life when so many of the day's finest thinkers beat a path to his door to hear him speak, had a multifaceted telescopic mind that seemed incapable of ignoring any psychological meteorite that swam into its ken. As a poet in collaboration with Wordsworth he practically launched a new Romantic movement with the publication of the *Lyrical Ballads* in 1798. But he was also a philosopher, a literary critic, a theologian, a political thinker, and a theoretician of the imagination.

One of the poems in the *Lyrical Ballads* was called "The Rime of the Ancient Mariner." It has had the genuine stamp and appeal of a classic from its inception: a blend of gothic imagery and classical, yet simple language hold the reader for 625 lines in a compelling aesthetic trance that demands interpretation even as swiftly as it eludes it.

The poem, which ostensibly deals with an ancient mariner, has a significant section about a pilot's boy, and I will attempt to explain why this child and his father make a sudden, almost uncanny appearance toward the end of the poem. It is my contention that certain childhood events suddenly erupted into the latter lines of the poem, disguised to be sure, but highly evocative of their genetic origins.

I

I begin by introducing the gist of the poem.

> It is an ancient Mariner
> And he stoppeth one of three.
> "By thy long grey beard and glittering eye,
> Now wherefore stopp'st thou me?"

The mariner has collared one of the wedding guests and forces him to listen to his story. Coleridge uses this dramatic device to great effect throughout the poem: a harrowing tale told to a listener who is reluctant to listen at first but gradually gets caught up in the web of the story. The mariner describes the journey from start to finish.

> "The ship was cheered, the harbour cleared.
> Merrily did we drop
> Below the kirk, below the hill,
> Below the lighthouse top."

[A storm drives the ship south into a region of snow and mist.]

> The ice was here, the ice was there,
> The ice was all around:
> It cracked and growled, and roared and howled,
> Like noises in a swound!

[Suddenly an albatross appears, coming through the snow-fog and brings good luck with it.]

> The ice did split with a thunder-fit;
> The helmsman steered us through!

The ship returns northward through fog and floating ice followed by the albatross. Suddenly the mariner in a seemingly inexplicable act kills the bird. His shipmates criticize him at first.

> Ah wretch! said they, the bird to slay,
> That made the breeze to blow!

[But when the fog clears, they reverse themselves.]

> 'Twas right, said they, such birds to slay,
> That bring the fog and mist.

[The fair breeze continues and all seems well for the voyage.]

> The fair breeze blew, the white foam flew,
> The furrow followed free;
> We were the first that ever burst
> Into that silent sea.

[But suddenly the wind dies down and the voyage comes to a standstill.]

> Down dropt the breeze, the sails dropt down,
> 'Twas sad as sad could be:
> And we did speak only to break
> The silence of the sea! . . .
> Day after day, day after day,
> We stuck, nor breath nor motion;
> As idle as a painted ship
> Upon a painted ocean.
>
> Water, water, every where,
> And all the boards did shrink;
> Water, water, every where,
> Nor any drop to drink. . . .
>
> The very deep did rot: O Christ!
> That ever this should be!
> Yea, slimy things did crawl with legs
> Upon the slimy sea.

It seems clear that the albatross is being avenged. The shipmates hang the dead sea bird around the ancient mariner's neck, highlighting his guilt rather than their own.

A skeleton ship suddenly appears, manned by a spectre-woman and her death-mate.

> And is that Woman all her crew?
> Is that a DEATH? and are there two?
> Is DEATH that woman's mate? . . .
>
> The Night-mare LIFE-IN-DEATH was she,
> Who thicks man's blood with cold.

[Death and Life-in-Death dice for the ship's crew and she wins the ancient mariner: the crew dies cursing the ancient mariner.]

> The souls did from their bodies fly,—
> They fled to bliss or woe!
> And every soul, it passed me by,
> Like the whizz of my cross-bow!

[The mariner's guilt is exquisite.]

> The many men, so beautiful!
> And they all dead did lie:
> And a thousand thousand slimy things
> Lived on; and so did I.

[The mariner is alone, accompanied only by "the curse in a dead man's eye." But he turns toward nature for consolation.]

> The moving moon went up the sky,
> And no where did abide:
> Softly she was going up,
> And a star or two beside—

[And he notices the animals of the deep.]

> Beyond the shadow of the ship,
> I watched the water-snakes:
> They moved in tracks of shining white,
> And when they reared, the elfish light
> Fell off in hoary flakes. . . .

> O happy living things! no tongue
> Their beauty might declare:
> A spring of love gushed from my heart,
> And I blessed them unaware.

> The self-same moment I could pray;
> And from my neck so free
> The Albatross fell off, and sank
> Like lead into the sea.

The tide turns for the mariner, so to speak.

Benign spirits inhabit the bodies of the crew and the voyage is able to resume. But the mariner's guilt requires further punishment, and less cooperative spirits comment, "The man hath penance done, And penance more will do." The mariner suffers another attack from the eyes of the dead crew before the curse is finally expiated.

> The pang, the curse, with which they died,
> Had never passed away:
> I could not draw my eyes from theirs,
> Nor turn them up to pray.

The mariner suddenly finds himself close to his native country. It is at this point that a pilot and the pilot's boy make a sudden entrance, accompanied by a hermit. They save the unconscious mariner after his ship suddenly sinks.

> But swift as dreams, myself I found
> Within the Pilot's boat. . . .
>
> I moved my lips—the Pilot shrieked
> And fell down in a fit;
> The holy Hermit raised his eyes,
> And prayed where he did sit.
>
> I took the oars: the Pilot's boy,
> Who now doth crazy go,
> Laughed loud and long, and all the while
> His eyes went to and fro.
> "Ha! Ha!" quoth he, "full plain I see,
> The Devil knows how to row."

The mariner is shrived by the hermit. He is relieved of guilt but not permanently. The repressed returns at "uncertain hours," as Coleridge puts it.

> Since then, at an uncertain hour,
> That agony returns:
> And till my ghastly tale is told,
> This heart within me burns.
> I pass, like night, from land to land;
> I have strange power of speech;
> That moment that his face I see,
> I know the man that must hear me:
> To him my tale I teach.

[The poem ends with the mariner's advice to the wedding guest.]

> Farewell, farewell! but this I tell
> To thee, thou Wedding-Guest!
> He prayeth well, who loveth well
> Both man and bird and beast.

[The wedding guest is so affected by the tale that he cannot rejoin the wedding ceremonies.]

> He went like one that hath been stunned,
> And is of sense forlorn:

A sadder and a wiser man,
He rose the morrow morn.

The poem is lush with imagery and symbolism and has been studied extensively. Themes of crime, punishment, death, rebirth, trauma, expiation, mourning, repeating, remembering, and working through make it an ideal hunting ground for interpreters of all persuasions, literary and psychoanalytic. Both have been well represented. I will choose the critiques of one literary critic and one psychoanalyst to suggest the flavor of aesthetic criticism that the poem has engendered.

Jonathan Livingston Lowes stands head and shoulders above all others. The *Road to Xanadu* by Lowes is such a creative study of Coleridge's imagination that subsequent scholarship, psychoanalytic and otherwise, must pale by comparison. Lowes, using Coleridge's notebooks as his guide, is able to immerse himself in the literary imagination of the poet so that he can come pretty close to what was on Coleridge's mind as he was putting pen to paper to create "Christabel" or "Xanadu" or "The Rime of the Ancient Mariner." "Pretty close" is the kind of yardstick that applied psychoanalysis has to settle for, since it is impossible to get the posthumous free associations of the artist to his creative product, the only kind of "evidence" that would really convince a psychoanalyst or any other investigator who seeks "aesthetic" truth, for that matter.

This is not meant to suggest that Lowes has had a monopoly on the Coleridge market. In fact, Coleridge scholarship has flourished since Lowes's time. For instance, whereas Lowes relied mainly on the famous Gutch notebook of S. T. C., Kathleen Coburn has unearthed several other notebooks which have now been published and have opened vast new vistas on the polymorphous imagination of the poet.

The poem has much to interest the psychoanalyst. The format of the poem is essentially a communication between two people: the one compelled to tell a story; the other, an unwilling listener at first, becomes later a sadder and wiser man. A comparison to the psychoanalytic situation is so suggestive as to be almost mandatory. There is trauma that must be talked about; there is reluctant listening that eventually becomes empathy.

David Beres (1951) contended that Coleridge's mother, significantly absent from his correspondence and other personal writings, may have entered indirectly into his literary life, leaving an imprint on his poetry in the form of preoedipal preoccupations. For example, according to Beres, the ancient mariner, guilty of a crime (the slaying of an albatross), is punished by being lost at sea without wind to move the sails, without water to slake his thirst, without sleep, without object relations (the crew dies). Beres argues that since the punishment has such a preoedipal ring to it (thirst, sleeplessness, abandonment), the crime must have been a preoedipal one—Coleridge's hatred of his depriving mother.

While Beres's interpretation of the text is not unconvincing, an alternate reading of "The Rime of the Ancient Mariner" occurred to me as I was reviewing Coleridge's autobiographical letters. I first give a brief sketch of Coleridge's life and then extract what I consider to be some key genetic moments from the autobiographical letters.

II

Samuel Taylor Coleridge was born October 21, 1772 at Ottery St. Mary, Devonshire, England. His father, a clergyman and schoolmaster, had 4 children by his first wife, 10 by his second. Samuel was the youngest. His relationship with his mother, as David Beres has argued, seems to have been cold and distant. He rarely mentions her in his writings. His relationship with his father is described in very warm terms. "I remember and never shall forget my father's face as he looked upon me while I lay in the servant's arms . . . for I was the child of his old age" (p. 224). This idyllic relationship was to be short-lived, the father dying when Coleridge was 10 years old. His mother sent him to London to complete his early schooling at Christ's Hospital, a famous charitable institution known as the Blue-coat School. His younger schoolmates Charles Lamb, in his essay "Christ's Hospital Five and Thirty Years Ago," and Leigh Hunt, in his autobiography, have given vivid accounts of their experiences. Memories of these years of sudden disenfranchisement from family occur frequently in Coleridge's writings.

At 19 Coleridge left London to accept a scholarship at Jesus College, Cambridge. He studied seriously for a short time, but soon his encyclopedic mind caught fire and he was reading everything except what he was supposed to read. "His mind was a ferment of newly discovered political and religious ideas," as Martin Gardner (1965, p. 10) has asserted.

There was revolution in France. Burke was writing his great political pamphlets. Coleridge's room at Cambridge was a beehive of intellectual activity; and there was no need to have the latest political tract on hand; Coleridge had always read it and would repeat whole passages word for word.

But his intellectual prowess, so clearly in evidence in Cambridge, would not discover its aesthetic birthright in the creation of "The Rime of the Ancient Mariner" and other brilliant works before two harebrained expressions of his psyche insisted on coming to the fore. To a psychoanalyst one sounds like suicide and the other an enactment of a family romance fantasy. But I have gotten ahead of myself. Let us return to Coleridge still in Cambridge, brilliant, scattered, irresponsible, and beginning to sink under the weight of his debts. When a plan to win the "Irish Lottery" did not materialize into the dream solution he had envisaged, he became despondent and suicidal. His next move was picaresque in the extreme. Under the name of Silas Tomkyn Comberbacke (thus preserving his initials) he enlisted in the 15th Light Dragoons, a cavalry unit of the King's Regiment. Hanson (1938) writes, "As a soldier of any kind, Coleridge would have been misplaced. As a cavalry man, he was a joke. He did not like horses: he could not ride: he was constantly thrown: he never learned to groom his horse: his accoutrements were never clean: he was constantly unwell" (p. 11).

Charitably, Coleridge's family obtained his discharge by providing a substitute, and in 1794 he was back at Jesus College. Soon he was hatching new schemes, one of which I have referred to earlier as an enactment of a family romance fantasy.

The plan was for 12 "gentlemen of good education and liberal principles" with 12 equally endowed ladies to leave England and establish a colony in North America on the banks of the Susquehanna. There, utopia would be established. Coleridge called it Pantisocracy, a newly coined Greek hybrid meaning government by all, as opposed to England's hated aristocracy!

Needless to say, this utopian dream was never realized. But it did lead to a marriage that in today's terms sounds more like a soap opera. Coleridge, in love with Mary Evans, decides to marry Sarah Fricker since Robert Southey, engaged to Edith Fricker, is one of the 12 who will accompany him to America.

"The first years of Coleridge's marriage were happy enough," according to Martin Gardner (1965). "He and Sarah lived mostly on money borrowed from friends, and small sums that Coleridge obtained from poetry" (p. 13). But tragedy and greatness were waiting impatiently in the wings of his life. Rheumatic pains were leading to increasing use of opium. (At Cambridge during an attack of rheumatic fever and jaundice he had been treated with small doses of opium and had slowly developed an addiction to the drug.)

But greatness was also imminent. In 1797, the Coleridges befriended the Wordsworths. Much has been written about Samuel, William, and Dorothy, and their mutual influences on each other. I would like to focus my attention on the triangular psychological climate that nourished the early creativity of Coleridge, neglecting all that came after which has been well documented. (I am referring to Coleridge's marital problems, drug dependency, medical treatment at Highgate, etc., all of which is beyond the scope and needs of this presentation.)

In July 1797, the Wordsworths, wishing to be closer to the Coleridges, moved to Alfoxden, an old mansion not far from Stowey. Coleridge was ecstatic. The next 12 months would be the most creative of his life. "The Ancient Mariner," the first part of "Christabel," and "Kubla Khan" were written (at fever pitch one imagines) before the middle of the following year.

The genesis of "The Ancient Mariner" is worthy of detailed description. John Cruikshank, a neighbor, had a dream about a "skeleton ship, with figures in it." This, coupled with some suggestions of Wordsworth, incites Coleridge to write a sea ballad. Dorothy, William, and Samuel go for a walk through the Quantock Hills. They decide to defray the expense of the tour by writing a poem to be sent to the *New Monthly Magazine*. They worked together on it, Wordsworth suggesting certain ideas about the killing of a bird and the revenge of the tutelary spirits. But soon their styles proved to be unalloyable, and Coleridge went on to write the ballad by himself. He worked on the ballad for 4 months before he read it to the Wordsworths in March 1798.

The poem seems different from anything Coleridge ever produced before or after. As Martin Gardner (1965) puts it, "It
seemed to spring out of Coleridge's skull with a fantastic life of
its own" (p. 18). I will end this brief biographical sketch at this
point and attempt to show that this poem that seems "to have a
fantastic life of its own" is indeed the brainchild of Samuel Taylor Coleridge and bears some indelible marks of his childhood
and the genius that was spawned there.

III

Now that I have reviewed the poem and reviewed Coleridge's
life, I would like to share with the reader that I have withheld
certain genetic events that in my opinion are crucial to an understanding of the poem from a psychodynamic point of view. I
have withheld them because they seem to get short shrift in most
biographies of Coleridge despite the fact that Coleridge himself
puts a certain emphasis on them in his autobiographical letters
written in 1797. I would like to suggest that S.T.C., like an analysand, was in a ferment of regressive and creative energies, remembering, sublimating, now one now the other.

The poem is an artistic product that is full of guilt, suffering,
masochism, repetition compulsion, murder, and retaliation, all
the elements of a classical neurosis, in other words, except that it
also happens to be a finely crafted creative act of genius. One is
permitted to speculate perhaps that the author of this masterpiece struggled with some unconscious imaginary crime which
he attempted to make sense of not only through the conduct of
his life, but also in his literary expressions. As sleuths of the
imagination, it would be neat indeed if we could at this point sift
through the pages of the suspect's childhood and find clues that
would help us to construct a hypothesis or two.

If Coleridge's father had a premonitory dream about his own
death a few hours prior to the event and if Coleridge himself, 9
years old at the time, also claimed some premonitory knowledge
of the event, we might be willing to consider the possibility that
the child's imagination would forever be unconsciously charged
with unresolvable oedipal angst. If the evening of the father's
death was coincidentally the evening that the father brought
Frank, Coleridge's rivalrous older brother, to begin his appren-

ticeship on board ship, we would feel sympathetic indeed toward the young Coleridge who in one fateful evening had dispatched two oedipal rivals with one blow, so to speak. If we add the content of Coleridge's father's premonitory dream, namely, that death came and touched him with his dart, we would have a plot that was thickening.

If there were documented evidence of a fight between the two brothers, in which Samuel Taylor Coleridge chased Frank with a knife until the latter fell down pretending to be dead, for instance, and then quickly revivified to tease the alarmed younger brother who fled from the scene, hiding out on a hill for many hours in an act of sullen sadomasochistic revenge until he was discovered by the townspeople; and if I could describe a similar event disguised in the imagery of the poem, my case would be strengthened.

Our vigilant minds would no doubt flash back and forth from the poem to the childhood, comparing and contrasting crossbow, dart, and knife in the poem with the dart-knife of childhood looking for fingerprints. The same vigilance would lead us back and forth from the significance of the ship in the poem— we know that Coleridge was inspired to write "The Rime of the Ancient Mariner" when a friend, John Cruikshank, made reference to a dream about a ship, "a skeleton ship with figures in it"—back to the significance of the ship of childhood which claimed his brother. It would also be helpful to our case if Coleridge had a screen memory which contained elements of the poem, a memory of inoculation in which he indignantly removed the bandage from his eyes so that he might see the lancet. A disavowal of the importance of this memory by the young defendant would only strengthen the case against him, negation, as Freud (1925) has taught us, being the most reliable index of repressed unconscious evidence. To make a long story short, if we could find the fingerprints of Coleridge's childhood, on the father's corpse, on the ship that banished his brother, on the dart in the dream that warned his father of his approaching death, on the doctor's lancet of inoculation that Coleridge insisted on seeing at age 3, on the knife with which Coleridge lunged at his brother—if we could find all those fingerprints in 1775 and find them again in 1798 in the mind of the great poet as he put pen to paper, our case would begin to stand on reasonably firm if speculative ground.

My case would be further strengthened by two documented pieces of information about the composition of "The Rime of the Ancient Mariner": not only was the poem inspired in part by a ship in a dream of a friend already mentioned, but we also know that Coleridge abandoned a project on Cain which he had planned to write in collaboration with Wordsworth. In other words, if ship and dream have a connection with the father's premonitory dream the night the father took Frank to the ship's captain for his apprenticeship, the turning away from the Cain and Abel story would seem to be a rejection of certain elements of his memory: a frankly fratricidal theme was being abandoned in favor of a much more disguised murder, the killing of an albatross.

What I have been building up as an imaginary case turns out to be the record of Coleridge himself. I have taken it largely from the autobiographical letters written to Thomas Poole in 1798. The record has its own significance inasmuch as it is a sort of confessional myth offered by Coleridge to his old friend and father figure and patron on the eve of his writing his masterpiece.

IV

The autobiographical letters that Coleridge wrote to his patron Thomas Poole, in February 1797, are significant for many reasons. This was clearly *the* poetic year of Coleridge's life. Unable to have him free associate in the present, we welcome the fact that at the time or around the time he was concocting his greatest poetry, he was reviewing his genetics with a friend and patron. The autobiographical letters stop short in 1782, a year after the father's death, as if Coleridge sensed that these 10 years were the formative ones. The letters to Poole begin:

Monday, February, 1797

My Dear Poole,

I would inform the dullest author how he might write an interesting book. Let him relate the events of his own life with honesty, not disguising the feelings that accompanied them.

What follows in subsequent letters sounds almost like an analysis, Coleridge the analysand offering his genetic past to his analyst patron.

These letters give a good sense of Coleridge's relationships with his brother Frank and with his father, and also of the first 3 years of his life. Coleridge tries to organize his memory describing in one letter the events from his first birthday to his second and from his second birthday to his third, and so on. He makes a parapraxis citing his birthday as October 20 rather than the correct date of October 21, 1772, suggesting that the birth of the last child of 10 was not devoid of conflictual significance.

Coleridge was inoculated between 2 and 3 and here is his description of it.

> I was inoculated; which I mention because I distinctly remember it, and that my eyes were bound; at which I manifested so much obstinate indignation, that at last they removed the bandage and unaffrighted I looked at the lancet, and suffered the scratch. . . . Here I shall end because the remaining years of my life all assisted to form *my particular mind*—The three first years had nothing in them that seems to relate to it.

As mentioned earlier, Coleridge's dismissal of the meaning of these childhood events does not rob them of the genetic significance that I am assigning them.

An earlier memory of trauma and rage also is dismissed as insignificant. Here is Coleridge's description of an event from the second year of his childhood.

> In this year I was carelessly left by my nurse, ran to the fire, and pulled out a live coal—burnt myself dreadfully. While my hand was being dressed by a Mr. Young, I spoke for the first time (so my mother informs me) and said 'nasty Dr. Young.' The snatching at fire and the circumstance of my first words expressing hatred to professional men—are they at all *ominous?*

Though Coleridge dismisses these early traumas, he is not completely ignorant of the uncanny, ominous, resurrectable force of the repressed!

The passages in the autobiographical letters that deal with his father and his brother Frank are most crucial to the thesis being proposed here and will be quoted at length, in Coleridge's own words. The ambivalent relationship with the older brother is graphically reported. At age 6 Samuel had "a dangerous putrid fever."

> My poor brother Francis, I remember, stole up in spite of orders to the contrary and sat by my bedside and read Pope's Homer to me. Frank had a violent love of beating me; but whenever that was superseded by any humour or circumstances, he was always very fond of me and used to regard me with a strange mixture of admiration and contempt.

Between Coleridge's seventh to ninth years an incident is described that sheds further light on the ambivalent relationship with his brother.

> October 16, 1797
>
> Dear Poole,
>
> From October 1779, to October 1781, I had asked my mother one evening to cut my cheese entire, so that I might toast it. This was no easy matter, it being a *crumbly* cheese. My mother, however, did it. I went into the garden for something or other, and in the mean time my brother Frank *minced* my cheese 'to disappoint the favorite.' I returned, saw the exploit, and in an agony of passion flew at Frank. He pretended to have been seriously hurt by my blow, flung himself on the ground, and there lay with outstretched limbs. I hung over him moaning, and in a great fright; he leaped up, and with a horse-laugh gave me a severe blow in the face. I seized a knife, and was running at him, when my mother came in and took me by the arm. I expected a flogging, and in struggling from her I ran away to a hill at the bottom of which the Otter flows, about one mile from Ottery. There I stayed; my rage died away, but my obstinacy vanquished my fears, and taking out a little shilling book which had, at the end, morning and evening prayers, I very devoutly repeated them—thinking at the *same time* with inward and gloomy satisfaction how miserable my mother must be!

Coleridge stays out all night. The family is frantic. The town crier announces his loss. His obituary is practically in print when a rescue party of townspeople in a last ditch effort finds him moribund beside the bank of a river. Coleridge dramatizes this childhood memory, milking every drop of childhood hysteria out of it in the autobiographical letters to his patron. This scene would crop up again in a more sublimated manner in the pilot's boy episode of "The Rime of the Ancient Mariner."

The theme of alive-dead-alive recurs throughout the poem most notable in connection with the mariner and the sailors. This passage back and forth could also relate to the brother who feigned death, then came alive. It could relate of course to deeper, earlier psychological strata of Coleridge's "death-in-life" character pathology.

The description of his father's death is perhaps the most moving portion of the autobiographical letters:

> Towards the latter end of September, 1781, my father went to Plymouth with my brother Francis, who was to go as a midshipman under Admiral Graves, who was a friend of my father's. My father settled my brother, and returned October 4, 1781. He arrived at Exeter about six o'clock, and was pressed to take a bed there at the Harts', but he refused, and, to avoid their entreaties, he told them, that he had never been superstitious, but that the night before he had had a dream which had made a deep impression. He dreamt that Death had appeared to him as he is commonly painted, and touched him with his dart. Well, he returned home, and all his family, I excepted, were up. He told my mother his dream; but he was in high health and good spirits, and there was a bowl of punch made, and my father gave a long and particular account of his travel, and that he had placed Frank under a religious captain, etc. At length he went to bed, very well and in high spirits. A short time after he had lain down he complained of a pain in his bowels. My mother got him some peppermint water, and, after a pause, he said, 'I am much better now, my dear!' and lay down again. In a minute my mother heard a noise in his throat, and spoke to him, but he did not answer; and she spoke repeatedly in vain. Her *shriek* awaked me, and I said, 'Papa is dead!' I did not know of my father's return, but I knew that he was expected. How came I to think of his death I cannot tell; but so it was. Dead he was. Some said it was the gout in the heart;—probably it was a fit of apoplexy. He was an Israelite without guile, simple, generous, and taking some Scripture texts in their literal sense, he was conscientiously indifferent to the good and the evil of this world.
>
> God love you and
>
>   S.T. Coleridge.

"How I came to think of his death I cannot tell," Coleridge states, somewhat naïvely it seems to me given the Freudian perspective on the lost innocence of childhood. My thesis, after all, suggests that the disavowals of childhood are the very molds out of which adult sublimations and convictions are fashioned. I shall sift the evidence again, holding the genetic experience of the poet in one hand, his sublimations in the other, comparing and contrasting with suspicious intent.

Samuel Taylor Coleridge was the beloved child of an old minister. His relationship with his father, destiny had decreed, would be short-lived. The oedipus complex of the fourteenth child of an aging father must have unique features. There are 13 siblings to intimidate him, not to mention the existential association between age and declining health. In other words, love and aggression ripen toward appropriate maturity in the imagination, when the objects they are addressed toward have average expectable dimensions. In simple English, parents should be healthy and survive long enough to assist their children through critical periods of development. I can only speculate as to how the death of his father, while Samuel Taylor Coleridge was still in his latency, played havoc with his resolution of his oedipal development. My reconstruction would suggest that the knife of imagination that every child plunges into the rivalrous father assists the development of reality testing when the rivalrous parent neither dies nor retaliates.

For Samuel Taylor Coleridge the irony must have been exquisite. His attack on his brother with a real knife led to a pretense of death; his attack on his father with the imaginary knife of premonition led to real death. What a trick reality had played on him. Perhaps it is little wonder that the knife of the 9-year-old would turn up again disguised as a crossbow in the poetic mind of the adult.

Let us attempt to reconstruct the creative ferment in Coleridge's mind on the eve of writing the "Mariner." By this stage of his life, he is a friend of Dorothy and William Wordsworth. He has an idolatrous view of Wordsworth's talents and a self-deprecating opinion of his own. He is planning to collaborate with Wordsworth on a work on the wanderings of Cain. That work describes Cain wandering with his son Enos, accosting the ghost of Abel seeking forgiveness. However, Coleridge abandons this guilt-ridden project and turns his attention to the "Ancient Mariner" where the guilt will receive a more disguised treatment. It is clearly a turning point in the creative individuation of a writer. Wordsworth drops out of an intended collaboration, and Coleridge is free to exercise his own imagination uninhibited by the creative genius of another. It is an exquisite exercise in curiosity to try to picture his conflicts at this moment in time and their expression in the creative act. He asserts himself, writing without his collaborator, turning away from the theme of fratricide and embracing instead a theme of murder, guilt, responsibility—the human condition, in other words, with all its oedipal, tragic, existential components. Coleridge has come of age; yet, on the other hand, the seeds of self-destruction are already stirring within him, seeds that will almost bring the whole edifice of his creativity to ruin in the next 40 years of his life. (I'm referring, of course, to the breakup of his marriage, the breakup of many of his friendships, and his almost total enslavement to opium addiction.)

We know that a casual comment about a ship in a dream of a friend was the spark that ignited a fire of imagination which had been waiting for it for perhaps as many as 20 years. My reconstruction would suggest that the unconscious had condensed certain images in the mind of the poet: ship, rivalry with brother, rivalry with father, knife, dart, crossbow, death, dream premonition, guilt, retribution, albatross.

The poem condenses and disguises, using fantastic images to represent the poet's seemingly forgotten childhood, but after 550 lines of verse, the repressed returns with such unexpected force that it almost ruins the whole architecture of the poem. After 550 lines of gothic disguise, the Mariner-sinner is saved by a man and his son and a hermit in a scene that is so human it is almost out of place amid the fantastic.

> But swift as dreams, myself I found
> Within the Pilot's boat.

> Upon the whirl, where sank the ship,
> The boat spun round and round,

And all was still, save that the hill
Was telling of the sound.

I moved my lips—the Pilot shrieked
And fell down in a fit;
The holy Hermit raised his eyes,
And prayed where he did sit.

I took the oars; the Pilot's boy,
Who now doth crazy go,
Laughed loud and long, and all the while
His eyes went to and fro.
"Ha! ha!" quoth he, "full plain I see,
The Devil knows how to row."

The sudden appearance of this "pilot's boy episode," as it has been called, has been interpreted in several ways.

Kenneth Burke (1941) argues that the presence of the pilot's boy in the poem "cannot be understood at all, except in superficial terms of the interesting or the picturesque, if we do not grasp his function as a scapegoat of some sort—a victimized vessel for drawing off the most malign aspects of the curse that afflicts the 'greybeard loon' whose cure has been effected under the dubious aegis of moonlight" (Gardner, 1965, p. 104).

I would agree with Burke, but I hasten to add that the "displacement" he intuits makes more genetic sense when the sibling rivalry of the autobiographical letters is given its appropriate weight in this context.

That siblings were on Coleridge's mind when he wrote "The Ancient Mariner" is confirmed by the sudden reference to a brother at line 341. Up to this moment in the narrative there is no mention of any brother of the mariner. At this point in the poem the dead sailors have been reanimated and they are helping to sail the ship.

The body of my brother's son
Stood by me, knee to knee:
The body and I pulled at one rope,
But he said nought to me.

The sudden appearance of a character not previously introduced in the list of *dramatis personae* suggests an unconscious script interfering with an aesthetic one. One is reminded of

Dickens's need to put rats in the basements of even the wealthy characters in his novels, so great was his need to drag in certain genetic personal traumas when they might seem least expected (Tyndall, 1982).

In other words, the mariner after his pilgrimage of suffering is saved by three people: a hermit, a father, and a son. The fantastic gothic imagery of Coleridge's imagination has finally come to rest in the ordinary existential language of everyday life. The hermit surely represents his pastor father, the old holy man who must shrive him for his oedipal crimes. The pilot falling down in a fit and his son going crazy at the mariner's unexpected return to life surely are condensations of multiple childhood images: the falling down (death) of his own pilot-father, his brother's crazy pretense of death, Coleridge's equally crazy attack on his brother with a knife and subsequent runaway episode which may have damaged his health permanently. The mad laughter of the pilot's boy at the mariner's ability to row represents not only Coleridge's struggle to row the ship of his ambition despite his father's death, but also the 9-year-old's wish that his dead father would open his eyes and spring into action and help him to continue his development.

What I am suggesting is that Coleridge uses an unusual *deus ex machina* to save his tragic hero, most unusual in the sense that the *deus* is not a god at all but a man and his son and a priest, a trinity if you will, but of human, not godlike dimensions. After a fantastic journey through a world of specters and phantom ships, Coleridge ends on the *terra firma* of human relationships as if the poet sensed that even if the imagination can be saved spiritually, only human hands can pull a body out of the depths: inside every ancient mariner there is a pilot's boy struggling to get out!

BIBLIOGRAPHY

Beres, D. (1951). A dream, a vision and a poem. *Int. J. Psychoanal.*, 23:97–116.
Burke, K. (1941). *The Philosophy of Literary Form*. Baton Rouge: Louisiana State Univ. Press.
Clark, K. (1981). *Moments of Vision*. New York: Harper & Row.
Coleridge, S. T. (1950). *The Portable Coleridge*, ed. with an introduction by I. A. Richards. New York: Viking Press.

FREUD, S. (1925). Negation. *S.E.*, 19:235–239.

GARDNER, M. (1965). *The Annotated Ancient Mariner*. New York: Bramhall House.

HANSON, L. (1938). *The Life of Samuel Taylor Coleridge*. London: George Allen & Unwin.

LOWES, J. L. (1927). *The Road to Xanadu*. Boston: Houghton Mifflin.

TYNDALL, G. (1982). Dickens and the blacking factory. Read at the International Association for Child and Adolescent Psychiatry and Allied Professions, Dublin, Ireland.

WOLFE, T. (1932). *The Letters of Thomas Wolfe*, ed. E. Nowell. New York: Scribner, p. 322.

Experiencing Music

EERO RECHARDT, M.D.

IN THE PSYCHOANALYTIC PSYCHOLOGY OF CREATIVE ART THE
share of music is a small one. Investigating music from the psychoanalytical viewpoint is less rewarding than investigating
other forms of art. Its language is abstract and difficult to grasp.
It creates experiences that swiftly pass by, not allowing themselves to be caught and held, unlike those of literature and the
illustrative arts.

Musical expression is nonverbal and nondiscursive. Now and
then, however, it seems to be narrating something to us. All the
moods and feelings that Shostakovich experienced are so clearly
expressed in his symphonies that the biography by Volkov
(1979) has few surprises. Mahler wrote: "My whole life is contained in my two symphonies. In them, I have set down my
experience and suffering, truth and poetry in words. To anyone, who knows how to listen, my whole life will become clear,
for my creative works and my existence are so closely interwoven
that if my life flowed as peacefully as a stream through a mead-
ow, I believe I would no longer be able to compose anything" (de
la Grange, 1973, p. 272).

As far as the arts are concerned, the psychoanalytic approach
always presents the kind of methodological problems to which
clinical psychoanalytic work has no direct answers. Attempts to
approach music have been made from different points of depar-

Docent of psychiatry, University of Helsinki. Training analyst in Finnish
Psychoanalytic Society.

Presented at the Finnish Psychoanalytic Society on September 27, 1984. This
is an elaborated version of a paper published in *Scand. Psychoanal. Rev.*, 8:95–
113, 1985.

Translated by Kirsti Aro.

ture (Feder, 1978, 1980, 1981; Friedman, 1960; Mosonyi, 1935; Kohut, 1957; Kohut and Levarie, 1950; Nass, 1971, 1975, 1984; Niederland, 1958; Spitz, 1965; Wittenberg, 1980): (1) introspective observation of the impressions evoked by listening to music—what can psychoanalysis say about these experiences? (2) psychoanalytic biographies of musicians and composers; autobiographies of musicians and their narratives of musical experience; (3) knowledge drawn from the analyses of musical people; and (4) psychoanalytic theory of childhood development utilized and extrapolated toward a psychoanalytic theory of music.

In this paper I look at the subjective musical experience with the purpose of showing that there exists an isomorphism (similarity in form, similar crystalline structure) that ties the psychic event and the musical language together from the primitive levels to current social relations. This perspective is the traditional one in the psychoanalytic literature of music. It forms the background for judging how musical language can be placed into the psychoanalytic concept of cognition. Finally, I examine the role that cognition as represented by music assumes in other branches of art and sciences. These latter approaches are of interest in the current psychoanalytic theory and point to possibilities of new developments.

ON THE ISOMORPHISM OF THE ELEMENTS OF MUSIC AND THE PSYCHOANALYTIC INDIVIDUATION DEVELOPMENT

It is reasonable to assume, along with Mosonyi (1935), that there is in music something that corresponds to the way our psyche deals with the experiential world. Musical thinking may follow along the same lines that we use when shaping an image of ourselves, our experiential world, and the relationship between these two (Kohut, 1957; Wittenberg, 1980).

In musical experience one can then find the same elements a psychoanalyst finds in the way a person deals with psychic contents, such as affects and feelings, childhood and later object relations, and irritating or pleasurable stimuli. It is this trait that is responsible for the appeal in music, whereas its absence makes it sound indifferent. Still, music always is like play, whereas life can be ruthlessly painful. Music is able to transform painful and overwhelming experiences into something tolerable and even enjoyable.

Man is born in a psychically formless state and with a rather limited equipment of functions. The experiential world is constructed only gradually, in part around innate traits and skills, but most importantly it is molded by the interaction with the environment. Psychoanalysis concerns itself with the way man forms a picture of himself and his surrounding world. The restlessness and pressure of our bodily being of which we can never rid ourselves are the object of the psychoanalytic theory of drives. In its most advanced form, Freud's theory of the drives is dualistic: on the one hand, there is the restless, insatiable desire to live, Eros; on the other, there is the passion for peace, order, and a static state of lifelessness: the death instinct (Freud, 1920). Together they create a binary system on the mutual interaction of which are constructed the most complex entities. Order is necessity so that life can find its framework (Ikonen and Rechardt, 1980; Rechardt, 1986). In the most comprehensive sense, the thinking process has this very function. Cognition is "grasping," "comprehending," and "perceiving." In many languages, including Finnish (*käsittää*, "to do something with hands") and Swedish (*begripa*, "gripa" = grasp), the concrete nature of understanding finds its expression in similar terms. Musical thinking, more than anything else, is primarily the process of bringing order into chaos (Kohut, 1957; Niederland, 1958), to "get a grip" on the formless (Bion, 1977).

On the Isomorphisms of Early Development and Rhythm

Even at the foetal stage the cosmic chaos of the infant's experiential world is influenced by rhythm: the heartbeats of the mother, and her walking rhythm. A musicologist finds nothing new in the idea that rhythm is the first form of organizing the experiential world.

For example: the home of a family had more than one story; as a consequence the daily life of the pregnant mother consisted of climbing up and down the stairs all day long. The significance of this for the baby was revealed in a surprising manner. During the first postnatal weeks, the baby would stop crying and invariably fall asleep in a few seconds the moment the person carrying him began to walk with a distinct rhythm, although all other means to pacify him had been in vain. This apparently brought back a pacifying and very familiar order into the baby's chaotic restlessness.

After birth the rhythmic alternations between good and bad feelings begin to take shape. If the infant is not helped in his restlessness by the person caring for him, he will soothe himself by lulling to and fro. A disturbed child will resort to compulsive head banging, whereas a healthy baby will lull himself to sleep in a pleasurable manner. A person in psychotic chaos makes catatonic rhythmic movements, and may add to the effect by banging his head on the wall. Rhythm brings order to chaos. It is the beginning of orderliness in its most primitive form. After the experiential world becomes more orderly, rhythm is no longer connected with chaos and pain, but begins to take on other qualities.

Experiences of some basic rhythmic elements are very much alike among different listeners to music. Depending on the rate of acceleration, it is felt as exciting to the degree of loss of control and even panic. A familiar, horrifying, tonal background effect in films is the echoing monotonic sound repeated with increasing speed and force. In the days when ether narcosis was used, many patients, on the verge of unconsciousness, experienced a similar sound and the accompanying feeling of horror. It was often described as a bell ringing with continuously increasing speed and sharpening sound. Such an experience may have been connected with the loss of cognitive control. It possibly contained the experience of the last and weakening effort not to lose grip on some primitive order. Now and then it happened that some unexplained deaths occurred at the preliminary stage of the ether narcosis. The reason might have been the traumatic horror experienced. Restlessness devoid of form, chaos, and loss of control are the most horrifying experiences one can go through (Ikonen and Rechardt, 1980). Even that experience has its acoustic counterpart.

The slowing down of the speed of the rhythm and its coming to a halt are experienced as the end of excitation, as being at peace, as pausing, and even as death. A pause always brings on the feeling of anxiety. Children playing an instrument find it very difficult to pause for the exact length of time indicated in the music notes. It cannot be accidental that the music of the adolescent culture knows no pauses. For young people, death does not exist. In primitive music the use of such rhythmic effects probably has the meaning of taking possession of mighty powers or being under their spell. They are used against spirits and cosmic forces to ward off evil powers. A funeral ceremony in New Guinea shown on television differed completely from any Western concept of a burial service. A wildly running group of people attending the funeral was drumming away with great excitement and screaming at the top of their voices. This ceremony expressed the paranoid fear of the spirit of the deceased. It was an attempt to master that fear by frightening the spirit permanently from disturbing the living and taking revenge on them. Music was used as a means of magical control.

Music can have similar experiential effects on the modern sophisticated listener. Music can invoke primitive cosmic-magical moods; it can be frightening or playfully exciting; it can relax tension; and by an abrupt pause, it can cause frightening suspense. It can also soothe and lull to rest.

ON THE ISOMORPHISMS OF SOUND QUALITIES AND EARLY DEVELOPMENT

Refuge from sounds cannot be taken by the use of the reflexes of withdrawal that are readily available against light and pain. The only protection is the stimulus threshold. Some infants have a lower threshold and are more easily irritated by loud or sudden sounds than others (Bergman and Escalona, 1949; Greenacre, 1956). Sensitive irritability may call for the specific need to control and to put in order sense stimuli, thus leading to the development of artistic talent. One stimulus toward musical skill could be certain sounds that are hated; a passionate need arises to order and control them (Niederland, 1958; Kohut, 1957). Psychoanalysis is quite familiar with compulsive repetition brought on by traumatic helplessness: the compulsive need to create out of weakness an overpowering ability to control. Perhaps it represents the biologically sensible compulsion to practice. The desire

to play with sounds even includes the wish to achieve pure pleasure, the love of sounds. The endearing and soothing sounds of
mother's voice, her cooing, prattling, and chattering are a source
of pleasure. Together with the experience of mother's body and
one's own, they are connected with the holistic bodily experiences that Spitz (1965) calls coenesthesia. It is a state of psycho-
physical integration beyond the reach of conscious and free voli-
tion that has significance throughout life. Endearing sounds
with the accompaniment of rhythmic elements evoke similar
states and moods. The boundaries of the ego fade away, the
feeling of separation disappears, experiences of *unio mystica*
arise, even sensations of bliss and mass hypnotic suggestion. All
of this may be the driving force behind ritualistic events. An
example of the integrative power of music is the person suffering from aphasia who is capable of singing the words of a song he
cannot utter without music.

As the experience of separation evolves, sounds increasingly
become meaningful in communication. They are a further
means to influence, demand, appeal, and command. The com-
manding quality of auditive sensations is especially strong. In
psychotic episodes, it is the sounds, the voices that dominate, not
the visual hallucinations. Music is imbued with the same meaning. Fantasies of the use of power, of experiencing majestic
greatness and submissive littleness, can be created by music.

The kind of music that is composed mainly for magical control
dispels evil powers and creates experiences of omnipotence. It
helps to call forth the presence of the omnipotently satisfying,
mighty person, of gods, of beneficial powers, and of the all-
gratifying mother. The features of ceremonial and ritual music
are enhanced, e.g., primitive music, ecclesiastical music, ceremonial music, but also the modern youth music with its rhythm,
decibels, and wattage. This close connection with magical and
collective psychology makes it understandable why music in ancient China and ancient Greece was a state-controlled institution. He that possesses music controls power, said Plato.

The work of Winnicott (1971) on the transitional experience
and transitional object has brought a new perspective to the
psychology of play and the arts. An infant less than 12 months
old is capable of creating the illusion of mother's presence by

making whimpering sounds, by sucking his thumb, or by cuddling a soft object. The child is soothing himself by the sounds he
produces himself; he crows, he plays with the sounds and enjoys
them. The transitional experiential world is the matrix of the
cognitive world of the mind. It creates a tranquil no-man's-land
and a protective distance between the subject and perceptible
reality. When mother is not present, an illusion of her presence
can be summoned instead. The mind's world makes it possible to
feel at home in one's life and to retain mental health. The mind
does not depend on the perceptible reality of each given moment, it can also be filled with what is absent. In severe states of
psychic disturbance such an ability is often very weak. One of the
ways by which music can influence mental health and have
therapeutic effect is perhaps its capacity to create transitional
experiences and a world of imagination and play.

Lehtonen (1986) showed how music could create a psychotherapeutic working relationship with very badly disturbed adolescents. His clients had been hospitalized for antisocial or
grossly disturbed behavior. Their social background consisted
of many, very severe, traumatic circumstances. They were
chosen for the music therapy experiment because the staff felt
totally helpless in treating them. As a means of establishing contact Lehtonen played records (mostly rock and pop music),
asked them to draw their experiences, played various instruments together with them, or played to them. Some of them had
been interested in music, some not. Music stimulated the world
of fantasy and feelings. It awakened the inner world which had
been inaccessible. Music probably functioned in creating transitional experiences, stimulating symbolic processes and acting as
a good self-object which is able to share the inner world. Music
created the necessary conditions for psychotherapy by opening
up the ability to share the world of the mind.

Winnicott showed that the laws of the world of reality do not
apply to the transitional world: nothing ever breaks there, loss
does not cause pain, there is no need to fear for one's self or for
others. The transitional object needs no protection: any kind of
play is possible. Music provides an opportunity to play with transitional experiences. Sound does not "break" altogether, a piece
of music is not shattered, music does not end with finality, it does

not "die." Music need not to be handled with care; nor does one have to be afraid for oneself when playing with music.

As the individuation process advances, the share of play in music is increased. Even painful experiences can be transformed into play and then be dealt with as such. Mother's leaving and returning, joy and sorrow, loneliness and companionship, increasing tension and discharge, fear and appeasing security can all be experienced in play. Important elements in experiencing music contain play with give and take, disappearing and reappearing, getting lost and safely finding the way back home. The time span of such play may be short, like playing in safety in the home yard. Musical experience calls for mother's familiar hand to give scope to experience. Play can take place both horizontally and vertically by rearranging and interlocking successive elements of rhythm, harmony, and themes (Friedman, 1960). The average listener longs for this playful element in carefully measured portions in such a way that what is familiar is dominating. The arrangement of classical music into popular forms is done by increasing or adding familiar elements of melody, rhythm, and harmony, and by eliminating the complex elaborations altogether.

Having successfully dealt with the challenging and even fearful elements of music gives the same kind of satisfaction that playing in general does. It should not be too trying but give pleasure and rouse the desire to continue so that even the difficult turns of the play may be found attractive. Competence and pleasure, love and hate in balance are at variance in different kinds of music. The composer endeavors to create a variety of states of balance between them by means of form. "Easy" and immediately satisfying music must be given an element that makes it exciting enough. Difficult music has to have an element inviting the listener to join and to follow.

Along with the continuing individuation process, the boundaries of self grow more distinct. The experiential world commences to contain the feelings, desires, disappointments, and passions of the individual. The mighty powers are no longer in one's possession, mother is not always present for companionship and playing. One's own capacities as well as limitations are more clearly outlined. One becomes conscious of the existence of one's world of emotions and its kaleidoscopic quality. In musical experience this is correlated with new elements. At a fairly early stage in the history of Western music secular music began to deal with personal feelings: with love, passion, longing, and disappointment. It was at first expressed more by the choice of words until later on musical expression took over. In baroque music the language of music itself contains many elements depicting whimsical moods within the network of complex rules. The affective expressions of musical means unfold: ascending and descending melodies, tonality, modulations, rhythm, pauses, harmony, and dynamic nuances. They represent the experience of the inner world: agitation and calmness, conflict and harmony, tension and discharge; controlled uprising in the emotional world. This no longer takes place as a collective event, as a play with the parents and playmates, but as an inner event. Dealing with affects, for the main part, has the aim of controlling inner restlessness that at the beginning of life and in the primary phases of musical experience was the responsibility of the environment. It could be said that the task baroque music had taken upon itself was to attempt to control the complexity of emotional life within the frame of balanced order, to be able to govern the drives supremely to the joy of oneself and the glory of God.

As rulers were overthrown by democracy, man's responsibility as an individual was stated with emphasis. This led to romanticism which meant iconoclastic deeds, to challenging accepted sets of rules, and the search for new, more universal laws. This transitional crisis has continued to the present day. At the turn of the century psychoanalysis was creating a tragic picture of man whose fate consisted of conflicts and the effort to solve them throughout his life. The main lines of our own time are more difficult to discern than those of the past. Is the tragic image of man about to acquire global forms? Does it contain antagonism between the will to live, and the forces of destruction that are being let loose? Is it reflected in the musical cognition of contemporary times?

MUSIC AS A CHALLENGE TO PSYCHIC WORK

John Cage, in a TV interview, told how he gradually realized that the essence of composing is to strive for peace of mind. The music offers a means of attaining a peace of mind in one's own way. There is no end to the forms of psychic work and the resulting solutions. Different composers represent different ways of psychic work and different tasks to work on. Gustav Mahler, contemporary of Freud and Jewish, simply hurled himself into the frenzy of introspection and drew into the open his inner tragedy in all its bareness. He was a modern, neurotic man of the Western culture, and this we apprehend in his music.

Anton Webern moved inner tragedy farther away into the balance of absolute tension by the means of his pointillistic music. Stravinsky vested his rootlessness and homesickness in the cosmopolitan irony which he combined with Slavic melodies. The struggles Shostakovich went through that are so clearly reflected in his music were quite obviously linked with the tragic circumstances of his personal life. His music evokes a tragic response in his listeners. It is not important whether the interpretation of his music by the listener is individual or ideological: whether it depicts an individual tragedy or the defiance and revolutionary reaction of a subjugated people in the universal language of music.

The contents and forms of the challenge for psychic work are countless, but the task should always be present in music, so as not to leave it at the stage of dallying with technical or intellectual games. The inner task is also absent when musical expression is constructed on the vogue of the day and on clichés. The number of clichés is quite limited, whereas the number of inner forms is boundless.

The compelling quality of some musical experiences can be reflected in neurotic symptoms. A young woman whose analysis revealed repeated experiences of intense exposure to the primal scene could not tolerate orchestra music without fainting. She was incapable of coping with the auditively transmitted excitation. Persons who find music neurotically intolerable and hateful are not especially rare.

This short tour into the isomorphisms of music and the stages and processes of the psychic world as understood by psychoanalysis has been superficial and biased. My aim has been to exemplify how the language of music can reflect not only the primitive and bodily experiential world of childhood but also the complex forms of culture. The latter are then understood as the frame and mold which offer the preferred forms of psychic work and its different solutions. Thus it seems that the world of music could contain or symbolize the whole picture of man's life.

The Enigmatic Nature of Musical Cognition

The approach to demonstrating isomorphisms of musical expressions and psychic processes on different developmental levels along psychoanalytic lines certainly adds something to our understanding of the psychology of music. Still, in some respects, it leaves one dissatisfied. It may be that psychoanalysis, by its very nature, is best equipped to treat different ways of working over psychic conflicts; and it is this aspect of musical experience that psychoanalysis, at its best, can illuminate. Should we accept that this is both the strength and the limitation of the psychoanalytic approach, or is it possible to go a step further into the complexity of the language of music with the help of psychoanalytic knowledge?

The working over of inner conflicts in the form of play certainly is an essential element in genuine musical experience, but it is not the only one. Composers are able to transmit great varieties of experience in music. They are prone to think about everything in terms of music (Nass, 1975). How is it possible, for instance, to transfer thoughts and feelings, and senses from different modalities such as muscular, visual, and visceral into the auditive sphere? Thus the extraordinary changeability of the structures of these experiences seems to be an enigma and a challenge to psychoanalytic understanding.

MUSIC AND ARCHAIC MEANING SCHEMATA

On closer inspection, this phenomenon really is related to psychoanalytic knowledge. As an instance of nonverbal bodily understanding of reality, I shall cite what Székely (1962) has written:

> A child not quite 2 years old is looking out of the window. Outside it is snowing, and a bird is hopping about on the window-sill picking up breadcrumbs. The child watches all this with interest. Suddenly the bird drops something. The child goes over and sees a white speck in the snow. 'Birdie do big,' calls out the child. There is nothing very remarkable in this. But the question arises: How does the child discover or know what the bird has done?
>
> . . . The product, the bird's faeces, resembles snow, since it is white, and not the child's own product, which is brown. Moreover, the child has never seen the act of defaecation, and consequently has no visual memory-trace to draw upon. He has only somatic and coenesthetic memory-traces of defaecation, for the child has experienced it only as a pleasurable bodily process in himself, and not as a visual event. How, then, did he identify what he saw? Let us recall Freud's thesis, previously quoted, that in order to understand the perceptual complex our own bodily sensations and motor images are necessary, and as long as these are absent, the elaborating part of the perceptual complex cannot be understood. It may perhaps at first appear surprising that the infantile mechanism should work with such extreme certainty and accuracy, and that the child should make his discoveries and apprehend his environment so correctly. Actually, the reaction is not so very exact. At this stage the child's mind works strictly according to certain schemata. If the child sees a parcel fall from a car in the street, he will also exclaim: 'Car do big,' i.e. he believes that the car is defaecating. In other words, the child tends at this stage, to interpret as faeces any small object falling from a larger object.
>
> . . . What the bird does, or a parcel dropped from a car passing by, or a small object becoming detached from a larger object, is apprehended and worked out by the child in the light of the body experiences with which he is acquainted; or, to state it differently, the child apprehends the visual world by incorporating his visual impressions into his body schema. Since this

incorporation takes place along definitely describable lines, I suggest that the result of these apprehensive processes be termed *archaic meaning schemata* [p. 302f.].

Székely here gives us a concrete example of the way comprehension really takes place without any verbal content, simply by way of form, a form that originates in the bodily functions but still is practical for use outside the self to a certain point. To what point? Of this Székely (1971) gives us another example in the young physicist doing creative research work. He describes how creative inspiration comes to his analysand in connection with a certain conflict. He is preoccupied by the movements of physical particles as movements of his body. He is running in the woods imagining himself being one particle and trying to catch another particle, which he has given the name of his girlfriend. He is able to arrive at certain new developments by this coenesthetic–intuitive thinking. He is then able to formalize mathematically the result of this bodily thinking. We come to realize that by nonverbal bodily thinking it is possible to deal not only with bodily realities and some of the realities of life but also with the realities of quantum physics! The thought model for arranging the physical scientific observations into a new explanatory theory is apparently sought from among a large store of coenesthetic, kinesthetic meaning schemes. After that its usefulness in explaining reality is put to test. This is what the 2-year-old was doing watching the bird, and later less successfully watching the car pass by. This is what the scientist accomplishes more or less successfully in his work.

The musical idiom does not appear to be so puzzling any longer. It provides the forms empty of content and the meaning schemas that have their origin in nonverbal bodily comprehension. It then remains for the listener himself to apply these forms to the experiential world of the moment, to invest them with contents of his own.

On closer inspection, however, the question arises how it is possible for the mind to operate in the manner described. The primitive, bodily, meaning schemas do not only represent some archaic preliminary forms of thinking, which are discarded later on as new cognitive operations develop. On the contrary, they are flexible, movable, and abstract schemes, which are able to shift from one sensory modality to another, from visual or muscular to auditive and so on. Such active maneuverability is best explained by the existence of the symbolic process, which however, requires closer explanation.

SYMBOLIC PROCESS AND BODY LANGUAGE

There is some ambiguity in the psychoanalytic literature with regard to the meaning of the term symbolic. Symbolic and linguistic are commonly linked together. The concept "linguistic," however, applies to an area much narrower than that of "symbolic." Susanne Langer (1951, 1953, 1967) bases her philosophy on the primary symbolic capacity of man that is reflected everywhere. Her words on the nature of musical experience are as modern as they were 30 years ago and are supported by recent psychoanalytic writings on nonverbal cognition. She has a broad conception of the symbolic: "Artistic conception . . . is a final *symbolic form* making revelation of truths about actual life" (1967, p. 81). And again on the same subject: "The nondiscursive form has a different office, namely, to articulate knowledge that cannot be rendered discursive because it concerns experiences that are not formally amenable to the discursive projection. Such experiences are the rhythms of life, organic, emotional and mental . . . which are not simply periodic, but endlessly complex, and sensitive to every sort of influence. All together they compose the *dynamic pattern of feeling*. It is this pattern that only *nondiscursive symbolic forms* can present, and that is the point and purpose of artistic construction" (1953, p. 240f.). Langer (1951) even says, "The real power of music lies in the fact that it can be 'true' to the life of feeling in a way that language cannot; for its significant forms have that *ambivalence* of content which words cannot have" (p. 206).

The poetic words of Langer now find a concrete basis in the psychoanalytic conception of archaic, bodily, meaning schemas and their use in artistic creations to scientific thinking. Instead of Langer's expression "ambivalence of content" I would suggest "emptiness of content," i.e., receptive to a variety of contents like a mathematical formula, to which Langer also compares musical expression. This partly equals the term "isomorphism" I have used earlier. Musical language is symbolic, but not discursive; it presents structures for cognitive processes, not contents.

Winnicott's observations of the transitional phenomenon have to do with those moments when the child takes possession of his innate ability to employ the symbolic process. He creates an illusion of mother's presence when she is absent, by giving this meaning to something else, such as his own voice, his thumb or some soft object. The most fundamental symbolic capacity is the *ability to treat the absent as being present.* By this means man is detached from the immediacy of the perceivable world, and on the foundation of this ability stands the world of the mind which is peculiar to man. Secondary derivatives of this capacity are, for instance, the ability to use arbitrarily chosen, designating signs, to make and use tools and weapons, and to advance languages common to all.

Research has so far not been able to answer the question: At what point in the development of the child does the symbolic capacity appear? Traditionally, this capacity is connected with the development of language, and placed between 18 months and 3 years of age. This is certainly too late. What Winnicott discovered was that this skill clinically manifested itself in the second half of the first year. It is possible, though, that symbolic ability is even more primary. In any case, it is quite clear that the world of the mind springs up before differentiation between subject and object. Consequently, the archaic meaning schemas contain a lot of *archaic interaction schemas,* where the roles of the object and the subject are confused. The notion of the early preverbal beginning of symbolic capacity thus lends some support to the Kleinian theory of early infantile fantasies. Recent research has indicated that newborn babies are able to perceive and to imitate facial expressions, to give some primitive "meaning" to their visual perceptions. As Field et al. (1982) put it, "there is an innate ability to compare the sensory information of the visually perceived expressions . . . with the proprioceptive feedback of the movements involved in the matching that expression" (p. 181). Furthermore, it appears to be clear that cognition begins prior to verbal skill, and that significant cognition takes place without any verbal forms both at the earlier stages of development and later on (Basch, 1976). Chomsky (1975), when speaking of the formation and use of concepts, states, "As techniques of investigation have improved, . . . so has the apparent sophistication of the infant's perceptual system" (p. 8). As a primary autonomous capacity the symbolic process thus seems to be more primary than the use of words and differentiation between self and object. Following that line of thought one could even consider the possibility of some intrauterine cognition. Vauhkonen (1986) presented the provocative hypothesis that the intrauterine activity of intending to put the thumb in the mouth may be the first form of psychic work of the foetus, thus becoming the very first bodily cognitive scheme in problem solving.

Auditory schemes derive from earliest childhood, possibly beginning with intrauterine experiences of the heartbeats and walking rhythm of the mother in the way described in the first part of this paper. There are even experiences of closeness, of playful, submissive, frightened, or rebellious interaction with the caretaking environment in connection with auditory stimuli. Put in musical form, they result in tender, excited, majestic, or religious qualities. Yet, in music there are other than auditive schemes. There are affective schemes and schemes pertaining to motion, which rather easily lend themselves to musical expressions and which the listener can invest with his or her personal experiential contents. When bodily schemas are interwoven with the symbolic process, the original border that is bound to different sensory schemas disappears. Thus they become interchangeable. For instance, visual impressions can be expressed in auditive form by creating with the aid of music images of scenery or variations of climates. Finally, musical cognition thus consists of bodily schemas from various sources, not only from auditive ones.

Investigation of musical thinking leads to the realization that the thinking process has a bodily foundation; when bodily experiences are interwoven with the symbolic process, they are also differentiated into abstract cognitive schemas at an early stage of development. They can then be used as cognitive tools in a variety of situations.

Preverbal, symbolic meaning schemas make it understandable

how a musical person using auditive elements is able to think in musical terms. Other schemas can be used similarly, e.g., motor, visual, proprioceptive. A scientist can, in similar fashion, use body language to represent complicated contemporary problems. He is looking for possible models, general abstract forms of reality in this coenesthetic language, and experimenting with their ability to describe and explain the actual problem. Nass (1984) gives clinical examples of these phenomena. Composers, mathematicians, and scientists, among them Einstein, very often—many say almost always—use nonverbal bodily cognition, e.g., muscular motility, when trying to solve problems.

Music Contained in the Psychoanalytic Language

The difference between science and arts lies in the fact that science tries to reach a general linkage, free of conflict, of the describing models on the basis of the numerous possibilities offered by archaic cognitive schemas. Different branches of science are at different stages in this striving. The farther away from abstract formalization they are, the more important it is that the specialists in the branch are in communication with one another to promote understanding of the idiosyncratic metaphors they use.

The linkage to actuality of the general meaning schemas in the arts is left to each individual participant to be dealt with moment by moment. Bodily meaning schemas are then transferred to the level of experiential reality. In science the endeavor is to raise it permanently to the level of theory.

The formalization process of psychoanalytic theory is at the same stage as physics was some centuries ago when the concept of "force" was still unclear and disputable. In a sense, psychoanalytic thinking is located in the no-man's-land between the arts and sciences. Noncontradictory patterns have not yet been reached; ever since Freud's day traditional usages have cropped up regionally in psychoanalytic language. In addition, each and everyone has the inclination—one could possibly say capacity—to use idiosyncratic meaning schemas, subconscious theories of more or less his own making which may function better than the "official" theory (Sandler, 1983). If psychoanalytic texts are read

with too strict expectations, one can easily be led completely
astray. In order to understand it, one has to find the "music" in
it.

Lesche (1981) has shown that the biological and physical models in the psychoanalytic theory are intended to be used explicitly
as empty models; he calls them "naked models." They must be
given a strictly psychoanalytic content. Freud (1920) speaks of
the inevitability of metaphoric thinking in psychoanalysis (p. 60).
He also says that even in resorting to the language of chemistry
and physics so familiar to us, we are doing it in the figurative
sense. His followers seem to have forgotten this.

Schafer (1976) criticizes psychoanalytic metapsychology for its
use of terms describing bodily functions. In his opinion, it is
archaic bodily language which is unsuitable in scientific discourse. It is, however, precisely these archaic, bodily meaning
schemas that we need in trying to cope with something unknown. And that is the main task of the psychoanalyst in his
work. These schemas provide more versatile choices of various
abstract models, if they are used in the same sense as Lesche's
naked models, than can be provided by models borrowed from
other branches of science.

If we take into consideration preverbal, archaic meaning schemas, the door can be opened for discussing the questions of
nonverbal communication and some telepathy-like phenomena
described in connection with projective identification. This can
help us to understand what in our work and practice still has no
verbal expression. We still are often in the same position as those
children in Piaget's (1973) experiment who were practically able
to comprehend more than they were able to explain themselves.

SUMMARY

I started with the paradox that music is the most nondiscursive
of all arts, yet it is said to contain "the whole human life" or
whatever subject can be expressed by musical means. I then
illustrated manifold isomorphisms which exist between the early
infantile experiences revealed through psychoanalysis and the
means of musical expressions and experiences. These isomorphisms exist in relation to various emotional states and have

been treated during various epochs and in different social conditions.

I then examined the subject from the perspective presented by Susanne Langer: music represents abstract forms of feelings without any specific content. These forms are based on preverbal bodily experiences, called "archaic meaning schemata" by Lajos Székely. These bodily schemas integrate with the symbolic process. This development probably starts very early and creates an almost inexhaustible store of affective-cognitive operations which can be used both in scientific and artistic work. The forms presented by the arts have to be connected with the here and now by the listener/receiver who thus finds his "truth." The task of the sciences is to use these archaic meaning schemas in order to build a model free of contradictions. Psychoanalysis is situated somewhere between these two. There are both "music" and attempts at formalized theories in it.

BIBLIOGRAPHY

BASCH, F. M. (1976). The concept of affect. *J. Amer. Psychoanal. Assn.*, 24:759–778.

BERGMAN, P. & ESCALONA, S. K. (1949). Unusual sensitivities in very young children. *Psychoanal. Study Child*, 3/4:333–352.

BION, W. (1977). *Seven Servants*. New York: Aronson.

CHOMSKY, N. (1975). *Reflections on Language*. New York: Pantheon.

DE LA GRANGE, H. (1973). *Mahler*, vol. 1. New York: Doubleday.

FEDER, S. (1978). Gustav Mahler. *Int. Rev. Psychoanal.*, 5:125–148.

——— (1980). Gustav Mahler um Mitternacht. *Int. Rev. Psychoanal.*, 7:11–26.

——— (1981). Gustav Mahler. *Int. Rev. Psychoanal.*, 8:257–284.

FIELD, T., WOODSON, R., GREENBERG, R., & COHEN, D. (1982). Discrimination and imitation of facial expressions by neonates. *Science*, 218:179–181.

FREUD, S. (1920). Beyond the pleasure principle. *S.E.*, 18:3–64.

FRIEDMAN, S. (1960). One aspect of the structure of music. *J. Amer. Psychoanal. Assn.*, 8:427–449.

GREENACRE, P. (1956). Experiences of awe in childhood. *Psychoanal. Study Child*, 11:9–30.

IKONEN, P. & RECHARDT, E. (1980). Binding, narcissistic psychopathology and the psychoanalytic process. *Scand. Psychoanal. Rev.*, 3:4–28.

KOHUT. H. (1957). Observations on the psychological functions of music. *J. Amer. Psychoanal. Assn.*, 5:389–407.

——— & LEVARIE, S. (1950). On the enjoyment of listening to music. *Psychoanal. Q.*, 19:64–87.

LANGER, S. (1951). *Philosophy in a New Key.* New York: Mentor Books.
_____ (1953). *Feeling and Form.* New York: Scribner's.
_____ (1967). *Mind.* Baltimore: Johns Hopkins Univ. Press.
LEHTONEN, K. (1986). *Musiikki psyykkisen työskentelyn edistäjänä.* Turku: Annales Universitatis Turkuensis.
LESCHE, C. (1981). The relation between metapsychology and psychoanalytic practice. *Scand. Psychoanal. Rev.,* 4:101–109.
MOSONYI, M. (1935). Die irrationalen Grundlagen der Musik. *Imago,* 21:207–228.
NASS, M. L. (1971). Some considerations of a psychoanalytic interpretation of music. *Psychoanal. Q.,* 40:303–316.
_____ (1975). On hearing and inspiration in the composition of music. *Psychoanal. Q.,* 44:431–449.
_____ (1984). The development of creative imagination in composers. *Int. Rev. Psychoanal.,* 11:481–491.
NIEDERLAND, W. G. (1958). Early auditory experiences, beating fantasies, and primal scene. *Psychoanal. Study Child,* 13:471–504.
PIAGET, J. (1973). The affective unconscious and the cognitive unconscious. *J. Amer. Psychoanal. Assn.,* 21:249–261.
RECHARDT, E. (1986). Die Interpretation des Todestriebs. *Psychoanalyse Heute,* ed. Hans Lobner. Wien: Orac, pp. 45–61.
SANDLER, J. (1983). Reflections on some relations between psychoanalytic concepts and psychoanalytic practice. *Int. J. Psychoanal.,* 64:35–45.
SCHAFER, R. (1976). *A New Language for Psychoanalysis.* New Haven & London: Yale. Univ. Press.
SPITZ, R. A. (1965). The evolution of dialogue. In *Drives, Affects, Behavior,* ed. M. Schur. New York: Int. Univ. Press, pp. 170–190.
SZÉKELY, L. (1962). Meaning, meaning schemata, and body schemata in thought. *Int. J. Psychoanal.,* 43:297–305.
_____ (1971). Über den Beginn des Maschinenzeitalters. In *Psychoanalyse in Berlin.* Meisenheim: Anton Hain, pp. 106–115.
VAUHKONEN, K. (1986). Presented at the meeting of the Finnish Psychoanalytical Society.
VOLKOV, S. (1979). *Testimony.* London: Hamilton.
WINNICOTT, D. W. (1971). *Playing and Reality.* Harmondsworth: Penguin Books.
WITTENBERG, R. (1980). Aspects of the creative process in music. *J. Amer. Psychoanal. Assn.,* 28:439–460.

Separation-Individuation in a Cycle of Songs

George Crumb's *Ancient Voices of Children*

ELLEN HANDLER SPITZ, Ph.D.

> Consciousness of self and absorption without aware-
> ness of self are the two polarities between which we
> move, with varying ease and with varying degrees of
> alternation or simultaneity.
> . . . gradual growing away from the maternal state of
> symbiosis, of one-ness with the mother . . . is a lifelong
> mourning process.
> —MARGARET S. MAHLER (1972, P. 333)

IT HAS BEEN REMARKED THAT WITHIN THE BODY OF PSYCHO-
analytic writing the art of music has received scant attention.
What has been said falls more or less into the category of patho-
graphy or psychobiography.[1] The thorny problems with that
general approach are well known and have been extensively
discussed by contemporary aestheticians, including Bouwsma
(1954), Tormey (1971), and Kivy (1980). It is my purpose here to

Special member, the Association for Psychoanalytic Medicine; adjunct assistant professor, Educational Psychology, New York University; Visting lec-
turer of aesthetics in psychiatry at Cornell University Medical College.

I wish to thank the following persons for their valuable comments: Maureen
Buja, Murray Dineen, James E. Gorney, Nathaniel Geoffrey Lew, Mitchell B.
Morris, and Brian Seirup. Special appreciation is due to soprano Barbara
Martin for her inspired performances of this piece at Juilliard under the aus-
pices of the Lincoln Center Institute.

A version of this essay, prepared for nonpsychoanalytic readers, will appear
in *Current Musicology*.

1. For some fine examples of this general approach, see Feder (1978, 1980,
1981, 1984).

demonstrate that the pioneering work of Margaret Mahler on preoedipal development gives rise to the possibility of quite a different psychoanalytic approach to music. My vehicle for this demonstration will be the description and interpretation of an extraordinary work of contemporary music which, when heard with the knowledge of early human development provided for us by Mahler, evokes that drama of early infant-mother interaction in all its nuance as an aesthetic experience.

Although I believe it may be possible to extrapolate from what is presented here a more general psychoanalytic approach to musical form, I shall leave that task to the future and limit this brief paper to the interpretation of one particularly relevant work.

In the summer of 1980 at Juilliard, soprano Barbara Martin gave two brilliant performances of George Crumb's 1970 composition entitled *Ancient Voices of Children: A Cycle of Songs on Texts by García Lorca*. This piece of music actually fuses several art forms into one, since it involves a special arrangement of instruments on stage, the strategically timed entrances and exits of certain performers, and the occasional vocalizing of instrumentalists as well as the changing of instruments by several performers during the piece. Consequently, as in the case of an opera, not even the finest recording (Nonesuch stereo disc, H-71255, featuring Jan deGaetani) can do justice to the full range of expressive possibilities offered by the work. I shall try to convey in what follows here that, with Mahler's developmental theory tacitly hovering in our minds, we cannot help but hear this piece as a complex musical metaphor not only for the ambiguities inherent in all our aesthetic experiences but for the varying degrees of alternation and simultaneity in our converging and dissolving experiences of self and other. I shall try to show, in other words, that *Ancient Voices of Children* lends itself with exquisite aptness to interpretation along the lines of Mahler's developmental formulations.

I

Ancient Voices is scored for soprano, boy soprano, oboe, mandolin, harp, electric piano, and assorted percussion instruments, including antique cymbals, tambourine, maracas, Tibetan prayer stones, sleighbells, and five Japanese temple bells. Its oversized score is a work of art in its own right, a festival for the eyes, with notes, markings, and poetic text that dance enticingly helter-skelter over its pages. Based on excerpts from five poems by Federico García Lorca, the text is, of course, sung in Spanish. I have, however, for the purpose of this essay, used the English translation provided in the score. My warrant for so doing comes directly from the composer himself who clearly indicates his desire that the meaning of the text he has chosen be understood by all his listeners: "N.B., both Spanish and English texts should be printed as part of the program notes" (see score, inside cover, *Ancient Voices*).

Examining the text, we find that poetic fragments by García Lorca are strung together into a five-part cycle by Crumb, who, with this arrangement, demonstrates his willingness to treat poetic text as material for assimilation and re-creation into a new totality of his own making. In so doing, he of course transforms and transcends it in ways that would have been impossible in earlier conventions governing the setting to song of poetry. He creates a synthesis of music and language, sound and voice, that embodies new meanings, reveals new interrelationships and sequential significance beyond those inherent in the original poetry.

He has, furthermore, given to his work a strong visual aspect, almost choreographic, by carefully designing the position of all instrumental groups on stage and by directing his performers to move about as they prepare to play different instruments. They turn away, depart to perform offstage, or come onstage after having been totally invisible to the audience. In fact, the entire piece possesses a theatrical aura, and the score actually states that it can be adapted to choreography or even to mime.

From the developmental perspective I am adopting here, one feature emerges as momentous: there is onstage from the beginning both a grand and a toy piano, and the visual relations (as well as the musical relations) between these instruments serve to underscore as well as to mirror the similar relations between the adult woman and young boy sopranos who perform central roles. Thus, as elsewhere throughout the piece, contrast and continuity are stressed by being presented in not merely one but at least two sensory modalities. Their intensity is magnified in a way reminiscent of the primitive "coenesthetic" experiences of our earliest (ancient) moments, described first by Spitz (1965) and more currently by Stern (1983), experiences which these authors both see as prototypic for our later experiences in the realm of the aesthetic.

Through an interweaving of unusual musical elements with poetry that has been partially deconstructed into its phonemic components, with visual counterparts including both objects and movements in space, *Ancient Voices* serves to juxtapose and oppose our notions of silence with absence, and of harmony and dissonance with congruent and incongruent size and shape, sex, and generation. *Ancient Voices* presents us with an experience in which only the "primary illusion" (Langer, 1953) is musical, but in which music is heightened by a drama that envelops us by engaging us cross-modally, as do perhaps not only the earliest but all the most intense dramas throughout our lives. And its dramatic action, illuminated by Mahler's developmental theory, importantly explores not only the perspective of the child but also that of the mother. By this extension, the piece becomes a complex metaphor for the mergings and separations that characterize all human relationships, for which this one is paradigmatic.

II

As a title, *Ancient Voices of Children* appears quixotic, even paradoxical, for how can it be that the youthful voices of children may be called ancient? The composer probes this strange theme by revealing with his haunting music that, for each of us, the old or former or ancient self is indeed that of a child, inextricably bound to the voice with which we once spoke, an ancient voice that we are fated to lose and mourn, along with all the quality of life and human relationship that once went with it, but which we can sometimes rediscover in the voices of other children. In art, in sound, George Crumb has fixed the central message of Margaret Mahler's inspired insights.

Ancient Voices is about the power, magic, ambiguity, and range of the human voice. It is about sounds created by human be-ings—about what they can be, what they can do, and what they can mean. The piece gives us two human characters, a woman (soprano), and a boy (soprano), who represent at least at times consciously, but on a deep level, unconsciously, a mother and her child. We are led by them to explore through the medium of voice but also of anthropomorphic instrumental sound the di-mensions of their changing relationship. The anthropomor-phism here moves characteristically back and forth; just as the voices of the two pianos take on the *personae* of adult and child, so also the plaintive oboe both imitates the human voice and is itself echoed, and likewise the soprano, vocalizing into an amplified piano, prefigures with clicking tongue the later percussive sounds of the Tibetan prayer stones. This intimacy and inter-mingling of human and instrumental sound thus characterize the piece, reinforcing its evocation of the ancient and the primitive.

Voice reaches out in all directions as a bridge across primal separateness. It is a mother calling ("When, my child, will you come?"), trying somehow to establish contact with the child with-in her body, with a child out in the world, and with the child who is her own partially forgotten self ("to give me back/ my ancient soul of a child"). But voice is also an affirmer of self, a confirmer of identity and self-sufficiency. ("The little boy was looking for his voice.") These two ways in which the human voice functions can be in painful conflict, as we hear in the occasional abrupt contrasts, juxtapositions, and interpenetrations of the music.

The painful separations of birth ("I'll tell you, my child, yes,/ I am torn and broken for you") and death ("a child dies each after-noon") are only the extremes of a spectrum of partial separations described by for us by Margaret Mahler in her writings on early child development. Such separations can be only partially over-come by music and the magical power of voice, which interpene-trates that surface between self and outer world ("como me pierdo en el corazón de algunos niños," as I lose myself in the heart of certain children). Thus, this music, through the regularities of its rhythms ("Todas las tardes en Granada," Each afternoon in Gra-nada) and "with a sense of suspended time," as the score directs, momentarily arrests our sense of life's evanescence.

III

As the piece begins, we see a young woman, the soprano, come onstage and walk over to the piano. Standing beside the great instrument, she is dwarfed by it, as our fleeting consciousness is dwarfed by the cavernous recesses of the unconscious into which it sends ever-widening ripples. She bends over and begins to sing into the sounding board. Her voice induces sympathetic vibrations in the piano strings. Rich vowel sounds vibrate and resonate throughout the hall as though in waves spreading out from her, echoing and reechoing. She is searching, exploring, questioning, exulting in what her voice can do. She does not turn to the audience, but seems to sing into the depths of her own psyche—letting the sounds of her own voice bring messages to her. She makes a compelling visual image, leaning over the piano as if it were a pool of water, an ocean, or a vast nothingness. She is perhaps the pregnant mother calling and listening to the unborn child within her who is still a part of her own body.

She sings sounds at this point—not words, but the inside stuff of words—sounds that suggest language unfettered to specific meanings, sounds evoking warmth and color unconstrained by outline. They are like the sounds with which the young infant practices, experiments, playing repetitively, joyously with his burgeoning power to make and simultaneously respond. In this opening section, by taking not words but the sounds of letters inside words as musical elements in his composition, the composer delves into the expressive tonal qualities of language—its internal values of sound. He isolates vowels, consonants, diphthongs. With this exploration, a vast richness of meaning opens, and associations multiply.

Margaret Mahler has beautifully described for us the symbiotic orbit that envelops infant and mother and exerts such powerful regressive pulls upon the latter. In *Ancient Voices of Children*, we experience through music the elaboration of this aspect of the dyadic drama. From the first notes, we are absorbed into the shimmering aura of the soprano's vocalise. The primeval quality of her voice as she renders these sounds loosened from word-shells is enhanced by the apparent freedom, spontaneity, and intense self-absorption with which she performs this opening section. Paradoxically, however, although the experience she conveys is almost improvisational in character, its every nuance is notated with consummate precision.

We do not hear these words at first, but the title of the first movement reads: "El niño busca su voz" (The little boy was looking for his voice). While it is the adult woman soprano who is singing, her voice merges in fantasy, as we listen, with the inarticulate experimentations of a small child perhaps too young to form words. Then, as if in confirmation, the child's own voice is heard remotely offstage at the close of the passage.

Or we might hear in this section (marked "very free and fantastic in character") the vocal expression of an adult overwhelmed by extreme emotion into incoherence, the strange and unpredictable sounds of ancient tribal music (which the composer suggests throughout the score by his markings, linking the history of individuals with that of cultures, as was also Freud's wont), the unfamiliar noises of some language we cannot comprehend, or perhaps at times just the fanciful, delirious liberation of sounds from the binding constraints of meaning.

As through the music, the earliest phases of the human drama of fusion and separation are evoked in us, we must struggle as the music pulls us into ourselves: we draw back, seeking to understand, to comprehend on another level, but are enveloped by the reverberating music, compelled by its primitive power that, in these listening moments, passes understanding.

Lorca's text continues:

> (The king of the crickets had it.)
> In a drop of water
> the little boy was looking for his voice.

All the ambiguity of these lines is embodied in the soprano's voice. As she clicks her tongue intermittently, flutters it, works with open and closed sounds (full-throated and nasal), varying dynamics and tempi, we can imagine that she is pretending to be the cricket king who has tried on a human voice, exploring all its possibilities, not certain what to do with it. Simultaneously, in these passages, she becomes the child trying to find his own voice, tentatively emerging from the fetal drop of water. She merges with and evokes the experience of the young toddler who tries on different pitches and rhythms like costumes to discover which feels comfortable, startling, useful, horrid, becoming. She becomes the child seeking a separate and unique identity in sound, a distinct voice of his own, and this theme is developed by the lines of the boy soprano's "after-song" rendered offstage softly through a cardboard speaking tube:

> I do not want it for speaking with;
> I will make a ring of it
> so that he may wear my silence
> on his little finger.

To find one's own voice is to be able also to choose silence. It is to be able to make a ring of inclusion and a ring of exclusion, and thus to become independent—of the voice of the mother.[2]

Associations from later developmental stages abound as well: a boy changing—on the brink of manhood, looking into the water, his memory, the sounding board, the vibrations—and seeking his former voice, his present one having grown unpredictable and strange. In singing, the soprano represents, perhaps, the voice for which the boy is searching and for which he will continue to search in all his relationships to come.

These meanings are all present in the music. As the soprano's voice reverberates in ever-expanding echoes, our own awareness of the possibilities of vocal sound expands. We become conscious of the multiple meanings released by this freeing of language from word and sound from poetry. We enter aesthetically into the recurring and layered dramas of early human development about which Mahler has taught us.

IV

The piece continues with an instrumental interlude, "Dances of the Ancient Earth," which is performed by oboe, strings, and

---

2. To introduce another perspective to interpret the place of the cricket king who *has* the little boy's voice might be to note that, according to Lacan (1977), it is "le nom/non du père" that intervenes and ruptures the child's symbiotic tie to the mother. Since, in symbiosis, symbolic communication is unnecessary, the father, by severing the bond with the mother, initiates the child into language and culture, suggested here, on one level, by the "king" who holds, possesses the voice of the child.

percussion. Although the composer disclaims this section as a commentary on the text (see score, *Ancient Voices*), the overarching theme of the human voice is developed and expanded here as the various instrumentalists vocalize in occasional shouts and whispers. As in later movements, the sounds made by the instruments themselves are often reminiscent of human voices—the raw wailing of cello bow on metal saw in section II, the antique toy piano's suggestive tinkling in section IV, the many different bells and touches of vibraphone, and, above all, the oboe's haunting abortive melodies which recapitulate qualities of the soprano's voice in section V. In this interlude and throughout the piece, the warmth and vitally personal quality of the human voice are present.

In section II, the soprano moves to center stage and, facing her audience with cupped hands, she proceeds to whisper the following lines of poetry, as if telling a secret:

> I have lost myself in the sea many times
> with my ear full of freshly cut flowers,
> with my tongue full of love and agony.
> I have lost myself in the sea many times
> as I lose myself in the heart of certain children.

These lines, not sung, but spoken quickly, quietly, confidentially, form almost a commentary on the preceding section as well as a further thematic development. We are, they suggest, always open to sound—to voice. Our ears are perpetual receptors unlike our eyes, and therefore we can be engulfed by sound: we can "lose" ourselves in it, for it has the power to surround and invade us. Music fills our ears with "freshly cut flowers," i.e., with notes or words that have been spoken or sung and that die soon or change once they have passed the lips of the singer. There is a wonderful irony in these lines expressed further in the following juxtaposition of "love and agony." For although voice creates an illusion of bridging the gulf between self and other, mother and child, this bridge is only an illusion.

A mother hearing her newborn infant's cry or an infant sensing his mother's voice and body-sounds feels a powerful urge to be reunited in that symbiotic prenatal and postnatal union (Mahler, 1968) which must gradually dissolve. The soprano's whispering words between cupped hands—words spoken but not sung—remind us that the transforming, reuniting magic of voice is but illusion; remind us of the paradox that to hear another's voice as one's very own (like "freshly cut flowers") is to be at once inexorably separate; hence, the love and agony together.

V

The next movement of the piece ("From where do you come, my love, my child?") is its centerpiece—musically, temporally, and even visually, in terms of the score itself. Its text, a block of richly imagistic poetry, comes from the song of Yerma—Lorca's unforgettable barren wife, who longs so desperately to bear a child. Her words become here a musical dialogue between the two soprano voices, the one adult, female, and present, and the other, youthful, male, and absent. For the child, whom we have already heard offstage in section I, continues to remain far away, remote, and invisible. Incorporated into this section are the "bolero" rhythms of the second dance, "Dance of the Sacred Life-Cycle," which is scored in a ring on the page (reminiscent of the "anillo" of voice and silence). Distinctly Spanish and melodic, this dance closely follows the skeletal structure of Lorca's poetry with its repeated, slightly varied yearning questions from the mother and vividly sensual and pictorial responses of the child and its thrice-repeated chorus. Against the rhythms and repetitions of this movement plays a rich variety of background accents produced by ingenious combinations of instruments and the composer's exploitation of their potential for creating new sound.

Visually and auditorily, the instrumentalists become almost a family to the major participants in the dialogue here as awareness of setting becomes more prominent both in the text and in the drama that is unfolding between mother and child and between mother and self. As background becomes foreground in the instrumental interludes, we grow more sensitive to the way in which all the noises that surround us—including those internal to us—have significance and hitherto unrecognized value. We begin to perceive these noises as relating us in subtle and heretofore unnoticed ways to life around us and to our intrapsychic and bodily selves.

VI

Section IV is preceded by a silence. Brief but deeply signifying, this silence symbolizes death, the ultimate absence, but also offers respite. Thus it prepares us for the complex and highly emotional threnody to come: "Todas las tardes en Granada todas las tardes se muere un niño." (Each afternoon in Granada, a child dies each afternoon.) Dominated by slow, unmeasured rhythms, this climactic movement evokes the death of children—not only loss of life but the death of childhood itself.

We are reminded of the first song in which the boy is heard offstage speaking of wanting his voice in order to make of it a "ring of silence." It is *this* silence, this distance, that the mother is mourning here—the kind of loss and death evoked by Margaret Mahler in the passage I have chosen as epigraph for this essay, and the toy piano's *perdendosi* rendition of "Bist du bei mir [Be near me]" addresses yet again and with special poignancy the theme of loss and separation.

But that the actual death of children is also lamented is revealed in the coda of this movement, aptly titled "Ghost Dance," as well as in the music of the final movement of *Ancient Voices* ("My heart of silk is filled with lights") by Crumb's quotation in his plaintive oboe solo of a melodic line from the final movement ("Der Abschied") of Gustav Mahler's *Das Lied von der Erde,* a piece written by that composer upon the death of his own 5-year-old daughter.

As the music evokes our sense of loss in these several dimensions, it conveys that "lifelong mourning process" of which Margaret Mahler speaks—that mourning for a special kind and quality of relationship that must irrevocably pass, and yet which is evanescently recaptured in our aesthetic moments with music.

Finally, in this concluding section of *Ancient Voices,* we hear voices—both human and instrumental—that reach with a progressive sense of urgency, as the soprano sings of traveling ("farther than those hills,/ farther than the seas,/ close to the stars") to span the distance, to close the gap between herself and "my ancient soul of a child." It is here that the oboe player, after performing his soulful motive, slowly rises and leaves the stage. Later, we hear him again, the oboe muted, distant, and somehow reminiscent in feeling of the soprano's voice. The oboist's physical departure is essential here, enabling us to experience fully and cross-modally the illusion: the power of voice to reach across the landscape, to attempt to heal the terrible anxieties of separation.

Then, after the last notes of the poem are sung, the child comes on to the stage for the first time. The "ring" is now closed as the soprano walks toward him, and, standing together in an exquisite cameo, they perform a series of wonderful, wordless sounds—a recapitulation of the first moments of the piece, but infused this time with shared serenity, joy, and resolution.

VII

By the conclusion of *Ancient Voices of Children,* we have experienced what Aristotle called a "catharsis of pity and fear" through music—through this extraordinary synthesis of music, poetry, and movement. With George Crumb's cycle of songs, we have relived our own ancient cycles of separation-individuation. Associations, impressions, partially formed ideas flood consciousness: that through the process of searching within herself for her own "ancient" childhood, a mother may ultimately find her child in a new way; that there must be death but also regeneration, agony, and yet love. The uncanny quality of the music fascinates and attracts us, inviting us to expand our sense of what music is and can be, just as it stretches and strengthens our sense of the open-ended possibilities of human relationship. After *Ancient Voices,* one can never again hear modern music in the same way, nor children's voices, nor any music, nor any voices. Hearing it in the context of Mahler's insights into the dawning phases of human development, we understand that the intense pleasure it affords derives in no small measure from its power to awaken in us that archaic experiential world of infant-mother dual union which lives on in the unconscious.

BIBLIOGRAPHY

Bouwsma, O. K. (1954). The expression theory of art. In *Aesthetics Today,* ed. M. Philipson & P. J. Gudel. New York: New American Library, rev. ed., 1980, pp. 243–266.

BURROWS, D. (1980). On hearing things. *Music. Q.*, 66:180–191.

CRUMB, G. (1970). *Ancient Voices of Children.* New York: C. F. Peters.

FEDER, S. (1978). Gustav Mahler, dying. *Int. Rev. Psychoanal.*, 5:125–148.

———— (1980). Gustav Mahler um Mitternacht. *Int. Rev. Psychoanal.*, 7:11–26.

———— (1981). Gustav Mahler. *Int. Rev. Psychoanal.*, 8:257–284.

———— (1984). Charles Ives and the unanswered question. *Psychoanal. Study Soc.*, 10:321–351.

KIVY, P. (1980). *The Corded Shell.* Princeton, N.J.: Princeton Univ. Press.

LACAN, J. (1977). *Écrits,* tr. A. Sheridan. New York: W. W. Norton.

LANGER, S. (1953). *Feeling and Form.* New York: Scribner's.

MAHLER, M. S. (1963). Thoughts about development and individuation. *Psychoanal. Study Child,* 18:307–324.

———— (1968). *On Human Symbiosis and the Vicissitudes of Individuation.* New York: Int. Univ. Press.

———— (1972). On the first three subphases of the separation-individuation process. *Int. J. Psychoanal.*, 53:333–338.

———— PINE, F., & BERGMAN, A. (1975). *The Psychological Birth of the Human Infant.* New York: Basic Books.

STERN, D. (1983). Implications of infancy research for psychoanalytic theory and practice. In *Psychiatry Update,* ed. L. Grinspoon. Washington, D.C.: American Psychiatric Press, 2:8–22.

SPITZ, E. H. (1985). *Art and Psyche.* New Haven & London: Yale Univ. Press.

SPITZ, R. A. (1965). *The First Year of Life.* New York: Int. Univ. Press.

TORMEY, A. (1971). Art and expression. In *Philosophy Looks at the Arts,* ed. J. Margolis. Philadelphia: Temple Univ. Press, 1978, pp. 346–361.

YANAL, R. J. (1981). Words and music. *J. Philos.*, 78:187–202.

Childhood Trauma and the Creative Product

A Look at the Early Lives and Later Works of Poe, Wharton, Magritte, Hitchcock, and Bergman

LENORE C. TERR, M.D.

TRAUMA IN CHILDHOOD MAY SET A THEME FOR THE SUBSEQUENT work of the artist. This comes about through the unconsciously activated mechanisms of play and reenactment. Although most children who are traumatized play out their "games" of trauma in a grim, monotonous way (Terr, 1981), the especially gifted child may do something special, something quite compelling. This special child, for instance, may tell a friend, "I thought up a verse, 'Ring Around the Rosie,'" as the Black Plague invades his medieval street. Or she may compose a little chant to express her terror of mechanized menaces, and everybody else will jump rope to the rhyme: "Polly on the railway, Picking up stones, Along came an engine, And broke Polly's bones. 'Oh,' said Polly, 'That's not fair.' 'Oh,' said the engine driver, 'I don't care.' How many bones did Polly break? One, two, three, four . . ." (a modern English grade-school jump-rope ditty, as quoted by Alison Lurie, 1985, p. 157).

We know that sometimes there is a delay between trauma and play. A child may wait to reenact—perhaps he has not found his metier yet, or perhaps a new and lesser external stress has not yet

Clinical professor of psychiatry, University of California, San Francisco School of Medicine.

This paper was presented at the Annual Meeting, American Academy of Child and Adolescent Psychiatry, October 17, 1986, Los Angeles.

sounded the unconscious call to action. Posttraumatic play and reenactment do not always follow traumatic events directly on cue (Terr, 1983a).

Furthermore, we know that playground games, creative as they are, do not reflect the competence, the probing understanding, the wit, the invention, and the industry of the mature artist. A clever little spoof, for instance, called "Gnaws," written in 1980 by a talented 13-year-old Chowchilla bus-kidnapping victim, tells the tale of panic in a town held at the mercy of a giant beaver; but it would not have entered the ranks of world literature unless our talented young writer could have gone on to develop himself further. The traumatic product in and of itself is not art. It takes a genius—someone creative enough to produce interesting works—to give us the art that expresses a trauma. This artistic product will reflect the trauma in two ways: in the literal re-creation of the artist's experience, and in the establishment of a tone of trauma—of helplessness, confinement, and panic.

In this paper I show that early trauma may function as a leitmotif in the grand opuses of the great—that terror experienced in the formative years may turn up in the products of artists, products that will, in turn, promote panic in the audience. Obviously a leitmotif does not make an entire opera, and so some of my explanations will indeed sound oversimplified. My purpose, however, is not to bring light to the meaning of everything an artist does, but rather to show how certain themes and old feelings, through the powerful posttraumatic compulsions to play and reenact, will appear and reappear in the traumatized artist's work.

This article will not explain how creativity comes about. Certainly Margritte was painting, Bergman was daydreaming, and little Edith Wharton was exhibiting a passion for storytelling long *before* they were shocked. It is the thing that is painted, the shots that are filmed and then saved from the editor's shears, and the tale that is eventually told in print that interests me here. As Freud puts it in his foreword to Marie Bonaparte's study of Poe (1933), "Investigations such as this do not claim to explain creative genius, but they do reveal the factors which awaken it and the sort of subject matter it is destined to choose" (p. xi). The reworking of childhood trauma is but one factor in creative work. It will influence content, subject matter, and tone—but it will not determine the creative process itself.

I have selected Poe, Wharton, Magritte, Hitchcock, and Bergman as my examples because (with the exception of Magritte) they have long been favorites of mine, although at certain times I have hated them.

I will briefly review the traumas these artists experienced in their childhoods. If there is evidence of behavioral reenactments in their later lives, I will give this. I will then describe, quote, or demonstrate the literal, specific reenactments these artists show in their works. Following this I will demonstrate how the pervasive tone in their art reflects their old traumatic anxiety from childhood—the sense of horror, panic, and overwhelming helplessness. Finally, I will discuss posttraumatic contagion—in other words, the effect of the traumatized artist's fears on the audience.

The questions which I cannot, will not, address are the most curious yet the most elusive ones of all. What creates the creative process? Why do most children re-create their traumas in a monotonous way, whereas a few geniuses can inject enough variety into their re-creations that audiences accept them time after time? What in these artists enables them to rise above their childhood ordeals, freeing themselves up enough to create great art? The mystery of genius-at-work along with the puzzle of genius that fails to produce—these dilemmas await more thought, more data, and perhaps a "genius" willing to tackle a task as formidable as this.[1]

POE

Edgar Poe was born January 19, 1809, the second son of impoverished and tubercular actors, David Poe, the son of a revolutionary war quartermaster, a man everyone addressed as "General," and Elizabeth Arnold Poe, the daughter of accomplished

1. There is a developing body of literature on the subject of creativity by such behavioral scientists as Guilford (1967), Feldman (1982), Gedo (1983), and Esman (1986).

London players. Because the young couple were so poor, they "farmed out" Edgar's older brother, William Henry, to the paternal grandparents in Baltimore. By the time Edgar was 18 months old, his father had abandoned the family, shortly afterwards, by at least one newspaper account, to die of TB. A baby girl, Rosalie, whose paternity still remains in question, was born 5 to 6 months after David Poe left. Neither of Edgar's siblings fared very well. William Henry died of TB in his early 20s; Edgar attended him in death. Rosalie's physical and mental development was arrested at age 12; one cannot even guess what could have happened to her at that time. Edgar and baby Rosalie, along with their actress-dancer mother, moved to various places on the Eastern seaboard—Boston, New York, Richmond, Norfolk, Charleston, and again, Richmond—swinging from high points, when Elizabeth Arnold was well enough to dance or to act, to the lows, when she was coughing up blood and there was barely enough food to eat.

As the unlucky autumn of 1811 rolled on, the lows outgained the highs. A few local ladies of Richmond heard of the terrible plight of the young actress and her two babes, sending over clothes or food and occasionally stopping by to visit. Mother and children shared a small, damp room in which there probably were a few chairs, Elizabeth's bed, a trundle bed for Edgar and Rosalie, and a chest full of clothes. Edgar most likely describes from a toddler perspective this awful little room in his story "Loss of Breath" as the hero is hanged, laid out in a room, and experiences Poe's well-known, often told sensation of living death:

> I was laid out in a chamber sufficiently small, and very much encumbered with furniture—yet to me it appeared of a size to contain the universe. I have never before or since, in body or mind, suffered half so much agony as from that single idea. Strange! That the simple conception of abstract magnitude—of infinity—should have been accompanied with pain. Yet it was so [Bonaparte, 1933, p. 392].

On November 29, 1811 a notice appeared in the *Richmond Enquirer* titled "To The Human Heart." "On this night," it says, "Mrs. Poe, lingering on the bed of disease and surrounded by her children, asks your assistance, and asks it perhaps for the last time. The generosity of the Richmond audience can need no other appeal. For particulars, see the Bills of the day" (Bonaparte, p. 6). On December 9, 1811, the young actress died. She left a miniature of herself, eyes glowing, to her almost 3-year-old son, Eddy. The luminous eyes show up all over Poe's works.

How would such a death appear to a toddler? First of all, probably no one but the tiny Rosalie was with Edgar at the moment Elizabeth Arnold died. People had been dropping in from time to time, but the little family lived by themselves. Perhaps no one came in for hours.

Poe never frequented the dissecting room, the funeral establishment, or the amputation disposal area—something that the young Ingmar Bergman *did* do. How then could Poe know so much about the disintegration and ugliness of death yet display such ignorance about the finality of the process? In my opinion, it is because his experience just short of age 3 with his dying and dead mother (without any adults to help him) left him with a permanently burned-in vision of death, a conscious verbal memory (Terr, 1986), a toddler impression, a traumatic one.

Poe talks about death like a late toddler. He gives us horrible, gruesome bodies with blood suffusing their faces and coming out of their mouths ("The Mystery of Marie Roget"), a death room that stretches out to infinity ("Loss of Breath"), women who are dead, yet somehow not dead enough to stay dead (Lady Madeline in "The Fall of the House of Usher," "Berenice," "Morella," and "Ligeia"), burials that are incorrect, premature, and unnatural ("The Colloquy of Monos and Una," "The Tell-Tale Heart," "The Pit and the Pendulum," and "The Premature Burial"), and bodies that simply gleam with corruption ("The Narrative of Arthur Gordon Pym"). The young Poe must have struggled with Elizabeth Arnold's body, shook it, talked to it, nestled into it, touched its hand, watched its eyes and mouth for minutes—perhaps hours—before anybody came to help him. The next day Edgar Poe was taken away by Mrs. Frances Allan, a Richmond lady of substance, who served as a kind foster mother to him and became the source of his middle name. But by then, the traumatic impression had jelled. Eddy must have been a genius to begin with—but this death, this horrible scene of quiet beyond all understanding and of disintegration beyond all belief, this set the subject and tone for Poe's works.

Poe's life itself was full of posttraumatic reenactment. He repeatedly achieved his own immobile deathlike states with opium or with the alcoholic binges that eventually killed him. He married a 13-year-old cousin, the frail, white-faced Virginia Clemm who of course was already destined to die, just like Poe's mother, of TB. As a West Point prank with overtones of death and bodily disintegration, Poe enlisted a colleague to throw a bleeding gander into a roomful of cadets, convincing his fellow cadets that they had just seen the axed-off head of one of their professors. Perhaps the strangest reenactment of all was his repeated need to see death—he felt absolutely cheated for missing the dying of his foster mother, Frances Allan, for instance. He wrote, "If she had not died while I was away there would have been nothing for me to regret" (Letter 24, Poe Museum, as quoted by Bonaparte).

Poe was a terrified, traumatized person. At 6 he became panicky while he and a foster uncle passed a graveyard. In adolescence he frequently hallucinated a cold, disembodied hand touching his face. He dreamed terrifying nightmares of white-robed women coming to get him, and shortly before his death, he hallucinated such women by day (bodies in the nineteenth century were ordinarily wrapped for burial in white shrouds, and women wore white nightgowns, even on their deathbeds). As for futurelessness which, along with repetition and fears, are, I think, three key findings that occur in the disorders of shock and extreme stress (Terr, 1987), Poe demonstrated this, too, in his lifetime. A girlfriend, Mary Devereax, commented 40 years after it had happened that the 20-year-old Poe told her several times, "there was a mystery hanging over him he never could fathom. *He believed he was born to suffer,* and this embittered his whole life" (Bonaparte, p. 68; my italics).

The tone of Poe is sad, horrible, and if humorous at all, only ironically so. Even in his poetical pieces there is a looming, a sense of "utter helplessness" (Freud, 1926)—the emotional tone of trauma. The "Raven" sits over the muser's doorway casting his long, black shadow. The hero of "Annabelle Lee" voluntarily lies down in a tomb next to his dead beloved. In "Ulalume," the hero's dead love prevents him from ever experiencing the carnal delights. His "Sleeper" is surrounded by worms. His Lenores (in "A Pean," "Lenore," and "The Raven") are always dead, always lost in the dark shadows. Poe felt that Death was necessary for art, for Beauty. He says in his "Introduction":

> I could not love except where Death,
> Was mingling his with Beauty's breath [Bonaparte, p. 61].

In "The Philosophy of Composition," Poe says, " 'Of all melancholy topics, what according to the *universal* understanding is *most* melancholy?' Death—was the obvious reply. 'And when,' I said, 'is this most melancholy of topics most poetical?' From what I have already explained at some length, the answer, here also, is obvious—When it most closely allies itself to *Beauty:* the death, then, of a beautiful woman is, unquestionably, the most poetical topic in the world" (Bonaparte, p. 45). Edgar says it is "poetical" and we must grant him that. But Poe's heroines are not all so beautifully poetic in their deaths—they die stuffed inside chimneys ("The Murders on the Rue Morgue"), strangled and floating down the Seine ("The Mystery of Marie Roget"), or suffering mysterious plagues ("The Masque of the Red Death"). As a matter of fact, Poe's plague imagery is so hysteria-provoking that I will return to his death "masquerades" when, at the end of this paper, I look at the response of the audience to trauma in art.

WHARTON

Edith Jones was born in 1862 to an aristocratic New York City family virtually untouched by the Civil War. After the war, the Joneses moved to Europe to escape the nose-diving American economy. By the time that she was 6 Edith obviously loved storytelling and classic mythology, but she never cared much for fairy tales. When Edith was 8 or 9 and her family was staying at Mildbad, a small Black Forest spa where her mother was "taking the cure," young Edith suddenly doubled over with a sharp pain in her stomach and was found to have typhoid. The doctor, a spa physician, knew so little about the disease that he treated Edith through a running correspondence with his son, an army doctor who barely knew any more than did his father. Between them, they failed miserably. The doctor told the Joneses that Edith was dying. Let us listen to what Edith Wharton (1985) herself tells us next:

> That very day they [the Joneses] happened to hear that the physician of the Czar of Russia was passing through Mildbad. In their despair they appealed to him, and on his way to the train he stopped at our hotel for five minutes, looked at me, changed the treatment—and saved my life.
>
> This illness . . . formed the dividing line between my little-childhood and the next stage. . . . When I came to myself, it was to enter a world haunted by formless horrors. I had been naturally a fearless child; now I lived in a state of chronic fear. Fear of *what?* I cannot say—and even at the time, I was never able to formulate my terror. It was like some dark undefinable menace, forever dogging my steps, lurking and threatening; I was conscious of it wherever I went by day, and at night it made sleep impossible, unless a light and a nurse-maid were in the room. But whatever it was, it was most formidable and pressing when I was returning from my daily walk (which I always took with a maid or governess or with my father). During the last few yards, and while I waited on the door-step for the door to be opened, I could feel it behind me, upon me; and if there was any delay in the opening of the door I was seized by a choking agony of terror. It did not matter who was with me, for no one could protect me; but, oh, the rapture of relief if my companion had a latch-key, and we could get in at once, before It caught me!
>
> This species of hallucination lasted seven or eight years, and I was a "young lady" with long skirts and my hair up before my heart ceased to beat with fear if I had to stand for half-a-minute on a doorstep! . . . But how long the traces of my illness lasted may be judged from the fact that, till I was twenty-seven or eight, I could not sleep in the room with a book containing a ghost-story, and that I have frequently had to burn books of this kind, because it frightened me to know that they were downstairs in the library! [p. 275f.]

Let us look a moment at what it was to have typhoid and almost die in the Black Forest of Germany in the late 1860s and early '70s. The disease was marked by diarrhea, lethargy, fever, and weakness. Nausea, vomiting, and a rash often went along with it. The emeritus chancellor of the University of California, San

Francisco, Dr. John B. D. C. M. Saunders, a noted historian of medicine, tells me that the child would have been "immured" at the far end of a wing of the hotel and confined in her room for weeks—in Edith Jones's case, for months—with few visits from parents who would not have dared come in because it was believed that direct contact with sick individuals would cause spread. A nurse with her own room nearby would have been hired, and she would not have left the area to which Edith was confined. No one but the doctor would have entered Edith's room from outside. And he (Edith spells doctor with a capital "D") would be robed in white with a gown covering his suit and a white mask over his nose and mouth. If the doctor were ordinarily allowed into the dissecting room, a white skull cap would have covered his head. But Dr. Saunders tells me, "ever since the sixteenth century, spa physicians have failed to distinguish themselves," so that we would have to guess that little Edith's doctor was robed and masked in white except for the very top of his head. He would pause at Edith's threshold—he rarely would enter the room because of the supposed risk of contamination to him—and he would talk to the child briefly, stop to chat with the parents in their quarters, and then leave as soon as he could. So much for Edith's daily visits at the time of her most terrible ordeal. Her doctor looked like a ghost. Her parents were absent. She was virtually alone.

As we know, Edith Wharton went on to write great books like *Ethan Frome, The House of Mirth,* and *The Age of Innocence,* for which she was nominated for the Nobel Prize and won the Pulitzer, the first woman ever to do so. Edith Wharton wrote ghost stories, too—some of the scariest ones ever written—at least after Poe. By the way, the critic R. W. B. Lewis (1975) says that Edith was influenced by Poe's tales of "trapped consciousness," which she brought into her story "The Bolted Door." She certainly treasured Poe enough, as a matter of fact, to bring the actual Edgar into her novella, *False Dawn,* written in the early 1920s.

How did a terrible illness, along with its accompanying feelings of entrapment and ongoing posttraumatic hallucination (Terr, 1986), express itself in Wharton's later life and work? She tells us herself about her ghost-hounded adolescence and of her aversion until age 27 or 28 to the ghost story. But she does not tell us of her nonphysical illness, something that felled her almost constantly for at least 4 years beginning at age 33 and which later brought her down on occasion. The illness, diagnosed as "neurasthenia," was characterized by "an occult, and un-get-at-able nausea," terrible fatigue requiring 6 to 7 rests a day, loss of weight, frequent headaches, and incapacity to make decisions (Lewis, 1975). One wonders if these bouts were the kind of psychophysiological reenactment that comes after trauma or extreme stress (Terr, 1983a)—obviously, the often-repeated symptoms were quite similar to those of typhoid. At any rate, Edith's first ghost story, "The Lady's Maid's Bell," was written in 1902 just before one of her many neurasthenic bouts and the tale begins with a literal, direct reenactment of Edith's childhood ordeal with the fever. "It was the autumn after I had typhoid," are her first words.

In her ghost stories and in many of her tales of the real world, Edith Wharton indulges in literal repetitions. In "Afterwards" (1909), for instance, she says, "There were even moments of weariness when, like the victim of some poison that leaves the brain clear, but holds the body motionless, she saw herself domesticated with the Horror, accepting its perpetual presence as one of the fixed conditions of life." Her sense of confinement is restated in "Afterwards": "These moments lengthened into hours and days, till she passed into a phase of stolid acquiescence. . . . She had come to regard herself as part of the routine, a spoke of the wheel, revolving with its motion; she felt almost like the furniture in the room in which she sat, an insensate object to be dusted and pushed about with the chairs and tables" (p. 71). R. W. B. Lewis considers "Afterwards" overly "melodramatic." Trauma and extreme stress can indeed strike one so— that is, until one knows it.

Wharton's first story, composed at age 12 and revised at age 15, tells of a heroine "Georgie" (Edith's brother called Edith "John") who contracts pneumonia at a ball and goes off to Nice to die. Thirty-five years later she writes "The Triumph of Night" (1910) about a dying young man with tuberculosis who is wrongly confined in New Hampshire through bad medical advice. In "Miss Mary Pask" (1925) the hero is recovering from "a nervous collapse supposed to be the result of having taken up my work again too soon after my touch of fever in Egypt." Miss Mary Pask, by the way, is a woman confined all by herself in a small European house. She is, as the little Edith was in her illness, quite alone.

Not only does Edith's latency-aged brush with death recur in her stories, but her ghost-at-the-threshold does so as well. "Mr. Jones," written in 1928, is probably the most striking example that she gives us. Mr. Jones, an unseen ghost, refuses to let people enter a young woman's house. Thirty years before, Mr. Jones had kept someone else out—someone who can still remember the experience (the young Edith, wouldn't you say?). The heroine of "Mr. Jones" feels strange at the entry way to her house, "She recalled the uneasy feeling which had come over her as she stood on the threshold after her first tentative ring." Finally, the heroine finds an old letter from a now-dead young lady, protesting, "I yet fail to conceive how anything in my state obliges that close seclusion in which Mr. Jones persists—and by your express orders, so he declares—in confining me" (Wharton, p. 192f.).

In her semiautobiographical "Mr. Jones," Edith Wharton gives, perhaps entirely conscious, homage to her fellow victim of traumatic confinement, Edgar Poe. The housekeeper who guards entry to the spooky house is named Mrs. Clemm, the name of Poe's mother-in-law. "Muddy" Clemm cared for Poe the last half of his life, and it is she, alone, who communicates with Edith Wharton's menace, the ghostly Mr. Jones. "What can I do?" Wharton writes. "Mrs. Clemm says [Mr. Jones] has a doctor who treats him by correspondence. I don't see that I can interfere." There they are together in one sentence! That old helplessness at the mercy of an incompetent, letter-writing doctor, Edith's childhood trauma, and the acknowledged Wharton bond to Poe.

Doorways mean menace to Wharton. From her autobiographical statement about her terror of ghosts at the doorway (probably precipitated by the earlier usages of her threshold by the white-robed doctor), one can plainly see why Wharton's ghosts usually attack their victims at or near doorways. They do so in "The Lady's Maid's Bell" (1902), "Afterwards" (1909), "Mr.

Jones" (1928), "Pomegranate Seed" (1931), and "All Souls," published posthumously in the year that Edith Wharton died, 1937.

Leon Edel, the inventor of "literary psychology," thinks that "All Souls," a ghost story about an elderly lady immobilized with a sprained ankle who is left all alone for 36 hours without any household help, is a statement of Wharton's own presentiment of her soon-to-come death (Edel, 1982, pp. 36–41). I, on the other hand, see it as the same old thing, the trauma, perhaps stimulated into repetition this time by the current stress of Edith's anticipated death. Edith Wharton, already ill with the heart disease that was to kill her within a few months, was still primarily playing out a trauma that she had experienced at age 8 or 9. Her terror flared up with new stresses—similar to the terrors of World War II veterans who 30 or more years after the War experienced new posttraumatic symptoms with new life stresses (Van Dyke et al., 1985).

How does the tone of Wharton convey to us the terror from her childhood? I think that the matter-of-fact tone that Wharton employs makes the extreme stress, when it comes, more piercing, more surprising than it sounds from the mellifluous nineteenth-century voice of Poe. Wharton plays things matter-of-factly, and the entrapment that follows becomes the more palpable, the more real because of this crisp, precise style. Lewis points out that entrapment is a major theme in Wharton. It characterizes the novel *The Fruit of the Tree* (1906), the story "Souls Belated" (1899), and her best known work *Ethan Frome* (1911), a novel I despised when I was forced to read it in college. In *Frome,* Wharton, who easily shifts the sex of her central character away from her own, says, "The inexorable facts closed in on him like prison wardens handcuffing a convict. . . . He was a prisoner for life." I hate that. But that is the sensation of psychic trauma.

MAGRITTE

We should take a break from all these linguistic entrapments and consider some of the more graphic depictions of trauma instead. Poe, as usual, forms our link here. The surrealistic painter, René Magritte, born in Belgium in 1898, greatly loved Poe. He named his paintings *The Imp of the Perverse* and *The Domain of Arnheim* after Poe stories. He, like Poe, suffered the shocking death of his mother; but in Magritte's case, it came later in his life, at age 14, and by her own hand.

As do the majority of traumatized persons (Terr, 1983a), Magritte hated to talk of the past. He blocked his contemporary peers, the psychoanalysts, who were so fascinated by his work, from ever getting an interview with him (Torczyner, 1977), and he laughed, even in his sculpture, at psychiatry (see *The Thera-peutist*, a sculpture that shows a psychiatrist with an empty bird-cage for a chest and no head at all). Magritte told his biographer, Suzi Gablik, a few early memories that he had; one was of a large wooden chest that stood enigmatically by his cradle; a second, of the arrival at his house of two balloonists whose conveyance had somehow collapsed on his roof; and a third, a visit at age 12 to a cemetery where he often played and where he found an artist from the city painting among the broken columns and dead leaves (p. 18). This, for Magritte, represented the beginning of his career in art.

When Magritte was 14, his mother who had been depressed for some time left the house in the middle of the night and drowned herself in the Sambre River. The body was fished out a day or two after the tragedy and lay in state at the Magritte home. Once one has been trained as a physician, one does not have to stretch the imagination to picture how that maternal body must have appeared to this impressionable adolescent who by now was "destined" to be a painter. Gablik says, "Of his moth-er's death Magritte's only remembrance [at least the only re-membrance he was willing to tell Gablik] was, he imagined, a certain pride at being the centre of attention in a drama" (p. 19).

The Belgian poet, Louis Scutenaire, also describes the event as his friend, Magritte, supposedly told it to him:

> She shared the room with her youngest son who, waking to find himself alone in the middle of the night, roused the rest of the family. They searched the house in vain; then, noticing foot-prints outside the front door and on the sidewalk, they followed them as far as the bridge over the Sambre, the river which ran through the town [Chatelet]. The mother of the painter had thrown herself into the water and, when they recovered the

body, they found her nightgown wrapped around her face. It was never known whether she had covered her eyes with it so as not to see the death she had chosen, or whether she had been veiled in that way by the swirling currents [Gablik, p. 18f.].

Magritte hated to face his past. As reported by Viederman (in press), the painter "never spoke about the past or the future and would refuse to make plans even for the immediate future if he could avoid doing so" (suppression of painful affect and "futurelessness" are both important findings in trauma [Terr, 1983a, 1983b, 1987]). Despite his avoidance of the past, however, Magritte continually played out his past in his paintings. Wolfenstein (1973) sees this harkening to the past as "a splitting of the ego as the child both acknowledges and denies the reality of the parent's death" (p. 455). Long-lasting grief certainly is a factor in Magritte, but the traumatic shock and horror of actually seeing the maternal body cry out for repetition in his art.

First, Magritte draws fish people, as metaphorically close to bodies fished out of the river as one can get: a sleeping mermaid in *The Forbidden Universe* (1943), an illustration of a woman with fish head and female hips and legs in *Le Chants de Maldrodor* (1948), and a fish-headed, bloated-bellied female washed up on shore in *Collective Invention* (1953). Second, he paints a woman's face with the naked breasts, navel, and genitals functioning as her features—again gruesomely close to an adolescent view of the exposed, drowned body of his mother (*The Rape,* 1945). Third, he paints human figures with drapes over their faces, too close to Scutenaire's fable for comfort: *The Heart of the Matter* (1928) and *The Lovers* (1928). Fourth, he avoids faces altogether, a Magritte "trademark." There is every chance that Magritte's mother's face was ruined among the eddying currents, the fish, and the rocks. He chooses to insert bowler hats, apples, even sky instead of the human face—anything, as a matter of fact, but the face: *Familiar Object* (1927–28), *The Difficult Crossing* (1963), *The Great War* (1964), *The Idea* (1966), *The Pilgrim* (1966), and *The King's Museum* (1966) are but a few examples. Fifth, Magritte does coffins—one often finds a woman laid out: *The Threatened Assassin* (1926–27), *The Reckless Sleeper* (1927), *A Night's Museum* (1927), and *David's 'Madame Recamier'* (1967). Hammacher (1973) tells of a visit Magritte once made to a coffin maker, winding up actually spending the entire afternoon inside a coffin. Finally, Magritte dreams up bridges, rivers, and endless vistas of the water. As a matter of fact, he does this so many times that a list of paintings would do an injustice to the frequency. His well-known painting *Homesickness*, created during his homeland's occupation by the Nazis (1941), shows the Belgian lion with a forelorn bird-man who is leaning over a bridge contemplating the river—a sad and also a terrifying reminder of an old trauma and a present stress. The picture is quite aptly titled.

The overall tone of Magritte is that "moment of panic" which sometimes occurs "if one has been trapped by the mystery of an image that refuses all explanation" (Gablik, p. 10). How does the painter achieve this? First, time in Magritte is consistently "out of joint." I have described in two papers how time often becomes distorted by the trauma victim (Terr, 1983b, 1984). Magritte illustrates this same time confusion. According to Viederman (in press), Magritte mixed up the dates on his paintings and deliberately threw off his biographical chronologies. Inside of his paintings, Magritte fixes time so securely that everything appears to stand still in a scary way and, as Viederman puts it, "past, present, and future become merged." Another thing Magritte does to induce panic in his viewer is a trick at which Wharton and Hitchcock were also masters: he takes the everyday, the humdrum, and suddenly inserts into it an incomprehensible horror. One thinks one is gliding along, a little bored amid banal reality, and then shockingly—as in real trauma—the panic ensues. Magritte inserts incongruities and impossibilities into the most smoothly realistic style of painting. The shock lasts. One remembers the Magrittes long after one has left the museum.

HITCHCOCK

"Hitch," as he liked to be called, was born to a retail-wholesale greengrocer and his wife in lower middle-class London in 1899. Alfred, like Wharton and Magritte, was a Poe lover. "Very likely," Hitchcock said, "it's because I was so taken with Poe stories that I later made suspense films. I don't want to seem immodest, but I can't help comparing what I've tried to put in my films and what Edgar Allan Poe put in his suspense novels [sic], a completely unbelievable story told to the readers with such a spell-binding logic that you get the impression that the same thing could happen to you tomorrow" (Spoto, 1984, p. 41).

Hitch went to good Catholic schools, but had to drop out altogether at age 14 when his father became ill. His father died when Hitchcock was 15 years old, and the boy, at relatively loose ends and quite poor with words, eventually took an art class and went to work at age 16 as an advertising sketcher for a telegraph and cable company. Hitchcock had spent a considerable part of his boyhood as a "trolly-jolly," a child who knew and timed the schedules of every tram, train, and boat that he could watch. While many trolly-jollys eventually grow up to schedule, main-tain, and manage their own transportation systems, Alfred Hitchcock was different. Something else was motivating him; and when just before turning 21, he learned that an American film company was setting up a new studio in London, he asked for a job as a title maker and he got it.

Alfred Hitchcock's road to the very top of the film industry was fairly straight and clear from that first job on. His talents were quickly recognized and he developed the "cult" of the di-rector through both his clever gimmickery, such as walking on camera in every movie, and his genius photography, emphasiz-ing strange angles and entirely subjective shots. But from the time he reached the top, Alfred Hitchcock repeatedly told a story on himself, a story of psychic trauma for which his sister also vouched (Taylor, 1981). This is Hitchcock's story, quoted from a speech he gave at a Hollywood banquet, March 7, 1979: "When I was no more than six years of age, I did something that my father considered worthy of reprimand. He sent me to the local police station with a note. The officer on duty read it and locked me in a jail cell for five minutes, saying, 'This is what we do to naughty boys.' I have, ever since, gone to any lengths to avoid arrest and confinement" (Spoto, 1984, p. 7).

Hitchcock insisted for years that this single childhood event inspired a body of work with two recurring motifs: fear of prison and enclosure, and fear of the legal authorities. In his fear of entrapment Hitchcock shares a life theme with Wharton, Poe, and Bergman.

If Hitchcock is telling the truth about his innocent jailing, we should find this "truth" literally repeated in his movies—and so we do. Alfred Hitchcock repeatedly gives us the young hero hounded by the law. In *Thirty-nine Steps* (1935), the guiltless young man is pursued by the police for a crime that he did not commit. In *Young and Innocent* (1937), the hero, also wanted for murder, is hunted down by his girlfriend's father, the chief of police. *Saboteur* (1942) gives us Robert Cummings, a factory munitions worker, wrongly accused of arson and other traitorous stuff. In *I Confess* (1952), Montgomery Clift, a priest, finds himself booked, tried, and sullied by a "reasonable doubt" acquittal for a murder another man has admitted to him in the confessional booth. In *Dial M for Murder* (1953), a woman, Grace Kelly, "stands in" for the 5- or 6-year-old Alfred as she is thrown in prison, tried, convicted, and saved from execution at the very last minute (changing voices does not seem to bother the reenacting artist). In 1957, Henry Fonda, *The Wrong Man*, spends a night in jail, wrongly arrested for armed robbery. The "wrong man plot" is, in fact, Hitchcock's most common story line. It turns up in *Strangers on a Train* (1951), *To Catch a Thief* (1955), *North by Northwest* (1959), and *Frenzy* (1972).

In regard to artistic reenactment, I am especially intrigued by a camera shot in the second from the last film Hitchcock ever made, *Frenzy*. Filmed around the Covent Garden markets where, in the old days, the young Alfred and his father often had gone wholesaling their fish, the hero, a rather flawed, down-on-his-luck fellow, is thrown into jail. As he stands wrongly accused of a series of hideous sex murders, Jon Finch (playing the part of Richard Blaney) is photographed from so high above the jail set that the full-grown actor looks like an errant 5-year-old—alone, confined, and utterly overwhelmed in his cell. In this one lingering shot, we see the young Alfred's predicament, a predicament that never left him.

Hitchcock, despite Spoto's and Taylor's tendencies to doubt him, was telling an emotional truth. As a boy he had been shocked. For him, the surprise incarceration held no motive and no fixed duration, that is, until all was finished. This is trauma. Hitchcock needed to transmit his shock to others. We watch fascinated.

Hitch, in his lifetime, committed a number of terrible pranks that shocked and confused, perhaps even traumatized others. He and another boy led a younger schoolmate into the parochial school basement, took off the boy's trousers, and tied him to the boiler. After making some ominous scratching sounds, Hitchcock and his friend ran away and the boy found himself terrified as a series of explosions sounded from the regions of his underpants. Hitchcock, unbeknownst to the boy, had pinned live firecrackers to the young fellow's briefs. The Reverend Robert Goold lived to tell his tale to Alfred Hitchcock's biographer, Donald Spoto (1984). Goold claims never to have seen a movie made by Hitchcock. One need not wonder why.

Confinement spelled terror to Hitchcock. He tried to overcome the fear by confining others. Once an actress asked Hitchcock to disallow cigarettes on the set because she hated the smoke. Hitch contrived that she play a "scene" in a telephone booth, and once she was inside, he released great amounts of smoke into the booth. She left the set, sick and scared. Another time Hitchcock recognized an uneasy tension between Madeline Carrol and Robert Donat on the first day of shooting *The Thirty-nine Steps*. He handcuffed them together for the handcuff scene, conveniently losing the key and not letting them escape one another until the very end of the day. They did not like it.

The tone of Hitchcock, like that of Wharton and Magritte, is absolutely commonplace and banal until the shock comes. Then all hell breaks loose. Cary Grant lolls about near a wheat field in the most famous scene of *North by Northwest*. A crop duster drones at its work. Suddenly the duster is after Grant, and the actor is running for his very life. Such is the tone of trauma—of panic, of shock, and of utter helplessness. Guy Haines (Farley Granger) happens to be playing tennis while his adversary Bruno Anthony (Robert Walker) is "playing" inside a storm drain, trying to retrieve the evidence that should wrongly convict Guy of murder. A bright, rather mundane athletic exercise at Forest Hills is cross-cut with a gloomy procedure aimed at malevolent mischief (Spoto, 1976). The cross-cutting of bright and gloom, mundane and mean—this is what creates the panicky terror. Hitchcock knew how to do this, perhaps better than anyone. That is why, when Cary Grant, on an elevator with two assassins and his rather silly mother, tries to tell her that he is in trouble and she turns to the killers and says, "You men aren't *really* trying to kill my son, are you?" the audience smiles its strychnined grin. It waits. It knows that Hitchcock's blow will strike soon enough, but it also knows the blow will come when least expected.

Two of Hitchcock's mature films reenact absolutely nothing literal from his own 5- or 6-year-old terror, but they create such a tone of utter helplessness and entrapment that the audience experiences in miniaturized form the affects specific to psychic trauma. In both *Psycho* and *The Birds*, relatively innocent people (yes, Janet Leigh did embezzle from her boss, but did she deserve that horrible shower scene?) are attacked by forces so big, so violent, so unexpected, so intense, and so scary that the feeling of trauma infects the viewer, whether or not he seems to be resting easy in his armchair at the movie house. That Hitchcock, like Bergman, Magritte, and Poe, can see menace in quite ordinary birds—or, like Poe, can find shock value in a mother alive-in-death—this shows that terror is created not only through direct reenactment but by the establishment of a tone. The horror film is best made by the formerly horrified.

BERGMAN

Ingmar Bergman was a true master of horror, though this time no fan of Poe's. Bergman's father was a strict Scandinavian minister more in the mold of the pastor in *Winter's Light* than of the one in *Fanny and Alexander*. His mother, an intelligent, well-educated, upper-class woman, was the second cousin to her husband. Their first child, Dag, grew up to become a diplomat. The second child was Ingmar, born in 1918, and the third, Margareta, born in 1922, eventually achieved some success as a novelist. Early in his life Ingmar spent happy hours with his maternal grandmother in her 14-room apartment in Uppsala, the most historic city in Sweden. (There are echoes of Uppsala and that apartment in much of his work.) Bergman describes having hallucinations at his grandmother's place at around age 5. He spent long hours there, sometimes alone under the dining room table "listening to the sunshine," or watching grandmother's Venus de Milo move, or staring at the nursery window blinds while innumerable figures, "no special little men or animals or heads or faces, but something for which no words existed . . . crept out of the curtains and moved toward the green lampshade or to the table where the drinking water stood" (Cowie, 1983, p. 8).

Some children who have been traumatized tend to hallucinate or to experience visual illusions (Terr, 1979, 1985). Could psychic trauma have already struck Ingmar Bergman well before he turned 5 years? He tells us "yes," although his story of the event makes one wonder if a child less sensitive than Ingmar would have been so overcome. One day in Uppsala while Bergman's grandmother was looking after him, he locked himself inside a wardrobe. Ingmar says he was shocked and furious beyond anything he ever felt. While his grandmother rushed about looking for a key, the little boy tore through the hem of his mother's dress with his teeth. In *Hour of the Wolf*, the main character, Johan Borg, tells his wife the identical story, adding that while locked in he felt terrified that "a little man" would gnaw at his feet in the darkness (Cowie, p. 11).

It seems that after this lock-up, Bergman repeatedly courted weird experience. When he was 6 and his father was assigned to the Royal Hospital, Sofia-hemmet, the child sought out the hospital gardener, whose duty it was to bring the dead from the hospital to the mortuary. "I found it fascinating to go with him; it was my first contact with the human being in death, and the faces looked like those of dolls. It was scary but also very fascinating" (Cowie, p. 8). Ingmar also liked to hang out in the boiler room under the hospital where amputated limbs were being burned in huge furnaces. "For a child," Bergman says, "it was traumatic, and I loved it!" (Cowie, p. 9).

Here is a child-dreamer, then, with a taste for the macabre and a profound sensitivity. He experiences two horrors: one, the unexpected shock of confinement in a wardrobe; and two, the repeatedly asked-for thrills of watching the disintegration and disposal of bodies.

Peter Cowie, Bergman's "critical biographer" who, as he wrote his book (1983), knew that his subject was still quite alive, is careful not to say too much about Bergman himself. We hear about five marriages, numerous beautiful and famous lovers, but we cannot understand why all but the most recent relationship have ended in simple "friendships." We do know, however, that in his late teens Ingmar fought with his parents because he hated "the iron caskets of duty" to which they seemed bound. After he dropped out of the university, the elder Bergmans erupted with anger and the young Ingmar broke completely with his parents, an estrangement that lasted for 4 years. The Bergman of the postuniversity period was ambitious, intense, prone to tears, and rebellious. He began directing plays—and soon, cinema—never experiencing a real failure. His career was largely a move from local to national and international recognition.

He would shut himself in—sometimes into the bathroom for such long spells that friends like the actor Stig Olin wondered "if he was alive, dead, or just sulking" (Cowie, p. 20). He would watch his early play productions from the projectionist's booth, again seeking confinement at times of anxiety.

But it is the films, not the life, that give us the most literal reenactments that we find in Bergman. In *Hour of the Wolf* (1966) we get the whole story of the confinement in the wardrobe, told as a child might do it for elementary school "Show and Tell." In *Torment* (1944), the first film that Bergman directed, a schoolmaster, after murdering a young woman, conceals himself behind several coats—a closet scene, full of panic and malevolence, though not as closed in as the 4- or 5-year-old's ancient confinement. *A Ship Bound for India* and *Port of Call* gives us several ship cabins and a tiny apartment that "assume the dimensions of a prison" (Cowie, p. 64). In *Thirst* (known in the U.S. as *Three Strange Loves*) Bergman shuts up his two warring marital protagonists in a train compartment, again creating a stifling sense of imprisonment. Bergman's 1952 film *Secrets of Women* gives us another couple trapped, this time in a stuck elevator, as they discuss and reconcile their marriage right there and then. *Secrets*, a dusky comedy, was Bergman's first great hit, but the director would come to find new and more sinister ways to confine his people. In 1955 Bergman, in possibly his greatest movie, *The Seventh Seal*, locks his protagonist, the Knight, into a medieval confessional with the persona of Death. The tiny confessional, supposedly a place in which one achieves liberation, is thus turned by Ingmar Bergman into his old chamber of horrors, the nursery wardrobe. This time Death himself serves as key-keeper.

Bergman appends his own, often grotesque fantasy and his own, often grotesque misperception to his later scenarios of traumatic lock-up. In his unique and very personal 1973 stage production of Strindberg's *A Ghost Sonata*, Bergman has the Old Man dragged off stage to die in a closet from whence the audience hears the sound of his neck being broken.[2] The old closet scene of Bergman's actual preschool life here is expanded through fantasy so that the small, barely audible sounds of childhood incisors biting away at a hem have become magnified to the giant sounds of adult cervical vertebrae being snapped asunder. Bergman also puts an old childhood traumatic misperception, that of being in two places at once, into his films (Terr, 1984). When a child is actually locked up, he may so urgently want to be let out that, in his "captivity," he pictures himself carried away to safety. He can "see" it. I think this explains the most confusing scene in Bergman's semiautobiographical movie, *Fanny and Alexander* (1982). The children have been locked into a tiny room by their wicked stepfather. Their friend, Uncle Isak, shows up with a trunk. As the youngsters remain locked up in a room at the top of the house, they are simultaneously being carried outside in a trunk. An impossibility, yes. But not for the active imagination of a preschooler in trouble—a sensitive lad locked in a nursery wardrobe. Bergman does another variation on this "room trick" in *Persona*. Here a nurse (played by Bibi Anderson) is supposedly answering a summons to the doctor's office, but simultaneously enters her patient's room. In the *Magician*, the conjurer, Vogler (Max von Sydow), is confined under house arrest, but is eventually "magicked" out by royal proclamation. Vogler is to appear before the King on July 14, Ingmar Bergman's birthday. In *Hour of the Wolf*, a sinister man walks up the walls and across the ceiling

2. In my 1985 paper "Remembered Images and Trauma," I made an error reproduced on p. 503. I had wrongly cited the 1973 Bergman production of Strindberg as *A Dream Play*. The research I did for the paper written on these pages turned up my mistake. It was *A Ghost Sonata* in which the old man dies off stage, confined in a closet.

of the room, another visitation, perhaps, from the "little man" in the director's ancient closet.

Bergman also seems to need to reexperience his "enjoyable," self-perpetuated "traumas" from ages 6, 7, and 8 at the hospital mortuary and disposal furnaces of Sophia-hemmet. In *The Magician,* he gives us an eyeball in an inkwell and a dismembered hand. In *Shame,* a body lies on a floor to be tripped over, and bodies float in waters that are meant for escape. In *Hour of the Wolf,* an old lady drops her eyeball into the wine and rips the skin off her face with a terrible crackle. In *The Passion of Anna,* a horse is burned up, sheep slaughtered, and a dog tortured, all in the name of terror—and in the name of Bergman's ever-present death and disintegration obsession.

Bergman went to the hospital with a virus just before writing *Persona.* Upon his release, he made it clear that the old "corpses" were back with him. He told the press: "In hospital one has a strong sense of corpses floating up through the bedstead. Besides which I had a view of the morgue, people marching in and out with little coffins, in and out" (Cowie, p. 227). Although *Persona* gives us the same grim reenactive embodiments of bodily disintegration and death that Bergman so often forces on us—a hand being nailed to the cross, a dead body lying in profile, a boy beneath a sheet—he gives us something even worse, scarier, the sense of utter annihilation, the wipe-out of all boundaries. Mauritz Edstrom, in reviewing *Persona,* describes the film "as a confession of fear: fear of your fellow man, fear of your neighbor's strength and insight—and the wish to see the security of others shattered by a naked fear of death" (Cowie, p. 235). This is psychic trauma, trauma contagious as a plague.

The tone of Bergman's work, with the exception of a handful of dark "comedies," is the tone of psychic trauma—terror, horror, panic, and absolute helplessness. Bergman gives us much shorter escapes into banality and humdrum everyday life than does Hitchcock. He most often shoots his films in heavily contrasting black and white. He makes horrible, shocking sounds. He also establishes a tone of terror in the settings he chooses. Bergman often goes back to the Middle Ages for an almost hysterical way of life, or he takes us to the strangest of cities (*The Silence*) and the barrenest of islands (*Shame*). We are almost always confined, locked in, and ready to scream. Bergman, like Poe, Magritte, and Hitchcock, sees birds as sinister objects. He films his villain in *Hour of the Wolf*, Lindhorst, holding his arms out wide like a bat as hundreds of little birds fly around him. He emphasizes fences (as in the fenced-in rape in *The Virgin Spring*) or walls or barriers (in *The Touch*). Sometimes he shows menace out in the open spaces (*Shame*), but more often he encloses us in the most painful, claustrophobic way (Karin's room in *Through a Glass Darkly*, for instance). Man's helplessness is emphasized again and again—ranging from a quick glimpse at a self-immo- lating monk (*Persona*) to a hopeless chess game on the beach with Death (*The Seventh Seal*). An evening with Ingmar is not easily forgotten. The aftertaste can be incredibly unpleasant.

THE AUDIENCE AND THE TRAUMATIZED ARTIST

Traumatized artists pick up fans. As a matter of fact, the pull of posttraumatic reenactment is so strong that traumatized artists may make and keep more fanatically faithful audiences than do geniuses who arrive at their art in entirely different ways. There is something about trauma that beckons the nontraumatized person to taste. The Cujos and the Christines may be far more popular than the Othellos or the Madame Bovarys.

Why is this so? Hitchcock thinks the audience, safe in its arm- chair, likes the vicarious thrill of a suspense film, knowing for certain that it will be safe no matter what horrors come out of the projector (Spoto, 1984). This is quite similar to Freud's (1900) explanation of the examination dream—the dreamer creates an unpleasantly suspenseful situation in his dream in order to real- ize in the relief of awakening that all is the opposite. The dream indirectly serves as a reassurance in the same sense as Hitchcock sees the suspense film serving the purpose of reassurance.

One wonders, though. Poe does not reassure us at all about death; rather, he gives us new information, compelling lessons in what happens to bodies in their corruption, in what horrible ways one might die. One may be safe in one's chair—but It's coming. Poe does not soothe. Rather, he stirs up. His action upon us is more in the mode of Freud's "traumatic dream"— creating new anxiety with every repetition.

Take two of Poe's tales, "The Masque of the Red Death" and the "Cask of Amontillado." One can just about see those masquers in that vast castle with its variously colored rooms, so vividly are they written. Poe's masquers are wearing the costumes originally adopted in Europe as protections against the Black Plague (people thought if you could just cover up enough, you could foil Death). There is a terrible plague—the Red Death—at hand. Good Lord, how they revel and dance their wild bacchanalias. But they are doomed, and the absolute hysteria of this final dance is almost too much for the reader to bear. So it is with the merry, masqued, and unsuspecting Fortunato. His death walled up in the basement vaults of his adversary creates hysteria, not calm. We learn that killers get away with their crimes—that wild revels may presage wilder attacks from Mother Nature herself; that color and costume cannot fool the blackest Death. There is no escape. We may be one of the unlucky ones. The teeth start to chatter. The audience is being sucked out of the armchair of reassurance. Traumatic art creates panic, not just the discomfort of a momentary impediment on the road to relief.

Parenthetical to my original studies at Chowchilla, I began to find (entirely by accident, in a sense) that the symptoms of childhood trauma were highly contagious—that these symptoms "infected" a certain number of nontraumatized youngsters who were exposed to the victim. Rather than finding the comfort inherent in looking at the horror from the "Hitchcockian armchair of reassurance," a good number of "normals" would join right into the symptoms of the traumatized. They would enter the reenactments, play the playground games of kidnap, rape, and death, and even pass them on to other normals. One Chowchilla girl, Leslie, as a matter of fact, even passed the horror of her burial in the "hole" to her toddler sister's dreams (Terr, 1979). The little girl screamed out one night in terror, about a year after the kidnapping, "I in a hole. In a hole."

I have observed the transmission of posttraumatic illusions, time skews, play, reenactment, fears, and dreams. I have already presented a bit of this hands-on contagion when I mentioned Poe's and Hitchcock's behavioral reenactments—their terrible "pranks" for which live accomplices and live victims were required. It does not take too much stretching of the imagination, I think, to broaden the idea of "accomplices" to the audience itself. A large pool of vicarious accomplices (and of vicarious victims) sit in those armchairs, walk through those galleries, and read those books. Some can hang tightly enough onto their own boundaries to "enjoy" the vicarious thrills of a horror well told. But some cannot. Those who cannot may be the modern brothers and sisters to the Children's Crusaders, the flagellants, and the masquers—those hysterical mobs who could not stand the traumatic anxieties inherent to the Plague. Plagues of birds do not differ that much from plagues of rats and their parasites, the bacilli. If one gets into the spirit of the thing, one may feel just a shade away from screaming.

I will finish this paper on a personal note. I have not been traumatized. But as a young child I saw a newsreel at the Saturday afternoon matinee the weekend after the atomic bomb was dropped on Hiroshima. I cannot forget how it looked there—bleached white and leveled to the earth. A cameraman had shot the shadow of a vaporized person on a footbridge near ground zero, and somehow I knew what that meant. I realized that the man's shadow had protected the bridge from bleaching out at the instant of the flash, but that the man had disintegrated almost at once. I see that "picture" now. I also admit to one posttraumatic symptom. If tonight you suddenly switched on my bedroom light at 2 or 3 A.M., or if you made a sudden loud sound, my heart would start to pound before I could help it. I would breath hard and sweat—and for a second or two, as I came to consciousness I would say to myself, "This is it. It's all over. The Bomb."

Last night as I finished correcting and editing these words, I did not sleep well. My mind was overloaded with snapshots of Tippi Heddren trying to beat off her feathered attackers, of Death eating his sandwich on Bergman's film set, of a Magritte lady gorging herself on a live bird (*Pleasure*), and of Ethan Frome trapped forever with that awful wife of his. I know I may have brought some of you nightmares with the pictures I have created as I write. But I also know something that you do not—you have already had your revenge! Last night I had three dreams, all the same. At the sound of a horrible piercing electronic beep, my death was announced. Three times—from sleep—I spoke aloud. "I'm dying," I said. I am here, yes. And a little reassured. But I have noticed today as I make these final corrections—every electronic watch or beeper that has gone off here at Lane Library, Stanford, has made my pen hesitate, has made it stay just a bit. I am one of you—that panicky part of the audience that thinks to itself, "Yes, it's not that far out. It happened to Poe, Wharton, Magritte, Hitch, and Bergman. It *could* happen to *me.*"

BIBLIOGRAPHY

BONAPARTE, M. (1933). *The Life and Works of Edgar Allan Poe.* London: Imago, 1949.

COWIE, P. (1983). *Ingmar Bergman.* New York: Scribner's.

EDEL, L. (1982). *Stuff of Sleep and Dreams.* New York: Avon Books.

ESMAN, A. H. (1986). Giftedness and creativity in children and adolescents. *Adol. Psychiatry,* 13:62–84.

FELDMAN, D. (1982). A developmental framework for research with gifted children. In *New Directions in Child Development,* ed. D. Feldman. San Francisco: Jossey-Bass.

FREUD, S. (1900). The interpretation of dreams. *S.E.,* 4 & 5.

———— (1926). Inhibitions, symptoms and anxiety. *S.E.,* 20:77–175.

———— (1933). Foreword to M. Bonaparte's *Poe.* London: Imago, 1949, p. xi.

GABLIK, S. (1985). *Magritte.* New York: Thames & Hudson.

GEDO, J. (1983). *Portraits of the Artist.* New York: Guilford Press.

GUILFORD, J. (1967). *The Nature of Human Intelligence.* New York: McGraw-Hill.

HAMMACHER, A. M. (1973). *Magritte.* New York: Abrams.

LEWIS, R. W. B. (1975). *Edith Wharton.* New York: Harper & Row.

LURIE, A. (1985). *Foreign Affair.* New York: Avon.

POE, E. (1971). *Poems.* Norwalk, Conn.: Heritage Press.

———— (1941). *Tales of Mystery and Imagination.* New York: Heritage Press.

SAUNDERS, J. B. D. C. M. (1986). Personal communication on the handling of contagious disease in Europe in 1860–1870.

SPOTO, D. (1976). *The Art of Alfred Hitchcock.* New York: Dolphin Books.

———— (1984). *The Dark Side of Genius.* New York: Ballantine Books.

TAYLOR, J. R. (1981). *Hitch.* London: Sphere Books (Abacus).

TERR, L. (1979). Children of Chowchilla. *Psychoanal. Study Child,* 34:547–623.

———— (1981). "Forbidden games." *J. Amer. Acad. Child Psychiat.,* 20:741–760.

———— (1983a). Chowchilla revisited. *Amer. J. Psychiat.,* 140:1543–1550.

———— (1983b). Time sense following psychic trauma. *Amer. J. Orthopsychiat.,* 53:244–261.

———— (1984). Time and trauma. *Psychoanal. Study Child,* 39:633–666.

—— (1985). Remembered images and trauma. *Psychoanal. Study Child,* 40:493–533.

—— (1986). Memories of preschool psychic trauma. Read at the annual meeting, American Psychiatric Association, Washington. D.C.

—— (1987). The trauma-stress disorders. Read as the Samuel B. Hibbs Award Lecture at the annual meeting, American Psychiatric Association, Chicago.

TORCZYNER, H. (1977). *Magritte.* France: Draeger.

VAN DYKE, C., ZILBERG, N., & McKINNON, J. (1985). Posttraumatic stress disorder. *Amer. J. Psychiat.,* 142:1070–1073.

VIEDERMAN, M. (1987). René Magritte. *J. Amer. Psychoanal. Assn.,* 35 (in press).

WHARTON, E. (1985). *The Ghost Stories of Edith Wharton.* New York: Scribner's.

WOLFENSTEIN, M. (1973). The image of the lost parent. *Psychoanal. Study Child,* 28:433–456.

PSYCHOANALYTIC EDUCATION

Supervision of Child Psychoanalyses

JULES GLENN, M.D.

THE FIRST SUPERVISION

FREUD (1909) WAS THE FIRST SUPERVISOR OF A CHILD PSYCHO-
analysis, the treatment of Little Hans by his father (see Glenn,
1980; Silverman, 1980). Hans's father, Max Graf, wrote letters
to Freud describing his son's phobia and seeking guidance, and
talked to him about the case. Freud not only provided the ana-
lyst/parent with confirmation and amplification of Hans's dynamics and suggested interpretations. He also appears to have
restrained the analyst's impatience. In addition, he arranged to
see the boy and offered him interpretations directly.

Freud had known the patient and his family before the outbreak of the phobia. He had analyzed Mrs. Graf and worked
with Mr. Graf. He had even met Hans previously. He thus knew
a great deal about the family interaction and Hans's life. This
knowledge was supplemented by the history Hans's father provided. Before Hans became ill, Max Graf had told Freud details
of the boy's sexual life and interests which confirmed some of
Freud's theories of psychosexual development.

The relationship between analyst and supervisor was collegial.
Max Graf, a music critic, had been a member of Freud's Wednesday evening group and had contributed to their study of creativ-

Clinical professor of psychiatry, New York University Medical Center.
Training and supervising analyst, The Psychoanalytic Institute, New York
University Medical Center.

I thank Drs. Isidor Bernstein, Helen Beiser, Roy Lilleskov, Heiman Van
Dam, and Stanley S. Weiss for their critical reading of this paper and their
helpful suggestions.

ity (Nunberg and Federn, 1967). The two men respected each other. Although Freud was expert in the analysis of adults, he had no experience with child analysis, which did not exist prior to this treatment. Graf, although he had never treated anybody before he analyzed his son, knew a great deal about analytic theory and technique. Freud and Graf were pioneers exploring new ground together.

Many of the elements of this first supervisory relationship are—or should be—true of later supervisions. A more experienced and a less experienced but knowledgeable analyst engage in a collegial relationship and discuss a particular case. The supervisor encourages the supervisee to conduct the analysis as his own, but offers insight, guidance, and support. For each it is a new adventure. Never before has this patient been analyzed. Each will learn things from the experience. Theory will be elucidated and extended. New techniques, or at least adaptations and modifications of known procedures, will be developed as the analyst struggles to understand his patient and convey his insights.

There were of course important aspects of the supervision that differ from usual contemporary supervision. Graf was not being trained to be a child analyst; Hans was his sole patient. Freud should probably be considered the analyst, in that he directed the case rather than taught the technique, as well as the supervisor (Isidor Bernstein, personal communication). In addition, the technique of child analysis has changed markedly. Fathers no longer analyze their own children, contrary to Freud's belief in 1909 that only parents could carry out an analysis. Current child analysts pay more attention to defenses, reality factors, transference, and countertransference. During Hans's visit, Freud (1909) made a remarkably probing interpretation: "Long before he was in the world, . . . I had known that a little Hans would come who would be so fond of his mother that he would be bound to feel afraid of his father because of it" (p. 42). Hans responded after he left his session, which his father had attended as well, by asking, "Does the Professor talk to God . . . as he can tell all that beforehand?" Freud recognized that his "joking boastfulness" (p. 43) had provoked this comment.

Even without such an overt narcissistic expression, supervisor and supervisee (or analyst and analysand) can enjoy the belief that one member of the dyad is superior, all knowing, and perfect. A kind of supervisory transference-countertransference myth may be propagated. Such a fantasy may temporarily facilitate the transmission of knowledge, but may eventually lead to disillusionment, a severed relationship, and a renunciation of the acquired knowledge. Indeed, years later Max Graf did break with Freud! Such a failure may be based on an oedipal rebellion of the son/supervisee against the father/supervisor or on a more primitive narcissistic blow. In this instance the fact that Freud had analyzed Mrs. Graf who later was divorced from her husband added to the difficulties.

Freud's description of Little Hans's analysis contains many of the basic issues of the supervisory experience. It is typical of Freud's clinical papers that his brilliant descriptions transcend his theoretical intentions. I will in this paper discuss the issues that appear in Freud's case study and other issues relevant to optimal child analytic supervision.

Discussion of child analytic supervision is particularly important because the scant literature on the subject (American Psychoanalytic Association, 1978; Becker, 1985; Deutsch, 1977; Francis, 1978; A. Freud, 1922–1980; Lewin and Ross, 1960) focuses for the most part on requirements and statistics, and does not include a systematic study of supervisory practice. Inevitably many of the problems and proposals will apply as well to the supervision of psychoanalysis and psychotherapy of adults and the psychotherapy of children.

The Elements of Child Analytic Training

Supervision is but one element in learning to practice child analysis. Before starting an analysis the student should have undergone (or be undergoing) a personal analysis and should have extensive didactic preparation. This should include courses in psychoanalytic theory and facts, including child development. The student's experience with children, including direct observation, should continue throughout his training, indeed optimally throughout his professional life. The student should also participate in courses in child and adolescent psychoanalytic technique and, to extend his experience, attend and present at continuous case seminars and other clinical conferences.

There has been some debate as to whether the prior practice of adult psychoanalysis is essential for the practice of child psychoanalysis. It would appear that since purely child analytic training programs exist, prior training is not necessary. Nonetheless, the American Psychoanalytic Association requires that at least some adult analytic training precede child analytic training. Perhaps this is justified. It may be that the flexibility required for child analysis interferes with the formation of a firm conception of adult analytic technique with a minimum of parameters. It may also be true that the discipline of carrying out an adult analysis in which the main instrument is interpretation strengthens the student's determination to adhere to an interpretive stance in treating children.

As I stated, Max Graf was well versed in the basics of psychoanalytic theory, even though he did not take formal courses. He did not treat adults. Interestingly enough, the Wednesday night study group—with Freud and Max Graf participating—discussed aspects of the case of Little Hans in their consideration of the sexual enlightenment of children on May 12, 1909 (Nunberg and Federn, 1967), a year after the termination of the analysis.

SUPERVISION OF THE CONSULTATION

Both analyst and supervisor must join in determining the child's diagnosis and his analyzability. This requires an extensive history of the child's life and the framework his family provided. Supervision of the assessment is invaluable. The consultation provides the background material that will help one to understand the child as a human being in his changing and throbbing environment. Whereas the therapist of adults does not have the details of his patient's development available—his birth and feeding history, for instance—the child analyst can acquire these data from his patient's parents. Nor does the analyst of adults get to know the parents directly and perceive their actual characteristics, as does the child analyst. This extra-analytic information can be a burden, but the student, with his supervisor's help, may learn to use it constructively. I shall discuss this further when I get to the problems of working with parents.

At this point, I want to emphasize that one should not accept the historical data at face value. Parents make errors in their anamnesis, which they may correct later, and often are inaccurate in their assessment of the child's inner life. The child's perception of reality is quite different from that of the adults. It is shaped by his immature cognitive capacities as well as by fantasies related to developmental stages and other inner forces and conflicts. In analysis we deal with the child's psychic reality as well as with external circumstances, a fact that the supervisor may help the student to appreciate. Nevertheless, knowledge of the child's experiences as he grows up can enrich the analysis.

Not all cases brought to the supervisor for discussion are suitable for child analysis. The supervisor must help the supervisee to make an appropriate decision about the proper form of treatment. He may have to discourage an overzealous desire to analyze an inappropriate child. On the other hand, the supervisor may have to encourage undertaking analysis when the student demurs. He may have to help the student take proper steps to convince the child's parents that analysis is the optimal treatment when it is, and to help the child join in the analytic work.

SUPERVISION OF THE ANALYSIS

Once the analysis itself starts, the supervisor and student continue to work together to understand the patient. To accomplish this the analyst provides a running description of the treatment—what both he and the patient said and did, what the parents told the analyst. Most often the supervisee refers to process notes taken after the sessions with patients. Some read the notes verbatim. Some are able to describe the analysis without notes. Ideally the supervisee eventually describes the flow of the material in less detail. Most often the supervisory sessions occur weekly at first and less frequently later.

What the supervisor helps the analyst to understand varies in accordance with the personal characteristics and needs of the participants. Some students quickly grasp the dynamics of the case and the unconscious wishes and fantasies that are defended against, but do not appreciate the surface manifestations or the environmental pressures. Other emphasize reality factors. Still others are attuned to the patients' more or less conscious thoughts and feelings and their defensive maneuvers, but have difficulty surmising the unconscious urges.

While appreciating the supervisee's understanding of his patient, the supervisor must help the student to broaden his perspective and perceive the many facets of the patient's personality and conflicts.

Inevitably different supervisors emphasize different aspects of the patient's pathology. Their personal ways of thinking about analytic cases and their individual technical propensities and styles influence the supervision. (Because of this diversity, it is wise for students to have several supervisors.) I—and many others—prefer to start at the surface and first construct a picture of the patient as a human being rather than a bundle of mental mechanisms. I prefer to view the patient in his family setting and see how he reacts to those about him early in the analysis, and indeed throughout the analysis. At the same time I early on concentrate on the patient's defenses while I allow my guesses about deeper strata to remain in the background of my thinking. As the analysis proceeds, I get to understand hidden conflicts better and to interpret these to a greater extent. I never attempt to ignore the surface and defensive aspects. Usually unconscious material becomes more and more conscious as the analysis proceeds. My students get to see my approach and frequently emulate it.

Perhaps I am being too cautious in suggesting that my approach is but one of many. Actually the principles I have stated are generally accepted as the proper approach. There may be differences in emphasis, but the basic technical procedures remain the same.

A student with a propensity to emphasize unconscious fantasies correctly saw the appearance of birth symbolism in his 10-year-old patient's play with clay early in the analysis.[1] The pa-

1. In the illustrations I have, for convenience and disguise, referred to all students and supervisors as male.

tient excitedly constructed flowers which multiplied within womblike enclosures. Pointing the symbolism out to the patient increased his excitement and anxiety. The supervisor helped the candidate to see that the patient, growing up in a seductive environment in which his parents openly fought and had affairs, was trying desperately to control his excitement. The analyst could then appreciate that he had best interpret the patient's attempts to cope with his overwhelming emotions.

In this example the analyst, in his quest for deep understanding, focused on the symbolism in the child's play. He deemphasized the role of the child's environment, the patient's conscious feelings of excitement and anxiety, the child's defensive attempts to cope with these. As it turned out, not only was the external stress important in his pathology. In addition, the child suffered from ego deficits which made it difficult for him to master inner urges and outer pressures.

Analytic Styles: Theoretical Conceptualization and Empathy

Some analysts rely heavily on theoretical constructs in picturing their patients' difficulties. Others use their intuition and empathy to a greater extent when they attempt to understand their patients. Both approaches are necessary and, again, the student should optimally reach a proper balance (Fenichel, 1941). An emphasis on empathy has the advantage of sensitizing one to the patient's reactions to possible interpretations.

A student observed that his 8-year-old patient's play with paper airplanes increased during his sessions. He sometimes made the plane crash with a combination of elation and dismay. At other times he grasped the flying machine, preventing it from taking off. The analyst realized that the patient's father was about to leave on a trip to Europe. He recognized the child's concern about his father being injured and the hostile wish that lay behind it. He also realized that the boy wanted to rescue his father, keep him alive, not allow him to leave, out of love and guilt. He chose to interpret the defensive aspects of the material by pointing out that the boy was worried about his father being hurt and therefore wanted father and his plane not to leave. The

boy immediately recognized that his play depicted these concerns. Later the analyst interpreted the patient's hostility to his
father for leaving him and his wishes that he die so that he could
be alone with his mother. Even here descriptions of defenses
were incorporated into the interpretation.

In this case the candidate understood the patient and his conflicts very well. The supervisor had nothing to add to the analyst's insight and technique. They did discuss the general principles involved: starting from the surface; generally interpreting
defenses before drives.

In a classical paper Bornstein (1949) described what interpretation would be most suitable. Frankie, her 5-year-old patient, repeatedly used dolls to play a scene in which a child sits in
a hospital lobby while his father visits his mother who is ill or has
given birth. A fire breaks out burning all the babies in the hospital. The child, at first in danger, joins the fire department and
rescues only lady patients who had no babies. In the course of the
play Frankie several times addressed one lady as "Mommy." She
was killed in the fire. Frankie's disturbance started after the birth
of his sister, and it was apparent that he was struggling with his
fury at her and his mother. Bornstein decided not to interpret
the rage or even the defenses at first, but to focus on the sadness
and loneliness the little boy experienced. This feeling was the
surface emotion which needed attention. Bornstein wrote, "before the defense proper could be dealt with, it was necessary to
have the child recognize and experience such affects" (p. 187).

In other cases the supervisor may encourage the student's use
of empathy by suggesting that he temporarily put himself in the
patient's place and imagine how he would feel. There is of
course the danger that the analyst's and the patient's reactions
may be quite different. It is necessary to examine the patient's
communications to ascertain whether the analyst's tentative conclusions are correct. "Empathy" without reality verification is
not empathy at all.

A student was puzzled by a patient's anger at him. She cursed
him as insignificant and threatened to stop seeing him. He knew
that the little girl was repeatedly neglected by her parents who
placed her in the care of a housekeeper. He also knew that the
mother deprecated the father, proclaiming him a weak and inef-

fectual man whose income was less than hers. Mulling over how he would feel in that situation, he concluded that the girl was angry at her parents for their neglect and desertion. He decided that her attacks on him were demeaning and that the girl directed her anger at him who, like her father, was considered an inferior being. The analyst also recognized that the girl's threats to leave him were a reversal of her feelings that she was left. These interpretations were verified. Later it developed that the mother not only demeaned the father in front of the patient, she also derogated the analyst and talked of switching to a woman therapist.

Supervisory Styles

As indicated above, supervisors vary in their approaches to their task. Some tend to encourage autonomy, while others guide their students' analyses. Some tend to emphasize short-term trends, while others focus on the longer haul. Some emphasize internal conflict, while others are more interested in development, sometimes in its nonconflictual aspects. Some underline reality, some the transference.

Ekstein and Wallerstein (1958) suggested that the best supervisors promote growth through identification with their own ideals and behavior rather than with their technical suggestions and beliefs. I subscribe to the belief that the supervisor optimally stirs the student's imagination and curiosity and spurs his creativity.

Although no studies of styles of supervisors of child analysis have appeared, Beiser (1982) compared the characteristics of male and female supervisors of adult analyses who had child analytic training and those who did not. "It was found that child-analyst supervisors, as they were when they were students, tended to be more oriented to the immediate supervisory situation. Non-child analysis were more oriented to the process in the patient. Women supervisors were more open about themselves and more supportive of the student, and men were somewhat more managing and task-oriented. Women were also more aware of situations outside the dyadic situation, and had fewer personal biases" (p. 68).

MEANS OF COMMUNICATION

Understanding the patient allows the analyst to provide the material and atmosphere that will encourage the patient to communicate in the way most appropriate for him. It will also enable the analyst to communicate to the patient on his terms and on his level.

Students usually learn during their coursework what types of toys to have available in the analytic playroom so as to provide a source of materials for communication: simple toys like blocks, dolls (large and small), and possibly a dollhouse, some vehicles, guns, crayons, and paper. (There is no firm list. Some children may utilize special tools for special needs.) But frequently the student becomes interested in the supervisor's storehouse of playthings and facilities. This becomes a basis for identification with the supervisor and a source of knowledge. Some analysts do not have playrooms but allow the child to use the consultation room for play. In the latter case, does the analyst have to restrain the child's activities excessively? The student may wonder about this and other questions. Should the analyst have paints and water available? What about board games or other organized games? These issues can be discussed in a nondogmatic way and experiences traded.

I for one generally do not provide organized games, including Chutes and Ladders, Monopoly, cards, checkers, and chess. At times, however, a particular patient may require simply organized games. And, of course, patients may bring their own games and toys to the sessions, sometimes to communicate their own conflicts, sometimes to hide them.

The child one student treated took advantage of the presence of organized games to reveal his competitiveness as well as to hide the amplifications of his thoughts and feelings that freer play would have allowed. The supervisor suggested that it might be best not to have such games available in the playroom, but the student vehemently opposed this idea. He pointed out that this child (and others) did express himself in the board games. Another supervisor, he said, had approved of such playroom material. In addition, the very act of removing the games would complicate the treatment. Although the reasons for doing so could be discussed with the patient, the anger at being deprived of the play the boy enjoyed might not be analyzable.

With time, the student changed his views and eventually the board games disappeared from the consultation room. The supervisor did not know when or how this was done or what the patient's reactions were. The student had maintained his autonomy in making the decision and executing the measure suggested by the supervisor. One cannot be certain that the course of the analysis was altered decisively by the change in arrangements. Suffice it to say that the analysis went very well.

Children do not free associate (except possibly for brief periods), but do communicate through play, drawing, and speech. The child analyst in turn must communicate to the patient. In order to make interpretations understandable and palpable the therapist must find appropriate means of expression. The supervisor can be helpful here.

Helping the student understand children of different developmental stages, aiding the children to find appropriate means of communication and the analyst to talk to the child in his language are essentials of child analytic supervision. Even in adult analysis the therapist must adapt the form and style of interpretation as well as its content to each patient's needs and capabilities. Nevertheless, the gap between the adult and child analyst's requirements in this area is much wider than in totally adult analytic practice. So too is the chasm between communication with children of different ages.

Getting the feel for how one should talk to children derives from many experiences: memories of one's own childhood; contact with one's own children and others that one meets outside of psychiatric, psychotherapeutic, and psychoanalytic encounters; children seen professionally. Often many experiences of this nature are not in the relatively young student's ken. In any case, although these contacts are important and helpful, they do not fully prepare the student for the special communications with analytic patients which attempt to reach the child in an extremely personal way, touching on subjects that are often painful and often forbidden.

The supervisor can help the candidate by telling him how *he* would talk to the patient and even by describing other analytic situations. When Bornstein supervised me, she did this repeatedly, and I often tried to emulate her. She would, for instance, describe her enthusiasm for the child's revelations of secret wishes. I understood her avoidance at times of a neutral voice tone as an attempt to bypass the child's normal narcissism which makes such revelations deflating and embarrassing as well as contrary to superego mandates. She would also depict her attempts to supply the emotion that a child omitted from his speech. The analyst might say with more heat than expected in an interpretation to an adult that he can see how angry the patient is even though he feels he shouldn't be. "So angry that you feel like ripping paper and cutting people who stop you from having pleasure," the analyst might say with emotion.

The supervisor may point out certain conceptual capacities of children which the analyst might not realize. They often understand the concept of the unconscious when it is explained to them in topographical terms, as Freud did in 1910. The analyst can tell the child that the mind consists of two rooms, one that contains conscious thoughts and feelings and one with unconscious thoughts and feelings. A closed door between the rooms keeps the unconscious thoughts and feelings out of awareness. But they appear in disguise in dreams and symptoms. Using this model, the analyst can offer a simple explanation of how treatment works through making the unconscious conscious.

Children also appreciate the role of conflict in their life so that the analyst can tell them that "a part of you would like to hurt me, but another part says you shouldn't."

Children are more frequently aware of their bodily sensations than many adults, thus enabling the analyst to say, "Your body wants to push things out, but you want to keep it from coming out of you," as I told a 4-year-old obstipated child in analysis (Glenn, 1978). Mary O'Neil Hawkins "was not only interested in children's emotional feelings, but also their physical feelings. . . . Concerning boys who . . . wet their pants in the day time, she would ask, 'What sensations do they have in their penis?'" (Becker, 1985, p. 4). The supervisor may thus help a student focus on the patient's bodily experiences.

The child analytic patient generally requires more talking to than the adult analysand. This may take the form of a "running commentary" (Kramer, 1960). The supervisor can help the analyst to gauge the appropriate degree of verbalization as well as appropriate content.

A student, aware that his talkativeness probably would further rather than hinder his work with his patient, made interpretations in a vigorous machine-gun style. This seemed to be so much a part of his character that the supervisor was gentle perhaps to a fault in calling it to his attention. The fact that the patient tolerated this style well and that the analysis was going well fortified his view that forceful intervention by the supervisor would be unwise. Toward the end of the analysis the student, satisfied with his work and confident of his skills, appeared quite capable of tolerating criticism and of altering his behavior. The supervisor thereupon emphasized more vigorously that his rapid-fire manner might gratify the patient's desire to be bombarded and that a change in approach could be helpful in eliciting more verbal expressions of conflict. The supervisee then made his interventions in a calmer way, with gratifying analytic results.

Nonpsychoanalytic Tendencies

Many students practice psychotherapy prior to entering child psychoanalytic training. They may apply techniques which, although helpful in other forms of treatment, are inimical to the development of a psychoanalytic process. They may reassure the child when it is not necessary or educate him inappropriately. They may encourage repression or, contrary to that, advocate catharsis as the prime mode of treatment. In such cases, the supervisor can help the student differentiate psychoanalysis from psychoanalytically oriented psychotherapy and other treatments and adapt this technique to the treatment he is learning.

Every time an 8-year-old patient became anxious, his analyst pointed out that realistically he had nothing to fear. The patient responded by becoming calm, and did not reveal what he was afraid of. After the supervisor observed this reassuring technique, the analyst altered his approach. The patient gradually became aware of his fear of being punished for masturbating.

THE ANALYST'S EMOTIONAL COUNTERREACTIONS

The child analytic student's personal characteristics may hinder his analytic work. Although some regard all such interferences countertransference, I prefer to restrict the term to the emergence of the analyst's transferences in response to the patient's transferences. Countertransferences should be differentiated from transferences to the patient and his parents, identification and counteridentification with them, empathy and the appearance of signal emotional response to the patient's behavior (Bernstein and Glenn, 1978).

The supervisor may strongly suspect a countertransference interference, but is usually not in a position to ascertain the exact type of counterreaction or its content. He may point out the student's unanalytic interventions or inhibitions that interfere with the analysis, but he cannot interpret them. It is up to the student to scrutinize his behavior with his own analyst or in the course of self-analysis.

The mother of an 8-year-old boy became pregnant and was considering aborting the child. The patient, who supposedly was unaware of this state of affairs, started to draw pictures that his analyst (and the supervisor) clearly saw were wombs containing fetuses. It was obvious that the patient knew of his mother's pregnancy, but was loyally silent about it or defensively denied its existence. Although the analyst knew all this, he could not make the appropriate interpretations. The supervisor pointed out this failing rather vigorously and the student presumably discussed it in his analysis. I would suspect that the analyst was reacting to feelings about the boy's parents, who he felt opposed the child's knowing about the pregnancy, and was identifying with the child who had to hide his knowledge.

RELATIONSHIPS WITH PARENTS

Relationships between the analyst and his patient's parents are quite different in child and adult analysis. The adult analyst deals directly only with his patient. His counterreactions to parents are not based on direct contact, but on his patient's descriptions, sometimes embellished by his own fantasies (Jacobs, 1983).

The child analyst sees and talks to the parents in person when he does the original consultation and during the course of the analysis. The extent of the contact varies with the age and communicativeness of the patient and with the propensities of the analyst and his supervisor; parents of younger analysands are seen more frequently than those of older children. In some geographical areas seeing parents at all is frowned upon. The frequency and type of interaction will to a great extent depend on the views of the training institute the student attends, and in particular the supervisor's approach. It is a rare student indeed who insists on behaving contrary to his supervisor's opinion.

For clarity's sake, I wish to emphasize that most Freudian child analysts find it important to see the parent. The reasons for seeing parents during the course of the analysis are: (1) to maintain a working alliance with them so that they will not disrupt the treatment; (2) and, related, to support the parents who have difficulty having their children in analysis; (3) to receive information about present and past events in the child's life; (4) at times providing advice and information to parents is necessary to sustain the treatment through alteration or stabilization of the environment.

These parent-therapist interactions provide a supervisory arena specific to child analysis. Analyst and supervisor must discuss the aims of parental contact and whether they help or interfere with the progress of the analysis. As we saw in the preceding section, possible counterreactions to parents must be monitored and discussed. The student may be helped by the supervisor's describing his own and others' emotional responses to parents, the usefulness of observing one's reactions, and the possible maladaptive effects of counterreactions. Sometimes observing one's own reactions to parents may help the analyst to understand how the child feels.

When the parents supplied a child analyst with contradictory information about their behavior and the child's, the analyst became confused about the events of the child's life. The father and mother not only contradicted each other, each was inconsistent in his or her own descriptions. The analyst, observing his own difficulty in understanding the family reality, realized that the child's reality confusion was in part a reaction to his parents, and could interpret to the patient how the child struggled with his parents' uncertainties and how he sometimes was not sure of what was real.

SUPERVISEE-SUPERVISOR RELATIONS

The relationship between analyst and teacher is central to the supervisory situation. Optimally the student and teacher are sufficiently mature so that the primary aims of learning and teaching are achieved. A collegial relationship is enhanced by the fact that most child analysis candidates are more or less experienced analysts of adults. Indeed, a number of my supervisors were remarkably hospitable during our meetings together. Becker (1985), writing about Mary O'Neil Hawkins, stated: "Supervision with Hawkie was unhurried. She served tea and sandwiches. In the winter one might help get the fire burning in the fireplace. One soon felt a colleague and became a friend" (p. 3). The ideal of friendly and collegial supervision is often achieved.

The supervisor must empathize with the student and employ tact in his comments. This had best not be done in a contrived way, but from a truly human and friendly base. The correct timing and tact of the supervisor may serve as a basis for the student's identification which aids his work with his patients. On the other hand, the supervisor should not lean over backward and avoid telling the student of deficiencies when that would advance his training.

Usually candidates in training are in analysis while they are in supervision. Such concomitance may help clarify and enhance the student's relationship with his supervisor. Sometimes displacement from analyst to supervisor—the split transference— may produce irrational reactions, transferences toward the supervisor. Students of child analysis have often completed their analysis and deal with the analyst more or less rationally. But this need not be the case, especially since the supervisory situation may produce a flaring up of the transference now directed toward the supervisor.

One student, no longer in analysis, complained to his supervisor that his analyst had mistreated him as his mother had when he was a child. She had died when he was a teenager. Soon his feeling of trust for the supervisor turned to suspicion. He began to feel that he too was behaving like a bad parent, was unreliable. He feared his graduation was in jeopardy. The supervisor decided not to direct the student's attention to the obvious dynamics, lest the transference intensify if he acted like the student's analyst. Rather, the supervisor remained his usual dependable self. The excessive suspicion disappeared when the patient was graduated. This student did not return to analysis, as some do.

In some cases returning to analysis during child training is sensible, not only because supervision may stir conflict and regression, but also because the very act of treating a child may do so. The supervisor, observing this, may suggest further analysis.

The supervisor may manifest counterreactions to his supervisee, especially when the student is displaying irrational transferences toward him. Antagonism may appear to be defended against. A sadomasochistic interaction may occur. The supervisor may become overly protective of the candidate and not provide proper advice. The supervisor should be on the lookout for his counterreactions and employ self-analysis when he observes them. In addition, the supervisor may share blind spots with the student, so that neither fully appreciates the patient's pathology.

A stalemate may occur for a number of the reasons already indicated and require a change of supervisor. The student's reactions to the supervisor may be intense and intractable. The supervisor may find himself unable to stop reacting adversely to the candidate. Shared blind spots may interfere with proper conduct of the analysis.

A particularly interesting form of student-supervisor interaction, labeled parallel process (Arlow, 1963; Ekstein and Wallerstein, 1958; Sachs and Shapiro, 1976), has been observed in child analyses. A student may repeat with the supervisor certain of the conflicts or defenses that appear in the analysis he is conducting.

An analyst of an intelligent child who acted stupid became inept and confused about his patient during many successive supervisory sessions. After the supervisor told the supervisee he was behaving with him in a manner similar to the patient's in the transference, the student realized he was identifying with his analysand. This led to his having a better grasp of the patient's dynamics and defensive profile.

The supervisor is also an evaluator of the student's capability to become a child analyst. He may have to tell the supervisee that he does not think he should continue child analytic training or inform the institute of this opinion and its justification. Sometimes the student progression committee comes to this conclusion, on the basis of several supervisors' reports, even though individual supervisors may disagree. The institute through its committee will then have the unpleasant task of relaying this information to the student, who may of course react to such a suggestion with anger and dismay. Some students find themselves relieved by being advised not to engage in treatment they do poorly.

Throughout supervision the teacher evaluates the student's capacities, achievements, and progress (Weiss and Fleming, 1975). Informing the student of his status at appropriate times will enable the student realistically to assess himself and strive for necessary improvement in essential areas. It will also help the supervisee to achieve a realistically based self-estimation.

Generally supervisors send written reports to the appropriate committee regarding students' work. It may also be helpful for the supervisors to meet together and compare their experiences. This may help them to observe the student's strengths as well as weakness, the types of reactions to different supervisory approaches. As a result impediments may be removed and training proceed more smoothly. Advice to the student will be sounder (Stanley S. Weiss, personal communication).

The repeated evaluations of the student by his supervisors and other faculty members may have an infantilizing effect. The child analytic student is often a more or less experienced analyst, a graduate of an adult program, more advanced in age than most candidates in adult psychoanalytic programs. He may feel he is being treated like a child well past the age when he is truly an adult out on his own, and may resent it. He may feel as though he is undergoing repeated initiation rituals (Arlow, 1969) in a never ending quest to become accepted as a peer by his older colleagues. Such feelings, which can foster regression and interfere with learning, can be countered by self-analysis if the supervisors truly recognize that the student is an adult learning advanced and sophisticated procedures. Subtle or gross depreciation of the supervisee will have a detrimental influence on such analyses and the achievement of a stable maturity.

DEVELOPMENT OF A CHILD ANALYTIC IDENTITY

The establishment of an identity as an analyst is a complicated matter which I can only touch on here (Joseph and Widlocher, 1983).[2] Although identifications are an essential part of one's identity, other conflictual and nonconflictual aspects of the personality participate. Historical factors and cultural expectations and demands are important too. Among the figures for identification that are integrated into the formation of such an identity are caretakers in childhood, including parents and physicians; psychoanalytic and psychotherapeutic pioneers such as Freud; mentors in adolescence and later psychoanalytic teachers and supervisors at the institute where one is trained. Prominent among those whom the candidate identifies with is his analyst. This may add a complication to one's analysis since identification can serve as a defense as well as an adaptive mechanism.

Sometimes analysts become child analytic candidates out of identification with their analysts, but frequently this is not the case. Candidates analyzed by nonchild analysts enter the field because of personal capacities and interests that antedate their analysis, contact with child analysts during their training, and for other reasons. (Of course, these same determinants will influence candidates treated by child analysts.)

Frequently the identification with child analytic supervisors and teachers plays a more important role in the establishment of an identity as a child analyst than identification with one's analyst. The student will identify with his supervisor's analytic (or even nonanalytic) stance, modes of interpretation, interaction with the child patient, and ways of thinking about his patients. Complex theoretical views may be based on such identifications. A child analytic identity may include a flexibility in behavior and thinking or a rigid adherence to a particular theoretical orienta-

---

2. See Solnit (1983) for a discussion of the child analyst's identity.

tion. As Anna Freud observed, those analyzed by Kleinians do Kleinian analyses and Freudian analyses are done by analysands of Freudians. Some analysts display a preference for oedipal interpretations, while others lean toward preoedipal insights including an understanding of separation-individuation. Optimally the analyst's mind is open to his patient's conflicts from all origins and interprets in accordance with his patient's needs.

Many factors enter into the development of theoretical and behavioral rigidity. Here I wish to emphasize that the approach of the supervisor may contribute. If the supervisor views each child analysis as an adventure, a new research project which will help not only the patient but our science to change, his student will more likely identify with his flexibility and open-mindedness. Encouraging students to seek new insights, even—if they are so disposed—to write scientific papers which expand our vistas, will help establish a child analytic identity that is broad and productive. A single supervisor is not likely to accomplish this, but a training program in which the faculty is devoted to curiosity, discovery, and insight as well as—really a part of—the proper care of patients is more likely to succeed.

A child analytic identity is furthered when the student conducts the analysis with a sense of autonomy. Spoon feeding the candidate throughout the treatment, directing his every interpretation, or providing insight excessively will hinder this development. Often, as the analysis proceeds and the student becomes more capable, the supervisor's activity diminishes, and the candidate's autonomous functioning increases. Diminishing the frequency of supervision can serve the same purpose.

Heiman Van Dam (personal communication) correctly asserts that in a good supervision the student, while describing a session, develops new insights even when the supervisor is silent. "The process of regression in the service of the work ego . . . broadens the skills of the supervisee." Identification with the supervisor is important here.

Students often read articles about patients similar to theirs in order to enhance their knowledge of issues that arise during the analysis. The supervisor may recommend papers which may further the analyst's insight and capacity. Reading will also help the development of one's child analytic identity by providing additional models for the understanding of patients, variations of technique, and research possibilities.

TEACHING SUPERVISION

There are no courses in the supervision of child analysis. Each supervisor generally creates his own method and his own style based on his understanding of psychoanalytic theory and facts. His methods of working with patients derive from his own teachers' concepts and procedures, from those practices of colleagues which he has learned about through reading, attending lectures and discussion groups, and conversations. Continuous case seminars also provide models for supervision. Some institutes run training analysts seminars during which supervision of adult analyses is discussed, but this is rather unusual, and I have not heard of such seminars regarding child analysis. Only recently has the Association for Child Psychoanalysis sponsored such workshops. Moise Shopper led a discussion group at the 1986 meeting and Robert L. Tyson ran one in 1987.

An innovative device grew out of the lack of sufficiently experienced supervisors at a number of institutes (Francis, 1978). A relatively inexperienced analyst discusses his supervision of a student with an experienced analyst. This method, called "piggy back" supervision, has proven useful in teaching the supervisory process as well as in monitoring the supervisor's understanding of the case under analysis and his technical suggestions.

SUMMARY

In addition to teaching procedures, supervisors of child psychoanalyses should facilitate the attainment of a child analytic identity and the development of an effective personal style. The analyst/student's interaction with his patients and their parents as well as the supervisor/supervisee interrelationship are important issues.

BIBLIOGRAPHY

AMERICAN PSYCHOANALYTIC ASSOCIATION (1978). Training Standards in Child and Adolescent Psychoanalysis.

ARLOW, J. A. (1963). The supervisory situation. *J. Amer. Psychoanal. Assn.*, 11:576–594.

–––––– (1969). Myth and ritual in psychoanalytic training. In *Training Analysis.* Pittsburgh Psychoanalytic Institute, pp. 104–120.

BECKER, T. E. (1985). Memorial for Dr. Mary O'Neil Hawkins. *Newsletter N.Y. Psychoanal. Soc. & Inst.*, 22:1–4.

BEISER, H. R. (1982). Styles of supervision related to child analysis training and the gender of the supervisor. *Annu. Psychoanal.*, 10:57–76.

BERNSTEIN, I. & GLENN, J. (1978). The child analyst's emotional reactions to his patients. In *Child Analysis and Therapy*, ed. J. Glenn. New York: Aronson, pp. 375–392.

BORNSTEIN, B. (1949). The analysis of a phobic child. *Psychoanal. Study Child*, 3/4:181–226.

DEUTSCH, B. G. (1977). Child analytic training today. *Cape News*, 7:2–3, 8.

EKSTEIN R. & WALLERSTEIN, R. S. (1958). *The Teaching and Learning of Psychotherapy.* New York: Basic Books; New York: Int. Univ. Press, 1972.

FENICHEL, O. (1941). *Problems of Psychoanalytic Technique.* Albany, N.Y.: Psychoanalytic Quarterly.

FRANCIS, J. J. (1978). The teaching of child psychoanalysis in the United States. In *Child Analysis and Therapy*, ed. J. Glenn. New York: Aronson, pp. 709–742.

FREUD, A. (1922–1980). *The Writings of Anna Freud*, vols. 1–8. New York: Int. Univ. Press.

FREUD, S. (1909). Analysis of a phobia in a five-year-old boy. *S.E.*, 10:5–149.

–––––– (1910). Five lectures on psycho-analysis. *S.E.*, 11:7–55.

GLENN, J., ed. (1978). *Child Analysis and Therapy.* New York: Aronson.

–––––– (1980). Freud's advice to Hans' father. In *Freud and His Patients*, ed. M. Kanzer & J. Glenn. New York: Aronson, pp. 121–127.

JACOBS, T. J. (1983). The analyst and the patient's object world. *J. Amer. Psychoanal. Assn.*, 31:619–642.

JOSEPH, E. D. & WIDLOCHER, D. (1983). *The Identity of the Psychoanalyst.* New York: Int. Univ. Press.

KRAMER, S. (1960). Running comments, confrontation and interpretation. Read at the Philadelphia Psychoanalytic Institute, Child Analysis Study Group.

LEWIN, B. D. & ROSS, H. (1960). *Psychoanalytic Education in the United States.* New York: Norton.

NUNBERG, H. & FEDERN, E.. eds. (1967). *Minutes of the Vienna Psychoanalytic Society*, vol. 2, 1908–1910. New York: Int. Univ. Press.

SACHS, D. M. & SHAPIRO, S. H. (1976). On parallel processes in therapy and teaching. *Psychoanal. Q.*, 45:394–415.

SILVERMAN, M. A. (1980). A fresh look at the case of Little Hans. In *Freud and His Patients*, ed. M. Kanzer & J. Glenn. New York: Aronson, pp. 95–120.

SOLNIT, A. J. (1983). Reflections of a child psychoanalyst. In *The Identity of the Psychoanalyst*, ed. E. D. Joseph & D. Wildlocher. New York: Int. Univ. Press, pp. 85–92.

WEISS, S. S. & FLEMING, J. (1975). Evaluation of progress in supervision. *Psychoanal. Q.*, 44:191–205.

Index